Clinical Methods in

OPHTHALMOLOGY

Clinical Methods in OPHTHALMOLOGY

A Practical Manual for Medical Students

Second Edition

Dadapeer K
MS DNB (Ophthalmology)
Associate Professor
Department of Ophthalmology
Hassan Institute of Medical Sciences
Hassan, Karnataka, India

Forewords
Ravikumar BC
Jyothi Swarup

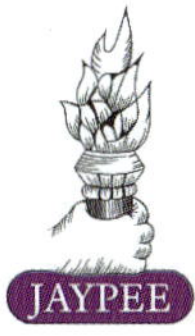

JAYPEE BROTHERS MEDICAL PUBLISHERS
The Health Sciences Publisher
New Delhi | London

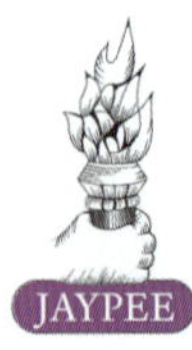

Jaypee Brothers Medical Publishers (P) Ltd

Headquarters
EMCA House, 23/23-B
Ansari Road, Daryaganj
New Delhi 110 002, India
Landline: +91-11-23272143, +91-11-23272703
+91-11-23282021, +91-11-23245672
e-mail: jaypee@jaypeebrothers.com

Corporate Office
4838/24, Ansari Road, Daryaganj
New Delhi 110 002, India
Phone: +91-11-43574357
Fax: +91-11-43574314
e-mail: jaypee@jaypeebrothers.com

Overseas Office
JP Medical Ltd.
83, Victoria Street, London
SW1H 0HW (UK)
Phone: +44-20 3170 8910
e-mail: info@jpmedpub.com

EU GPSR Authorised Representative
Logos Europe, 9 rue Nicolas Poussin
17000, La Rochelle, France
Phone: +33 (0) 6 67 93 73 78
e-mail: contact@logoseurope.eu

Website: www.jaypeebrothers.com
Website: www.jaypeedigital.com

Inquiries for bulk sales may be solicited at: jaypee@jaypeebrothers.com

Clinical Methods in Ophthalmology—A Practical Manual for Medical Students

First Edition: 2013

Second Edition: 2015

Reprint: 2023, 2025, **2026**

ISBN 978-93-5152-907-1

Printed at: Samrat Offset Pvt. Ltd.

Dedicated to

My parents
Mr Karimsab B and Mrs Babujan K
for their blessings

My uncle
Mr Emamsab B
for his encouragement
and

My wife
Dr Shama Taj KR
for her support

Preface to the First Edition

This book is basically written for the needs of undergraduate medical students. I have observed that the undergraduate medical students often find it difficult to understand clinical ophthalmology in spite of knowing theory part of it. The book aims to present clinical ophthalmology in a simplified, yet in a comprehensive manner with a lot of clinical photographs. Few chapters are discussed in more detail to provide complete information of the topic and this will be beneficial to the postgraduate students and residents in ophthalmology also. The book has the following key features thus making it, an easy-to-use guide for the students:

- History taking with clinically structured questionnaire for each case
- Detailed case discussion with explanation of clinical problems
- Comprehensive coverage with emphasis on clinical application.

While writing this book, I have gone through many books, enquired students regarding their common doubts and problems, recollected what my teachers had taught me and then I have presented all of them in a concise manner. I hope that the book will be a useful guide for the medical students during their course in ophthalmology. Efforts have been made to check for the accuracy of the matter and to correct the mistakes, if any. I will be happy to receive constructive comments, which will help in betterment of the book.

Dadapeer K

Acknowledgments

My wholehearted expression of gratitude to one and all who have contributed in many ways for completion of this book. I affectionately thank my parents Mr and Mrs Karimsab, my uncle and aunt Mr and Mrs Emamsab, my father-in-law and mother-in-law Mr and Mrs Abdul Razak, and my sister-in-law Ms Heena Kousar and brother-in-law Mr Waris, for their constant support and encouragement.

My special thanks to my wife, Dr Shama Taj KR, Assistant Professor, Department of Microbiology, SS Institute of Medical Sciences and Research Centre, Davangere, Karnataka, India, for her constant support, encouragement and cooperation without which this book would have never been a reality.

I would like to extend my heartful thanks to Dr Pratap VGM, Dr Dilip HR, Dr Gayathri V (Residents in Ophthalmology, Aravind Eye Care Hospital, Madurai, Tamil Nadu, India), Dr Lakshmi (Resident in Ophthalmology, AJ Institute of Medical Sciences and Research Centre, Mangaluru, Karnataka), for all the help in taking the photographs and preparing the book.

I thank Dr Lakshmi BR, Dr Sahana Mainpur, Dr Shwetha S, Dr Farah Zeba, Dr Divya Mishra, Dr Chaitra CM, Dr Archana K, Dr Anuraj, Dr Arpitha, Dr Ashish, Dr Nehla Tahim, Dr Moorthy TN and Dr Ashitha S, for helping me in proofreading the book.

I thank colleagues of my department Dr Kavitha CV, Dr Pavana Acharya, Mr Radhakrishna, Mr Nagesh and Mr Ishidhara Kumar (Ophthalmic Officer, Government Hospital, Alur, Hassan, Karnataka), for their help rendered to me.

I would like to thank Dr Ramamurthy D (Chairman, The Eye Foundation and Vice-President, All India Ophthalmic Society), Dr Ravikumar BC (Professor of Dermatology, Hassan Institute of Medical Sciences, Hassan, Karnataka), Dr Gangadhar (Professor of ENT, Shimoga Institute of Medical Sciences, Shivamogga, Karnataka), Dr Praveen G (Associate Professor of Community Medicine), Dr Niranjan (Associate Professor of Medicine), Dr Devraja R (Consultant Hepatologist), Dr Sudhanava (Associate Professor of Physiology), Dr Deepak (Associate Professor of Pharmacology, Hassan Institute of Medical Sciences), Dr Pradeep Kumar (Associate Professor of Ophthalmology, Shimoga Institute of Medical Sciences), Dr Sandhya (Professor of Ophthalmology, Sri Siddhartha Medical College, Tumakuru, Karnataka), Dr Rakesh (Consultant Ophthalmologist, CSI Mission Hospital, Hassan), Dr CV Andrews (Professor of Ophthalmology, Jubilee Mission Medical College and Research Institute, Thrissur, Kerala), Dr Prakash HM (Associate Professor of Pathology, Vinayaka Mission Medical College, Salem, Tamil Nadu), Dr Niranjan (Associate Professor of Biochemistry, Mahatma Gandhi Medical College and Research Institute, Puducherry), Dr Kavitha (Consultant Ophthalmologist, Vasan Eye Care, Bengaluru, Karnataka), Dr Narendra Shenoy (Consultant Ophthalmologist, Udupi Eye Center, Udupi, Karnataka), Dr Shailaja Shenoy (Associate Professor of Ophthalmology, Kasturba Medical College, Manipal, Karnataka),

Dr Venkat (Consultant Ophthalmologist, Globe Eye Foundation, Bengaluru), Dr Parivadhini AP (Consultant Ophthalmologist, Sankara Nethralaya, Chennai, Tamil Nadu), Dr Prashanth CN (Associate Professor of Ophthalmology, Dr BR Ambedkar Medical College, Bengaluru), Dr Rajashekar (Associate Professor of Ophthalmology, Karnataka Institute of Medical Sciences, Hubballi, Karnataka), Dr Nadeem (Assistant Professor of Ophthalmology, Raichur Institute of Medical Sciences, Raichur, Karnataka), Dr Shenoy (Associate Professor of Ophthalmology) and Dr Dinesh (Assistant Professor of Ophthalmology, Adhichunchanagiri Institute of Medical Sciences, Bengaluru), for their support.

I thank Dr Balasubramanya S, Dr Nataraj PL, Dr Shrimanth, Dr Madhusudan, Dr Chandan BC, Dr Sharan, Dr Abdul Qadeer, Dr Shashidhara, Dr Fahima Shakir, Dr Samarath, Dr Shobhitha, Dr Girish and Dr Prakash, who were of great help in preparing the first edition of the book.

I am grateful to the positive feedback and Foreword written by Dr Ravikumar BC, Former Director, Hassan Institute of Medical Sciences.

I am thankful to my teacher Dr Jyothi Swarup (Professor of ENT, Sri Siddhartha Medical College), for his encouragement and for writing Foreword.

I am thankful to Professor Chandrashekar Shetty (Former Vice-Chancellor, RGUHS), Professor Sriprakash KS (Former Vice-Chancellor, RGUHS), for their support and encouragement.

I am thankful to my postgraduate teachers, Dr Raviprakash D, Dr Ramesh TK, Dr Sriprakash KS, Dr Shivakumar, Dr Prabha AR, Dr Shivaprasad Reddy, Dr Dakshayani, Dr Suresh Babu and Dr Nagaraju (Bangalore Medical College and Research Institute, Bengaluru), for being an endless source of inspiration and guidance.

I affectionately thank my friends and relatives, for their support and encouragement.

My deeply felt gratitude to Shri Jitendar P Vij (Group Chairman), Mr Ankit Vij (Group President), Tarun Duneja (Director–Publishing), Mr Venugopal Vishnumurthy [Associate Director-South (Sales & Marketing)], Mr Vasudev (Commissioning Editor) and all staff of Bengaluru Production Unit of M/s Jaypee Brothers Medical Publishers (P) Ltd, New Delhi, India.

Contents

- Macular degenerations and macular dystrophies
- Diabetic retinopathy and other retinopathies
- Chorioretinal degenerations and dystrophies.

- Primary open-angle glaucoma
- Refractive errors
- *Optic nerve:* Hereditary optic atrophies, drug-induced optic neuropathies and toxic amblyopia.

Gradual painful diminution of vision

- Corneal ulcer
- Chronic iridocyclitis.

Sudden painless diminution of vision

- Vascular occlusions of retinal vessels, e.g. central retinal artery occlusion, central retinal vein occlusion, cilioretinal artery occlusion, branch retinal artery occlusion and branch retinal vein occlusion
- Optic neuritis, non-arteritic anterior ischemic optic neuropathy (NAION)
- Central serous retinopathy
- Vitreous hemorrhage
- Retinal detachment.

Sudden painful diminution of vision

- Mechanical or chemical trauma to eye
- Acute iridocyclitis
- Acute angle-closure glaucoma
- Endophthalmitis
- Giant cell arteritis with arteritic ischemic optic neuropathy.

Loss of Vision

Loss of vision refers to inability to perceive light, i.e. perception of light (PL)—'negative'.

Causes

1. Any disease involving retina and/or optic nerve only can cause total loss of vision.
2. Isolated diseases of lens or cornea can never cause PL negative vision unless there is a problem in retina and/or optic nerve such as optic atrophy, total retinal detachment.

Transient Loss of Vision

Transient loss of vision is also called amaurosis fugax. It is characterized by sudden, temporary loss of vision due to transient hypoxia of visual system. The attack lasts from few seconds to 30 minutes and it recovers completely.

Causes

Causes for transient loss of vision are:

- Migraine headache—aura
- Transient ischemic attack involving visual cortex
- Papilledema
- Prodromal symptom of central retinal artery occlusion, anterior ischemic optic neuropathy
- Hypoperfusion of the retinal arteries, which may be due to hypotension, cardiac failure, anemia
- Carotid artery disease and atherosclerotic cerebrovascular disease.

Floaters

A condition characterized by perceiving black spots in front of the eyes, which move with the movement of eyes, is called floaters. Any opacity behind the nodal point of the eye, i.e. behind the lens will cast its shadow on the retina causing floaters.

Causes

- Posterior vitreous detachment
- Vitreous hemorrhage
- Vitreous opacities such as muscae volitantes, asteroid hyalosis, synchysis scintillans

- Inflammations of the posterior segment such as vitritis, pars planitis, chorioretinitis.

Flashes of Light

A condition characterized by perceiving a sensation of flickering of lights is called flashes of light. It is also called photopsia. This occurs because of traction on the vitreoretinal attachments, irritating the retina and causing it to discharge electrical impulses, which are interpreted by brain as flashes of light.

Causes

- Posterior vitreous detachment
- Retinal tear
- Prodromal symptom of retinal detachment
- Papilledema.

> Sudden onset of flashes of light with floaters requires evaluation by indirect ophthalmoscopy to rule out retinal tear or retinal detachment.

Glare

A condition characterized by difficulty to see in bright light is called glare. Glare occurs because of diffraction of light caused by opacities in the refractive surfaces, cornea and lens. Hence, it is seen in diseases of cornea and lens such as corneal opacity, lenticular opacity/cataract.

Causes

- Corneal opacity
- Lenticular opacity.

> Normally everyone would have experienced glare, while driving during night or on seeing sun directly.

Photophobia

A condition in which person has difficulty to see/open eyes in normal intensity light. Photophobia occurs because of stimulation of sensory nerve endings of cornea.

Causes

- Corneal diseases, e.g. corneal epithelial defect, corneal ulcer, keratitis, corneal edema
- Iridocyclitis.

Distorted Vision

Distorted vision is a condition in which the person perceives objects to have altered size or shape:

- *Micropsia:* Objects are perceived smaller in size
- *Macropsia:* Objects are perceived bigger in size
- *Metamorphopsia:* Objects are perceived altered in shape.

Causes

Macular lesions such as macular edema, macular degeneration, etc.

Diplopia

Diplopia is a condition in which the person perceives double images of an object.

Binocular Diplopia

Diplopia is present only when both eyes are open and it disappears on closing one eye. Problem with nerve, neuromuscular junction or muscle can lead to binocular diplopia:

- Paresis or paralysis of nerves supplying extraocular muscles—paralytic squint
- Myasthenia gravis
- Fractures of orbit with entrapment of extraocular muscles
- Thyroid ophthalmopathy.

Uniocular Diplopia

Diplopia is present even with one eye (abnormal eye) being open. Problem within the refractive medium of the eye involving cornea/pupil/lens can cause uniocular diplopia because of double refraction:
- Corneal causes, e.g. keratoconus
- Causes in pupil, e.g. double pupil
- Causes in lens, e.g. subluxated lens, displaced intraocular lens and incipient cataract.

Colored Halos

A condition in which person perceives colored rings around lights. Colored halos are because of prismatic dispersion of light (breakage of light into seven colors because of abnormal collection of fluid) in the refractive media, i.e. in cornea and/or lens.

Causes

- Collection of mucus on corneal surface as in conjunctivitis
- Corneal edema because of bullous keratopathy or acute congestive glaucoma
- Immature cataract.

Differentiation of Causes of Colored Halos
The causes can be differentiated from another by the following methods:
1. Colored halos due to collection of mucus on corneal surface as in conjunctivitis will disappear if the mucus is removed manually or by eye wash.
2. Colored halos due to corneal edema and immature cataract can be differentiated by Fincham stenopaic slit test.

Fincham Stenopaic Slit Test
A stenopaic slit 2 mm wide is passed in front of the eyes. The colored halos, because of corneal edema, remain intact and lenticular opacity is broken into segments.

The appearance of colored halos can be demonstrated by asking the patients to look through Lycopodium powder enclosed between two glass plates.

Day Blindness

Day blindness is called hemeralopia. It is a condition in which patient has decreased vision in day light/bright light.

Causes

- Diseases of cones, e.g. congenital deficiency of cones
- Central opacities in the cornea and/or lens, e.g. central corneal opacity and polar cataracts (as the pupil constricts in bright light the opacity in the center will come in the path of light causing diminution of vision).

Night Blindness

Night blindness is called nyctalopia. It is a condition in which patient has decreased vision in dim light/night.

Causes

- Diseases of rods, e.g. retinitis pigmentosa
- Vitamin A deficiency
- Congenital stationary night blindness, Oguchi's disease and fundus albipunctatus
- Pathological myopia
- Choroidal dystrophies, e.g. gyrate atrophy and choroideremia.

Diminution of Vision for Near Only

A condition in which person is not able to see near things with distant vision being normal.

Causes

- Presbyopia because of decrease in accommodation due to aging

- Cycloplegia and ophthalmoplegia because of paralysis of accommodation.

SYMPTOMS NOT RELATED TO VISION (Box 1.2)

Box 1.2: Symptoms not related to vision

- Redness
- Watering
- Discharge
- Itching
- Pain
- Headache
- Deviation of eye
- Protrusion of eyeball (Proptosis).

Redness

Acute red eye is seen in:
- Acute conjunctivitis
- Acute iridocyclitis
- Acute congestive glaucoma
- Redness is a common symptom and it is seen in all inflammatory conditions of eye such as blepharoconjunctivitis, all types of conjunctivitis, keratitis, uveitis, endophthalmitis and panophthalmitis.

Watering

A condition in which eye appears wet with tears being overflowed from eyes.

Causes

1. Hyperlacrimation due to either central lacrimation or primary hypersecretion, or reflex hyperlacrimation.
2. Epiphora due to obstruction in the lacrimal drainage system to normally formed tears. The site of obstruction can be in punctum, canaliculi, lacrimal sac and nasolacrimal duct.

Discharge

Discharge from eye is seen in conditions associated with mucosal surfaces of the eye (conjunctiva and lacrimal sac). It can be mucoid, mucopurulent, purulent or serosanguineous depending on the type of inflammation:
- Conjunctiva, e.g. conjunctivitis
- Lacrimal sac, e.g. acute and chronic dacryocystitis.

Itching

Itching is mainly seen in allergic conditions associated with eye, e.g. allergic conjunctivitis.

Ocular Pain

Ocular pain is seen in inflammations of the eye or adnexal structures such as keratitis, iridocyclitis, orbital cellulitis, internal hordeolum, external hordeolum and in acute congestive glaucoma. Referred pain to the eye is seen in diseases involving the surrounding structures as in sinusitis and dental problems.

Headache

Ocular Causes

- Refractive errors (mainly mild, uncorrected refractive errors and astigmatism), extraocular muscle imbalance, deficiency of accommodation and convergence insufficiency
- Ocular inflammations
- Glaucoma.

Nonocular Causes

- Neurological disorders, e.g. intracranial space-occupying lesions, meningitis, subarachnoid hemorrhage
- Ear, nose and throat (ENT) diseases, e.g. sinusitis, rhinitis
- Psychiatric problems
- Primary headaches, e.g. migraine, cluster headache and tension headache.

Deviation of Eye

Deviation of eye is called strabismus or squint. Misalignment of visual axes of the two eyes because of deviation of eyes is known as squint.

Protrusion of Eyeball (Proptosis)

Forward displacement/protrusion of normal-sized eyeball beyond the orbital margins is called proptosis.

SYMPTOMS DUE TO ADNEXA OF EYE (BOX 1.3)

Symptoms due to adnexa of the eye are described in Chapter 2 'Ocular Examination'. 'Ptosis' is described in detail in Chapter 4 'Case Presentation'.

Box 1.3: Symptoms due to adnexa of eye

- Drooping of the upper eyelid—ptosis
- Retraction of the eyelids
- Inward or outward turning of the lid margin—entropion or ectropion
- Increased blinking rate of eyelids—blepharospasm
- Inability to close eyelids—lagophthalmos
- Inward misdirection of eyelashes—trichiasis
- Swelling in the lacrimal sac region.

Chapter 2

Ocular Examination

Chapter Outline

- Head Posture
- Facial Symmetry
- Abnormal Facial Symmetry and Ocular Posture
- Visual Acuity
- Eyebrows
- Eyelids
- Lacrimal Apparatus
- Eyeball
- Examination of a Patient with Exophthalmos
- Examination of Binocular Extraocular Movements
- Conjunctiva
- Examination of Conjunctiva
- Cornea
- Sclera
- Anterior Chamber
- Iris
- Pupil
- Lens
- Fundus: Vitreous and Retina

Ocular examination is done under diffuse illumination using torch light and focal illumi nation using slit lamp. Ocular examination should begin with the examination of head posture and facial symmetry as these can be altered by the patient voluntarily. They are best examined before the patient's realization that examination has begun.

HEAD POSTURE

Normal head posture: Normally head is kept in erect and straight posture without any tilt of the head or turn of the face or elevation/depression of chin or any abnormal movements of head.

There are three pair of extraocular muscles, two horizontal recti, two vertical recti and two oblique muscles. When the movement of the eye is affected because of paresis or paralysis of the extraocular muscles, head posture acts as compensatory mechanism to compensate for the restricted eye movements to avoid diplopia:

- Restricted horizontal movements are compensated by face turn
- Restricted vertical movements are compensated by elevation or depression of chin
- Restricted oblique movements are compensated by head tilt.

function concerned with the appreciation of form sense. Testing visual acuity involves testing both distant vision and near vision.

Testing Distance Vision

Bedside

In the absence of charts designed for testing visual acuity it can be assessed roughly by counting fingers by standing at a distance of 6 m and if the patient is not able to count fingers at 6 m, examiner moves towards the patient reducing the distance between him and the patient by 1 m each time till the patient is able to count the fingers:

- Counting fingers greater than 6 m
- Counting fingers at 6 m
- Counting fingers at 5 m
- Counting fingers at 4 m
- Counting fingers at 3 m
- Counting fingers at 2 m
- Counting fingers at 1 m
- Counting fingers at 1 feet
- Counting fingers close to face
- Hand movements
- Perception of light with projection of rays in all the quadrants
- Perception of light negative.

Counting fingers at 6 m is roughly equal to 6/60 (top most line) with Snellen's chart (Fig. 2.9). The size of the top most letters is roughly equal to the size of the fingers; hence by counting of fingers at bedside vision can be assessed up to 6/60 of Snellen's chart.

Visual Acuity Charts

Snellen's chart is the commonly used chart for measurement of visual acuity.

Two distant points can be visible as separate when they subtend an angle of 1 min at the nodal point of the eye. Snellen's chart consists of series of black letters arranged progressively decreasing in size. The letters selected are such that each letter will subtend an angle of 1 min at the nodal point of the eye. The top letter can be read from a distance of 60 m, the succeeding lines can be read from 36, 24, 18, 12, 9, 6, 5 and 4 meters respectively.

Procedure

1. Patient is seated at a distance of 6 m and the patient is asked to read the chart separately in each eye after closing one eye. Visual acuity is recorded as a fraction, of which numerator is distance of the patient from the chart and denominator is smallest letters, which the patient reads, which is written below the letters, i.e. 60, 36, 24.
2. If the patient is not able to read the top most line from 6 m he/she is asked to move by 1 m front till he/she can see the top most line clearly, then numerator becomes 5, 4, 3, 2, 1. If the patient cannot read from 1 m then check for:
   a. Counting fingers at 0.3048 m.
   b. Counting fingers close to face.
   c. Hand movements.
   d. Perception of light with projection of rays in all the four quadrants.
   e. Perception of light negative.

Why 6 Meters?

At 6 meters the rays of light are practically parallel and the patient exerts minimum accommodation. Hence 6 meters is chosen. The same can be achieved by placing a plane mirror at 3 meters and the patient is asked to read the reflected image in the mirror which makes it 6 meters.

The other visual acuity charts available other than Snellen's letter chart are:

- Snellen's E chart (Fig. 2.10)
- Landolt's C chart
- Allen's picture chart.

Testing Near Vision

Near vision is tested by near vision chart by asking the patient to read this from a distance

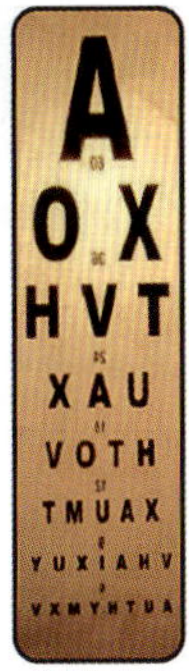

Fig. 2.9: Snellen's distance visual acuity chart

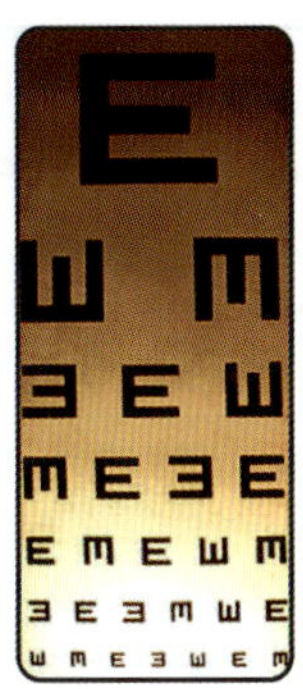
Figure 2.10: E chart

of 30 cm, the routine working distance in each eye separately. The smallest letters, which the person can read is recorded as the near vision of the person. Normal near vision is N6 (Fig. 2.11).

Near Vision Charts
- Jaeger near vision chart
- Roman near vision chart
- Snellen's near vision chart.

Testing Color Vision

Pseudoisochromatic charts (Ishihara's plates): The person is asked to read the numbers in the color plates. Normal people can read all the plates (normally six screening plates) correctly whereas people with color blindness will read it wrong as shown in the following Table 2.1 (Fig. 2.12).

Table 2.1: Interpretation of Ishihara's plates

Person with normal color vision		Person with red-green color blindness	Person with total color blindness
Plate 1	12	12	12
Plate 2	29	70	X
Plate 3	5	2	X
Plate 4	6	X	X
Plate 5	7	X	X
Plate 6	X	5	X

Note: X—not able to identify the letter will say as empty plate.

Other methods for testing color vision:
- Farnsworth-Munsell 100 hue test
- Nagel's anomaloscope.

Testing Visual Field

- Confrontation test
- Perimetry
- Visual acuity is recorded under the following headings:
  - Right eye left eye
- Distance vision:
  - With naked eye
  - With pinhole (if the visual acuity is less than 6/6)
  - With spectacles (if the patient is wearing spectacles).
- Near vision.

Pinhole Test
If the distance vision is less than 6/6 all patients should be asked to look through a pinhole and improvement if any in visual acuity should be recorded.
1. A pinhole cuts off all the peripheral rays and allows only central parallel beam of rays to enter eye and visual improvement is seen in cases of refractive errors.
2. If the cause for diminution of vision is not refractive error like cataract then improvement in vision is not seen. The results of pinhole test can be summarized as.

Contd...

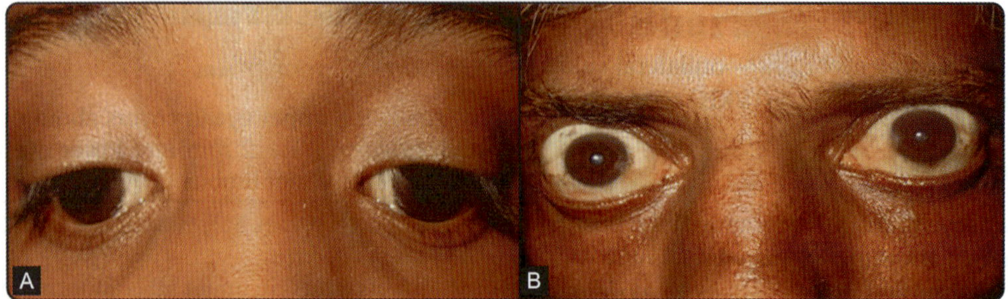

Figs 2.15A and B: Abnormal position of the eyelids. **A.** Bilateral ptosis (*Note:* Drooping of upper eyelids, upper eyelid covering more than 2 mm of cornea); **B.** Bilateral retraction (*Note:* Upper eyelid covers less than 2 mm of cornea hence upper limbus is visible scleral show).

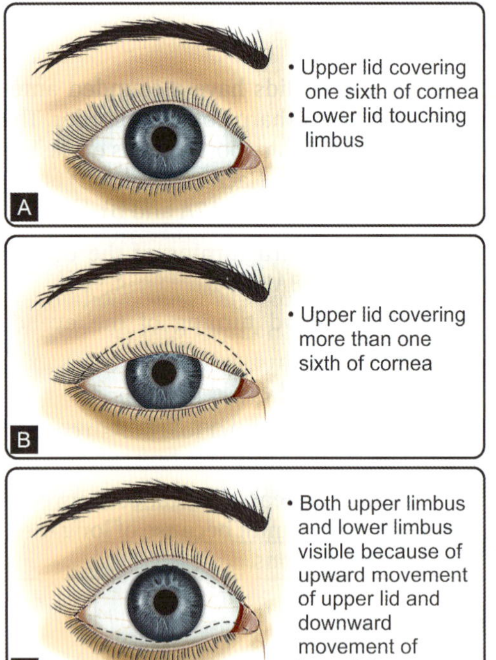

Figs 2.16A to C: Abnormalities of eyelid position. **A.** Normal position of eyelids; **B.** Ptosis of upper eyelids; **C.** Retraction of eyelids.

Palpebral Aperture Width

Normal palpebral aperture width is vertical 10 mm and horizontal 30 mm (Fig. 2.20).

All round narrow palpebral fissure width is seen in blepharophimosis (Fig. 2.21):

1. Horizontally narrow palpebral fissure width is seen in ankyloblepharon.
2. Vertically narrow palpebral fissure width is seen in ptosis, phthisis bulbi.
3. Vertically wide palpebral fissure width is seen in proptosis.

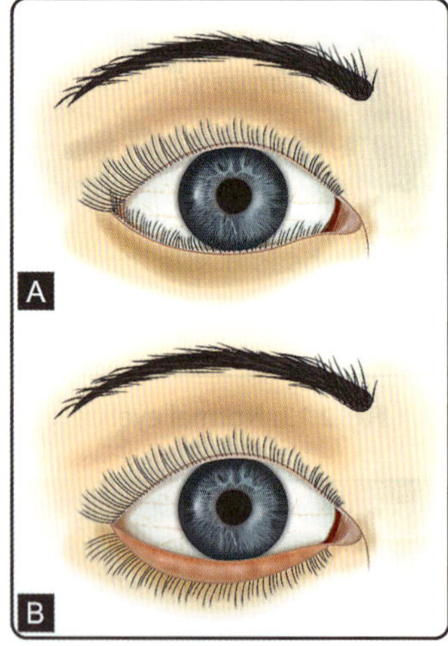

Figs 2.17A and B: Abnormalities of eyelid margin. **A.** Entropion (*Note:* Inward turning of lower eye lid margin with eye lashes touching the globe); **B.** Ectropion (*Note:* Outward turning of lower eye lid margin with exposure of lower conjunctival fornix).

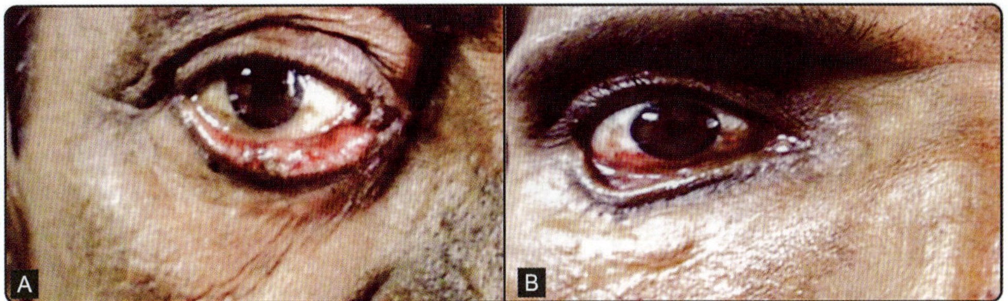

Figs 2.18A and B: Ectropion. **A.** Ectropion of the lower eyelid; **B.** Cicatricial ectropion of lower eyelid (*Note:* The scar over the skin).

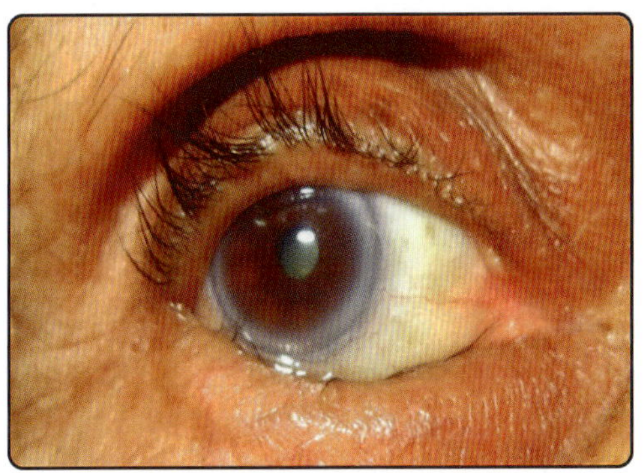

Fig. 2.19: Entropion of lower eyelid

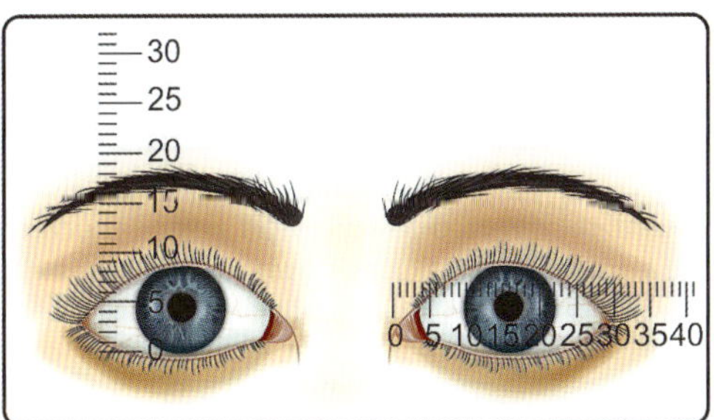

Fig. 2.20: Palpebral aperture width [measuring palpebral fissure width (vertical) and measuring palpebral fissure width (horizontal)].

EYELASHES

Normally eyelashes in the upper eyelid are directed forwards, upwards and backwards, and in the lower eyelid they are directed forwards, downwards and backwards.

Trichiasis: Misdirection of eyelashes toward the globe with normal position of eyelid margin (Fig. 2.22A).

Distichiasis: It is a rare congenital disorder characterized by the presence of a posterior row of eyelashes directed toward the globe (Fig. 2.22B).

Madarosis: Loss or decrease in the number of cilia of eyelashes and or eyebrows. The common causes include ocular causes such as blepharitis, trachoma, local trauma (mechanical, thermal or following radiotherapy or cryotherapy) of the eyelids, tumors of the eyelids and systemic causes like hypothyroidism, hyperthyroidism, hypoparathyroidism, hyperparathyroidism, hypopituitarism, leprosy, syphilis.

Poliosis: Presence of localized hypopigmented hair follicles involving eyelashes and or eyebrows. The common causes for poliosis are sarcoidosis, Vogt-Koyanagi-Harada syndrome, sympathetic ophthalmitis, blepharitis, vitiligo, side effect of topically administered prostaglandins.

Skin: Normally skin of eyelid is thin, smooth and elastic. Common eyelid swellings are, external and internal hordeolum (Figs 2.23A and B to 2.25), lid tumors, chalazion (Fig. 2.26).

Cryptophthalmos: Hidden eyeball, i.e. eyeball is covered by a layer of skin. It is a rare

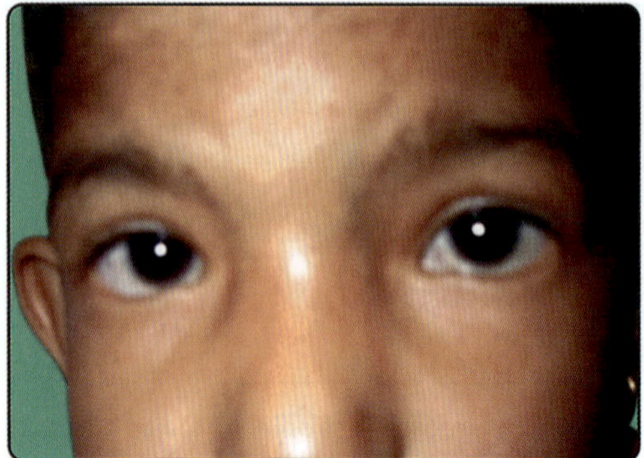

Fig. 2.21: Blepharophimosis syndrome consisting of ptosis, blepharophimosis, epicanthus inversus and telecanthus.

congenital anomalous condition resulting from failure of eyelid formation.

Reasons for easy swelling of the eyelids:

1. Skin of the eyelids is the thinnest in the body.
2. It does not have a subcutaneous fatty layer.
3. Layer of loose subcutaneous tissue gets distended easily by blood in case of injuries to head and by fluid in cardiac failure, which presents as puffiness of face.
4. The submuscular areolar tissue of upper eyelids is in continuity with subaponeurotic space of scalp allowing easy passage of fluid and blood to the upper eyelids leading to black eye or ecchymosis of upper eyelids in cases of head injuries (Figs 2.27 to 2.29).

LACRIMAL APPARATUS

Lacrimal apparatus consists of lacrimal secretory system and lacrimal drainage system. Lacrimal secretory system consists of main lacrimal gland situated in the anterolateral part of the roof of the orbit and accessory lacrimal glands situated in the subconjunctival tissue.

Lacrimal drainage system consists of puncta, canaliculi, lacrimal sac and nasolacrimal duct. Examination of lacrimal drainage system

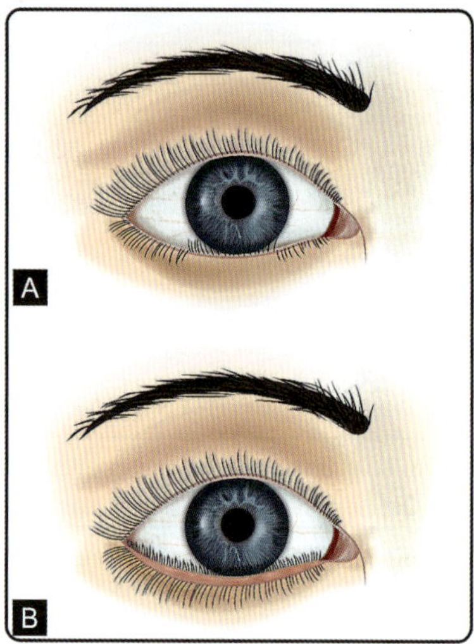

Figs 2.22A and B: Eyelashes. **A.** Trichiasis (Note: Inward misdirected lower eyelid lashes touching the cornea); **B.** Distichiasis (*Note:* Abnormal extra row of eyelashes in lower eyelid).

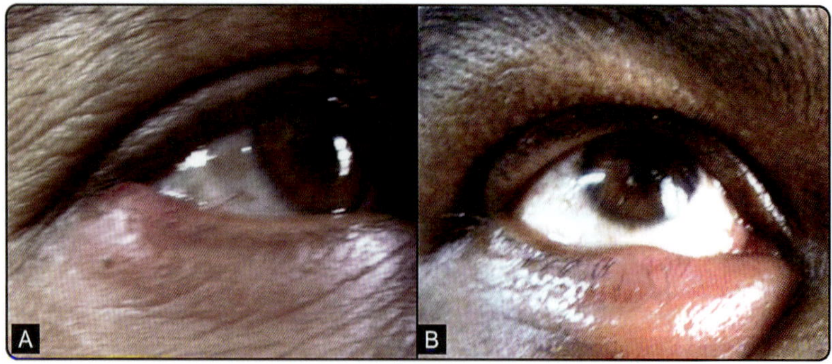

Figs 2.23A and B: Internal hordeolum (*Note:* Localized swelling presenting on the conjunctival side of the lower eyelid away from lid margin with inflammatory signs)

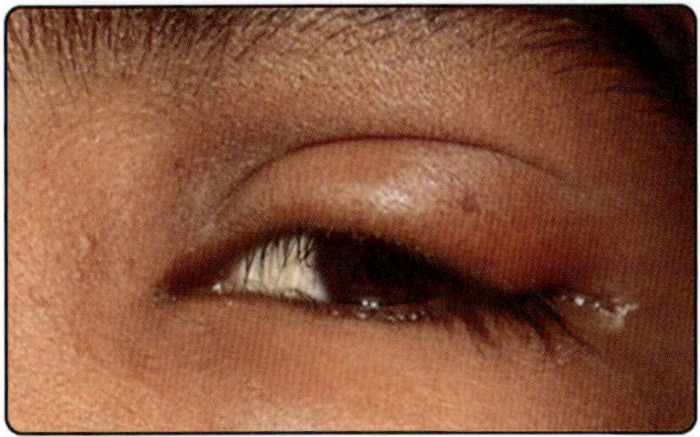

Fig. 2.24: External hordeolum (*Note:* Localized swelling presenting on the skin side of the lower eyelid at lid margin with inflammatory signs).

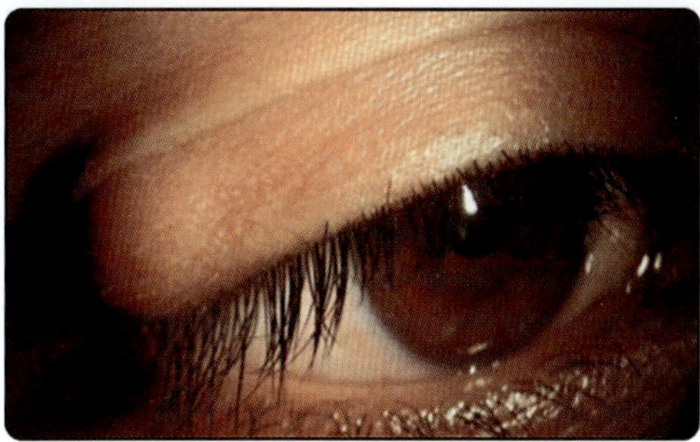

Fig. 2.25: Chalazion (*Note:* Localized swelling presenting on the conjunctival side, away from lid margin of upper eyelid with no inflammatory signs).

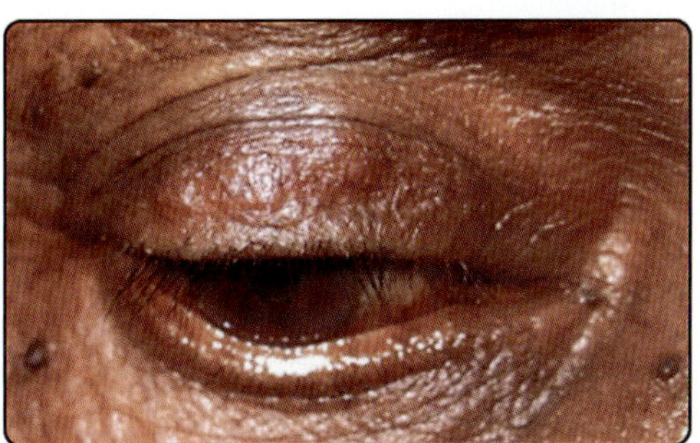

Fig. 2.26: Multiple chalazion of upper eyelid

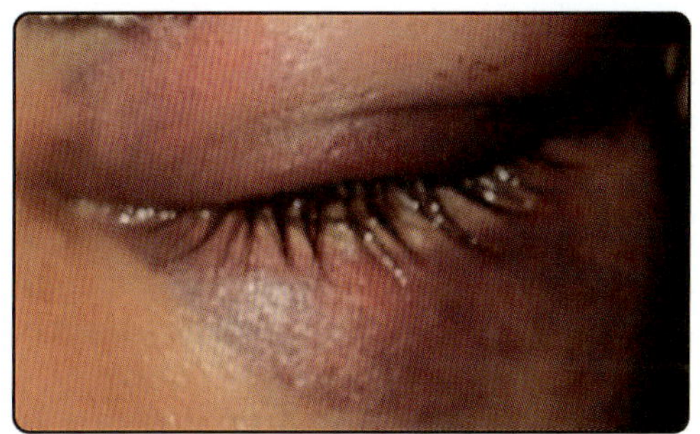

Fig. 2.27: Ecchymosis of eyelid (black eye)

is done by inspection of lacrimal puncta situated one each in upper and lower eyelids.

Abnormalities of lacrimal puncta can be absence, eversion and stenosis of punctum.

Inspection of skin over lacrimal sac area for redness, swelling, fistula.

Regurgitation Test

Apply pressure over the lacrimal sac area with either thumb or index finger and look for the regurgitation of fluid or discharge from upper or lower punctum:

1. Normally, it is negative, i.e. no regurgitation of fluid or discharge.
2. Regurgitation of fluid or discharge is called positive regurgitation test and it indicates chronic dacryocystitis.
3. In chronic dacryocystitis with encysted mucocele there is no regurgitation of the contents leading to false-negative test.

EYEBALL

Eyeball has to be examined under the headings, position, size and movements of the eyeball.

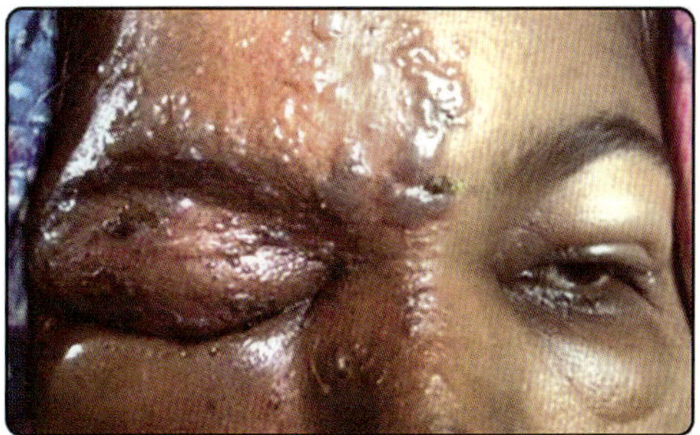

Fig. 2.28: Herpes zoster ophthalmicus (*Note:* Vesicular lesions strictly not crossing the midline with involvement of tip of the nose and involvement of skin of the eyelids; Hutchinson's rule—ocular involvement is present, if the tip of the nose is involved as both are supplied by nasociliary nerve).

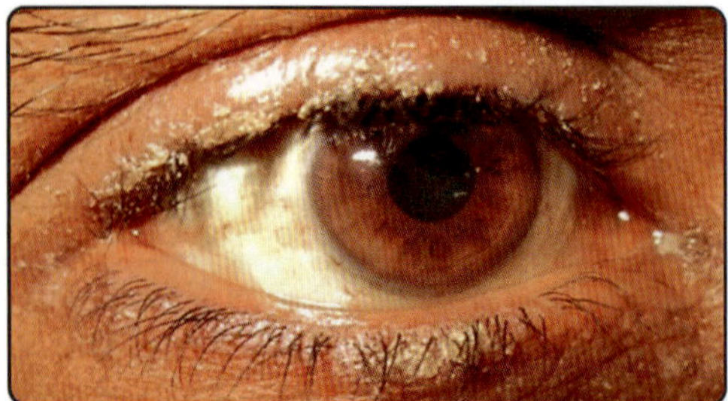

Fig. 2.29: Squamous blepharitis (*Note:* The presence of yellow crusts seen along the eyelashes)

Position

Normally two eyeballs are suspended in the orbit by four recti muscles and two oblique muscles.

Abnormalities in Position of Eyeball: Proptosis and Enophthalmos

Proptosis: Abnormal forward displacement/ protrusion of normal sized eyeball beyond orbital margins.

Proptosis caused by thyroid disease is called exophthalmos. It is the most common cause for unilateral or bilateral proptosis in adults. In children orbital cellulitis is the most common cause for unilateral proptosis and neuroblastoma or leukemia for bilateral proptosis.

Proptosis is because of mass lesions pushing the eyeball forwards. The direction of displacement depends on the direction of mass lesion. Axial proptosis is due to retrobulbar space occupying lesions, eccentric proptosis is due to mass lesion in the peribulbar space or surrounding structures (eyeball will be pushed in the direction opposite to that of mass lesion), e.g. mass in maxillary sinus will cause proptosis in upward direction (Figs 2.30, 2.31A and B).

Causes of Proptosis

Unilateral proptosis: These are as follows:

- Congenital causes like dermoid cyst, orbital teratoma
- Inflammations like orbital cellulitis, pseudotumor
- Vascular malformations like orbital varices, carotid cavernous fistula
- Cysts of the orbit
- Tumors such as hemangioma, rhabdomyosarcoma, optic nerve glioma, lymphoma, metastatic tumors
- Traumatic causes like orbital hemorrhage, orbital emphysema.

Bilateral proptosis: These are as follows:

- Anomalies of skull like craniofacial dysostosis
- Systemic diseases such as histiocytosis, amyloidosis
- Inflammations like cavernous sinus thrombosis
- Tumors such as lymphoma, leukemia, secondaries from neuroblastoma, nephroblastoma
- Exophthalmos.

Acute proptosis: These are as follows:

- Orbital infections like orbital cellulitis, fungal infections of the orbit
- Orbital emphysema
- Orbital hemorrhage
- Idiopathic orbital inflammatory syndrome
- Thyroid orbitopathy
- Systemic diseases such as Wegener's granulomatosis, lymphoma, leukemia and polyarteritis nodosa.

Pulsating proptosis: It is characterized by the presence of pulsations synchronously with the arterial pulse:

- True pulsating proptosis is seen in:
  - Carotid cavernous fistula
  - Aneurysm of internal carotid artery.

  Transmitted cerebral pulsations in proptosis are seen in:
- Congenital conditions with absence of orbital roof as in meningocele, meningoencephalocele

Contd...

Contd...

- Acquired conditions with destruction of the orbital roof as in neurofibroma.

Intermittent proptosis: It is characterized by presence of transitory proptosis. The causes for intermittent proptosis are:

- Orbital varices
- Recurrent orbital hemorrhage and orbital emphysema.

Exophthalmometry

Measurement of proptosis/exophthalmos is called exophthalmometry.

By plastic scale: A plastic scale is placed tightly on the lateral orbital margin and the level of the apex of the cornea is read from the scale:

- Normal 16 mm
- Borderline 16–20 mm
- Proptosis more than 21 mm or difference of more than 2 mm between two eyes.

Instruments to measure proptosis: Luedde exophthalmometer and Hertel exophthalmometer are used.

Ocular Signs in Exophthalmos (Figs 2.32)

- Dalrymple's sign: Lid retraction
- Von Graefe sign: Upper lid lag on down gaze
- Grove sign: Resistance of upper lid to downward traction
- Gifford sign: Difficult to evert upper eyelid
- Griffith sign: Lower lid lags behind the globe on up gaze
- Kocher's sign: Staring look of eyes
- Rosenbach sign: Tremors of closed eyelid
- Stellwag's sign: Infrequent blinking
- Jellinek sign: Increased pigmentation of upper eyelid
- Joffroy's sign: Decreased wrinkling on forehead on upgaze
- Enroth sign: Fullness of eyelids
- Mobius sign: Convergence weakness.

Enophthalmos

Enophthalmos is defined as posterior displacement or inward displacement of the eyeball. It is because of decrease in the contents of the orbit. The causes for enophthalmos are:

- Blow out fractures leading to loss of orbital contents
- Atrophy of the orbital contents following irradiation, trauma, infection, cicatrizing carcinomas, aging.

Pseudoproptosis

Pseudoproptosis is defined as a condition in which the eyeball appears to be proptosed, but there is no displacement of the eyeball. The common causes for pseudoproptosis are:

- Enlargement of the eyeball as in pathological myopia, buphthalmos, staphylomas
- Causes in the eyelid like lid retraction
- Causes resulting in false impression of proptosis as in the contralateral eye in unilateral ptosis, microphthalmos, phthisis bulbi, enophthalmos, globe retraction.

Size of the Eyeball

Normal dimensions:

- Anteroposterior diameter 24 mm
- Vertical diameter 23 mm
- Horizontal diameter 23.5 mm
- Anteroposterior diameter is measured by A-scan.

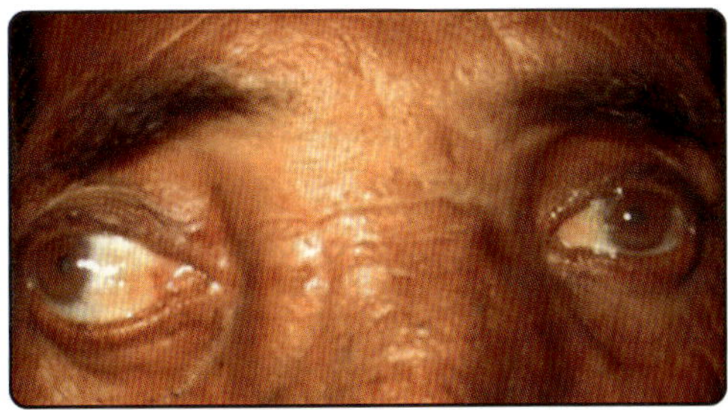

Fig. 2.30: Eccentric proptosis

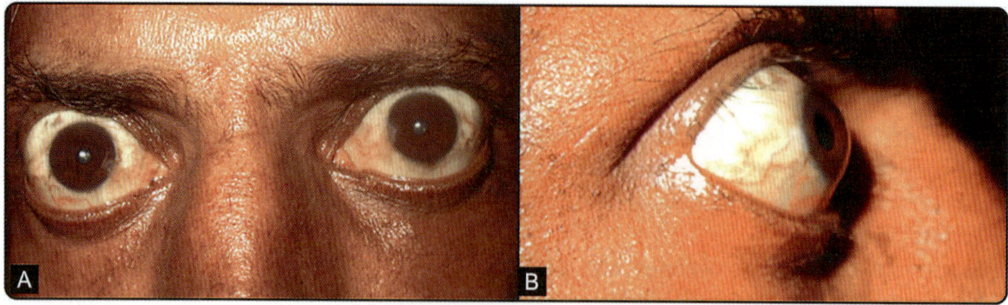

Figs 2.31A and B: Bilateral axial proptosis

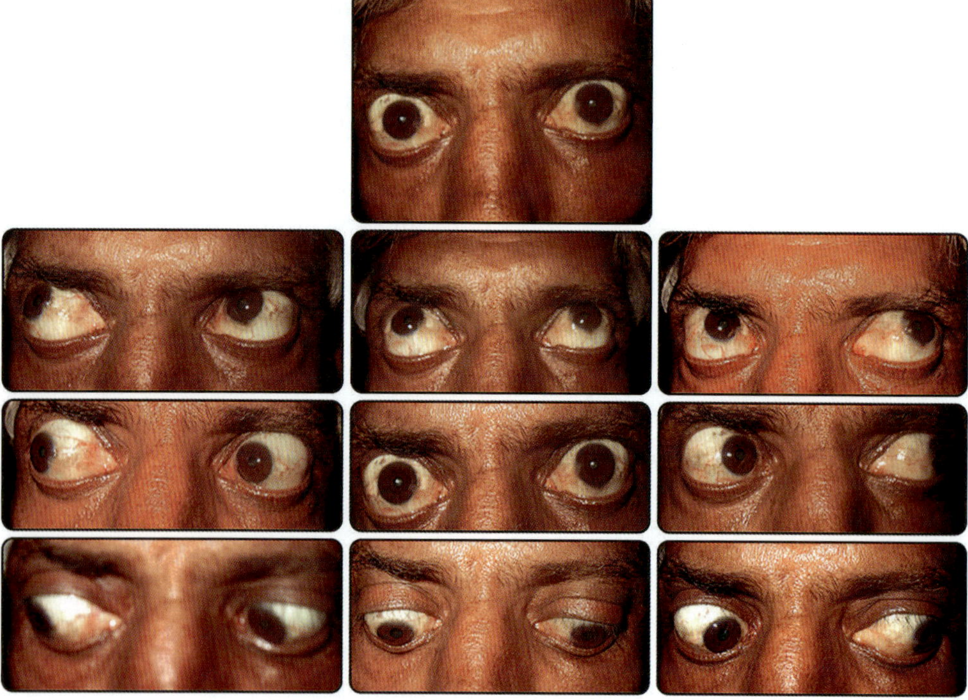

Figs 2.32: Examination of a patient with exophthalmos (*Note:* Lid retraction, scleral show, decreased wrinkling on forehead, staring look, upper eyelid lag on down gaze)

Increased Size of Eyeball:
- High myopia
- Buphthalmos.

Decreased Size of Eyeball:
- Microphthalmos
- Phthisis bulbi (Figs 2.33A and B)
- Atrophic bulbi.

Movements of Eyeball

Uniocular movements (ductions) and binocular movements (versions and vergence) have to be tested. Ocular movements can be limited or restricted.

Limited ocular movements are because of paresis or paralysis of the nerves supplying the

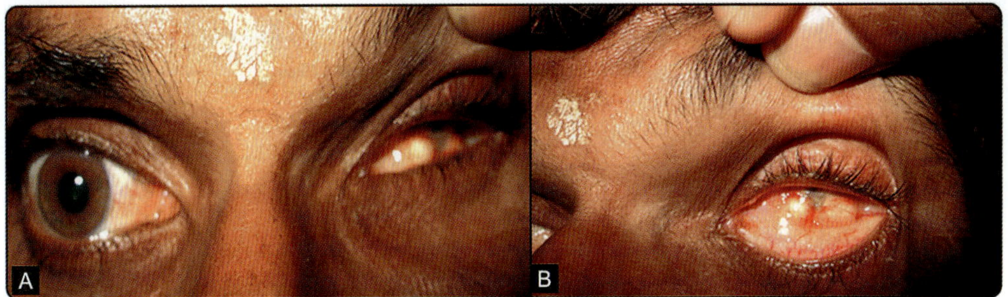

Figs 2.33A and B: Phthisis bulbi—sizeless, shapeless, sightless, soft and shrunken eyeball

extraocular muscles, e.g. third nerve paresis, fourth nerve paresis. Restricted ocular movements are because of mass lesions outside the muscle restricting the movement of the muscle. Examination of binocular extraocular movements as shown in Figures 2.34 and 2.35.

CONJUNCTIVA

Conjunctiva is a mucous membrane lining the posterior aspect of the eyelids and anterior surface of sclera. Conjunctiva is examined under the headings:

- Bulbar conjunctiva
- Palpebral conjunctiva
- Conjunctival fornices.

How to Examine Conjunctiva?

Bulbar conjunctiva, lower palpebral conjunctiva and conjunctival fornices (except superior fornix) can be examined by retracting the upper lid and lower lid with the index finger/thumb (Figs 2.36A to C, 2.37A to E).

Upper palpebral conjunctiva is examined by eversion of the upper lid. Eversion of the upper eyelid is done by everting the upper eyelid by holding the lid margin with one hand or using two hands.

Superior fornix is examined after double eversion of upper lid using Desmarres lid retractor (Figs 2.38A and B, 2.39).

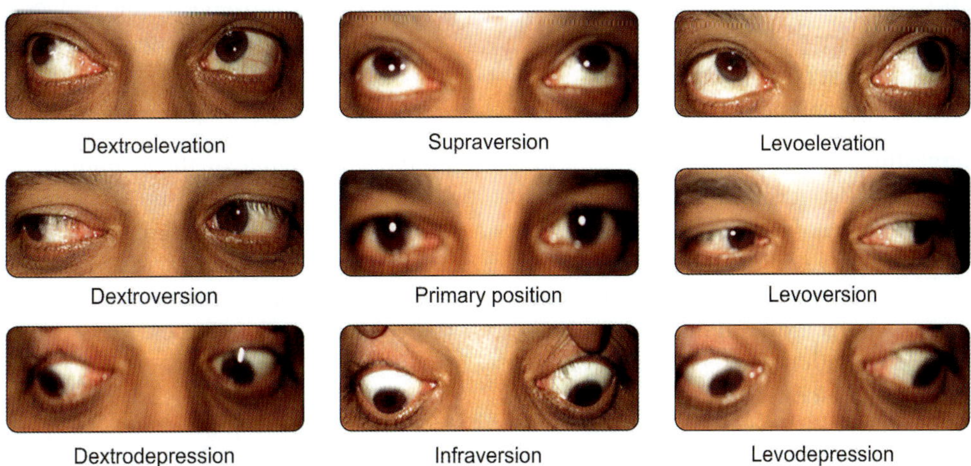

Figs 2.34: Examination of binocular extraocular movements

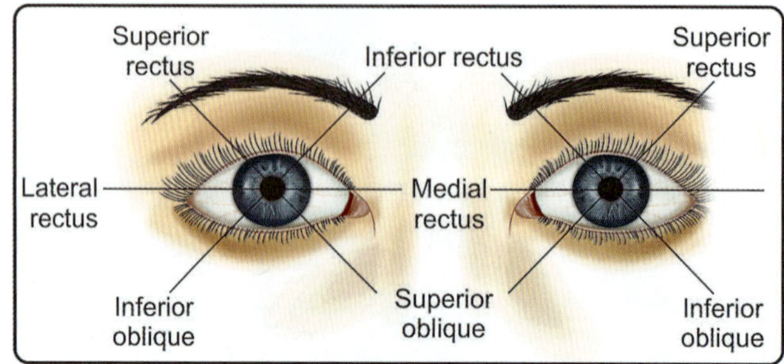

Fig. 2.35: Ocular movements

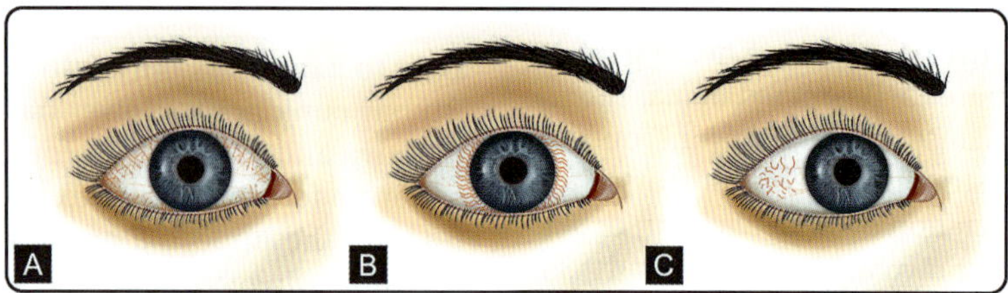

Figs 2.36A to C: Congestion. **A.** Conjunctival congestion; **B.** Circumciliary congestion; **C.** Scleral congestion.

Abnormalities of Conjunctiva (Figs 2.40 to 2.48A and B)

- Congestion
- Chemosis
- Discoloration
- Follicles
- Papillae
- Pterygium
- Pinguecula
- Conjunctival cysts and tumors
- Xerosis of conjunctiva.

Congestion

Conjunctival congestion: Because of conjunctival vessels seen in acute conjunctivitis, allergic conjunctivitis. Congested vessels are bright red in color, superficial and branching, move on moving conjunctiva; blanch with phenylephrine and more marked in fornices.

Ciliary congestion: Because of ciliary vessels seen in keratitis, iridocyclitis. Congested vessels are purplish red in color, deep and radiating, will not move on moving the conjunctiva, will not blanch with phenylephrine and more marked around limbus.

Scleral congestion: Because of ciliary vessels seen in episcleritis and scleritis. Congestion is limited to a sector or a quadrant, congested vessels are dull red in color, conjunctiva can be moved over the congested vessels and vessels will not blanch with phenylephrine.

Chemosis

Swelling or edema of the conjunctiva is called chemosis. Chemosis is because of collection of fluid under the loosely attached bulbar conjunctiva arising because of exudation from the abnormally permeable conjunctival capillaries.

Causes

- Ocular inflammatory conditions like conjunctivitis, keratitis, iridocyclitis, endophthalmitis, panophthalmitis and

Contd...

Contd...

allergic conditions of eye like allergic conjunctivitis.

- Systemic conditions like congestive cardiac failure, anemia, hypoproteinemia, nephritic syndrome, angioneurotic syndrome.
- Passive congestion due to mechanical obstruction to venous outflow as in exophthalmos, orbital tumors, cavernous sinus thrombosis.

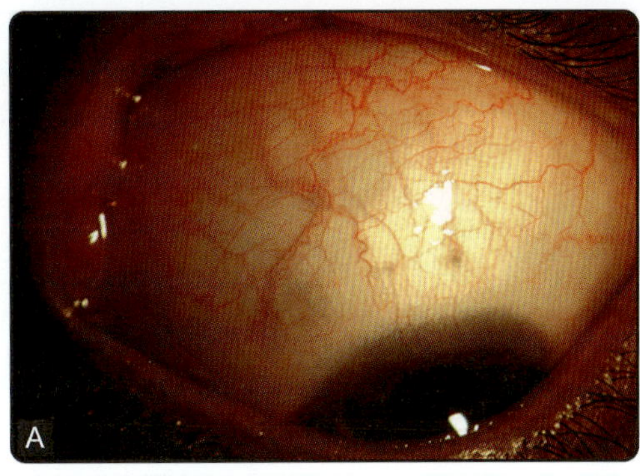

Fig. 2.37A: Examination of superior bulbar conjunctiva and superior fornix by asking the patient to look down.

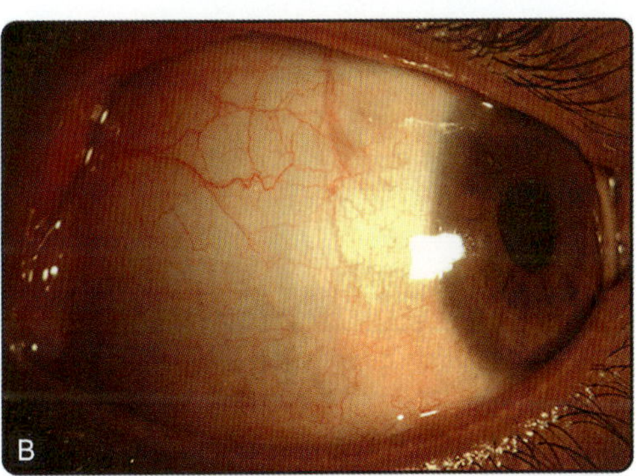

Fig. 2.37B: Examination of nasal bulbar conjunctiva and medial fornix by asking the patient to look temporally.

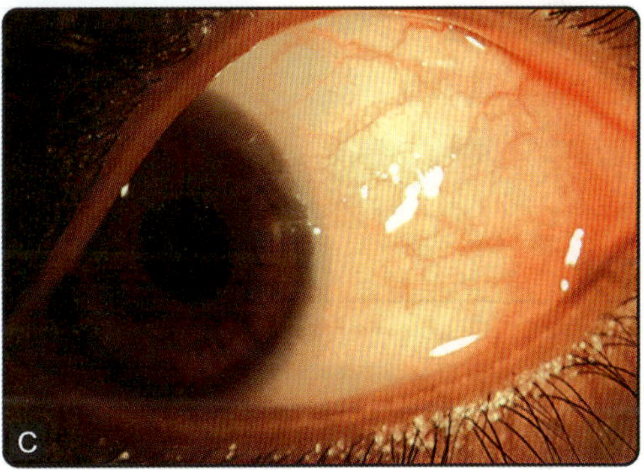

Fig. 2.37C: Examination of temporal bulbar conjunctiva and lateral fornix by asking the patient to look nasally.

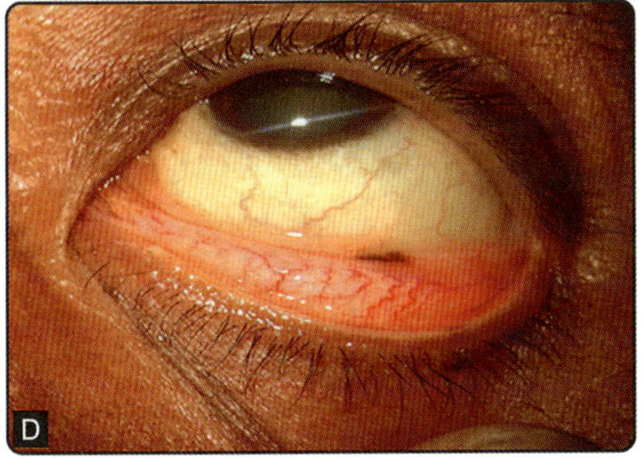

Fig. 2.37D: Examination of inferior palpebral conjunctiva and inferior conjunctival fornix by asking the patient to look up and pulling the lower lid downwards.

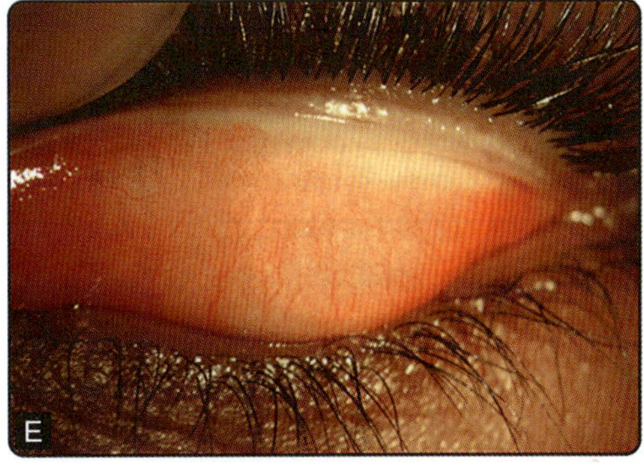

Fig. 2.37E: Examination of upper bulbar conjunctiva by eversion of the upper eyelid

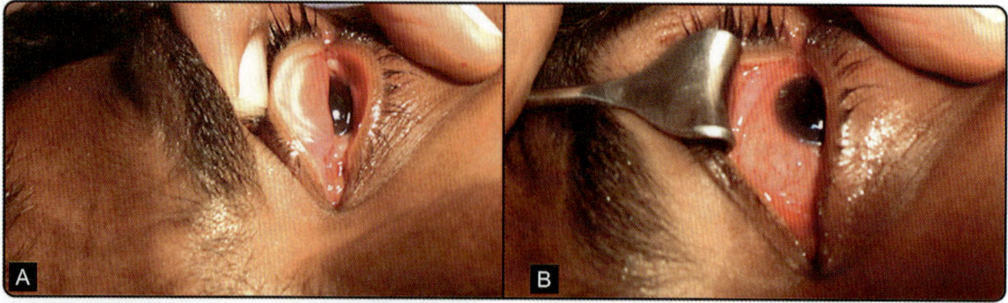

Figs 2.38A and B: Examination of superior fornix by using Desmarres lid retractor

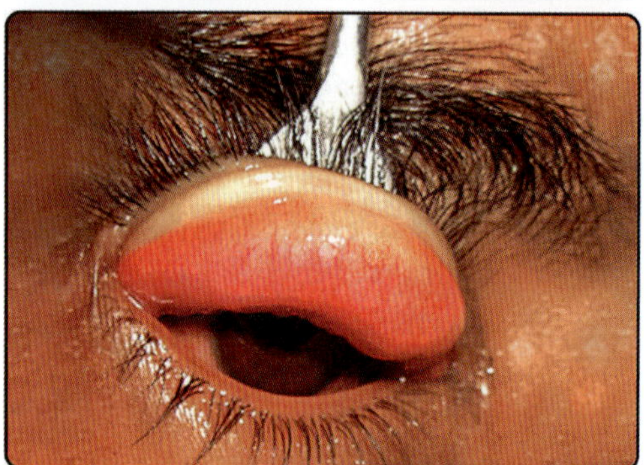

Fig. 2.39: Double eversion of the upper eyelid using Desmarres lid retractor

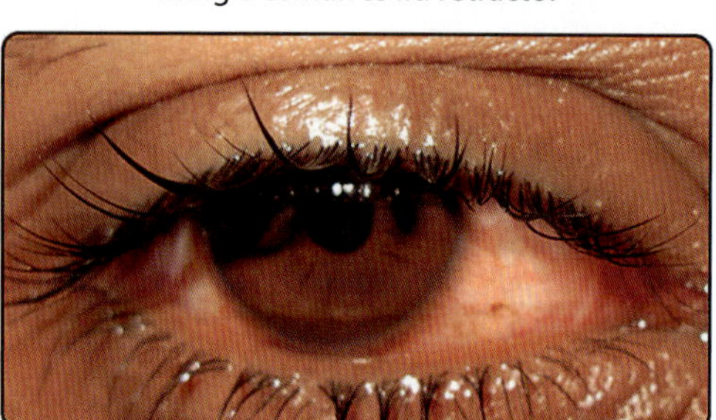

Fig. 2.40: Conjunctival congestion in a patient with acute conjunctivitis

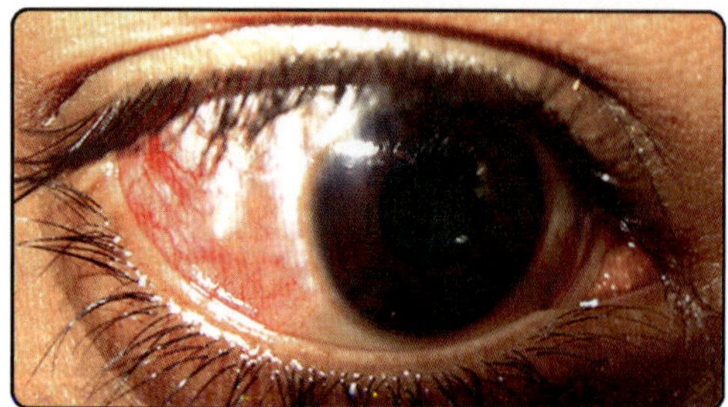

Fig. 2.41: Sectoral congestion in a patient with episcleritis

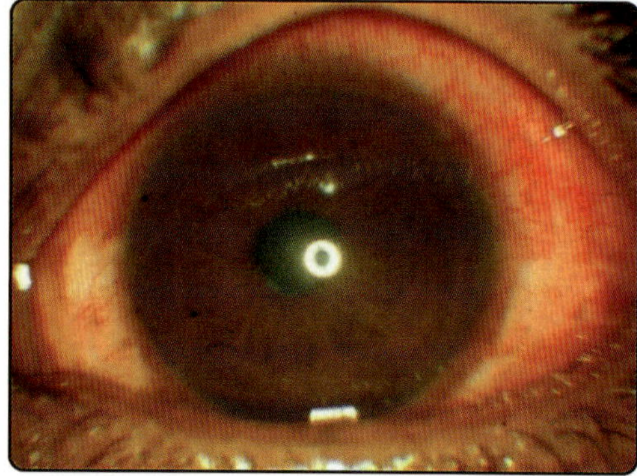

Fig. 2.42: Ciliary congestion in a patient with anterior iridocyclitis

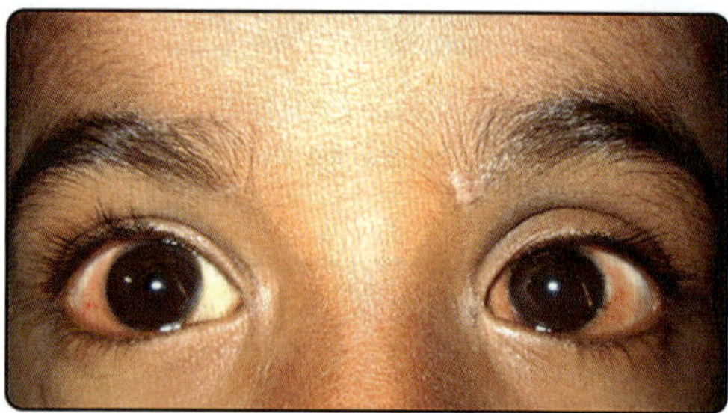

Fig. 2.43: Dusky red congestion seen in allergic conjunctivitis

Ecchymosis

Collection of blood under the bulbar conjunctiva is called ecchymosis.

Causes

1. Trauma is the commonest cause for subconjunctival hemorrhage. It may be because of direct trauma to conjunctiva resulting in rupture of conjunctival

Contd...

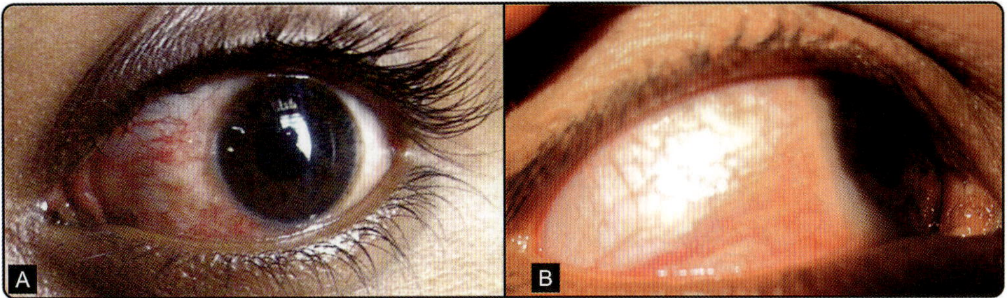

Figs 2.44A and B: Gelatinous thickening around limbus seen in bulbar form of vernal conjunctivitis

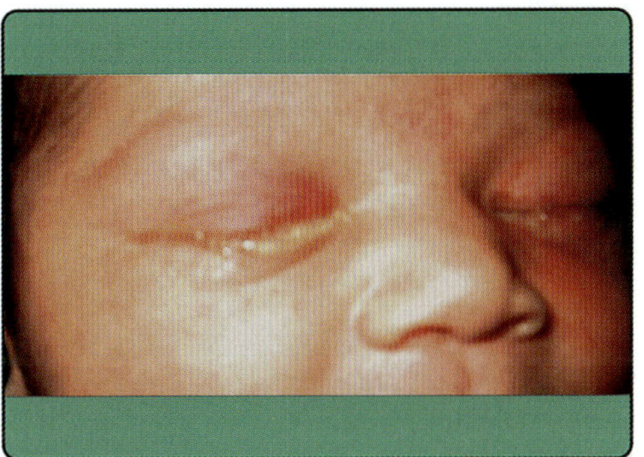

Fig. 2.45: An infant with ophthalmia neonatorum

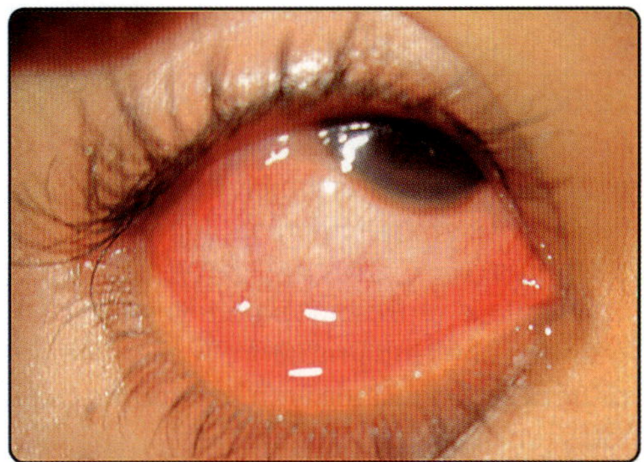

Fig. 2.46: Chemosis

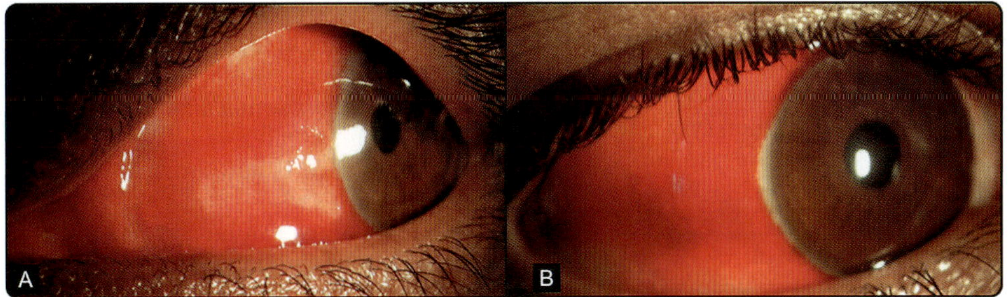

Figs 2.47A and B: Subconjunctival hemorrhage

Contd...

capillaries or because of seepage of blood along floor of the orbit as in fractures of base of skull and head injuries.

2. Hemorrhagic conjunctivitis caused by enterovirus, pneumococci.
3. Vascular diseases because of spontaneous rupture of the capillaries, e.g. diabetes, hypertension and arteriosclerosis.
4. Bleeding diseases like hemophilia and blood dyscrasis like leukemia, anemia.

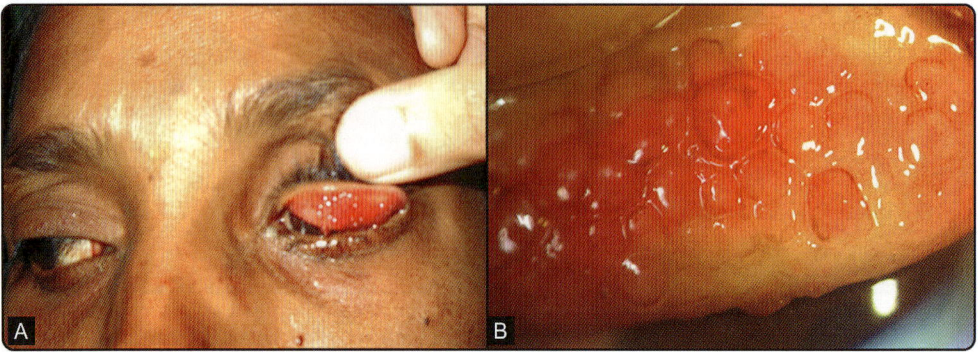

Figs 2.48A and B: Examination of upper palpebral conjunctiva by eversion of the upper eyelid— showing papillae

Follicles and Papillae

Follicles are aggregation of lymphocytes, which present as elevated lesions with pale centers, seen in follicular conjunctivitis, trachoma.

Papillae represent blood vessels surrounded by inflammatory cells, which present as flat lesions with hyperemic center, seen in allergic conjunctivitis.

Pterygium and Pinguecula

Common degenerative conditions of conjunctiva are described under pterygium.

Conjunctival Cysts and Tumors

- Common conjunctival cysts are cysticercosis cyst, retention cyst
- Common tumors are papilloma, squamous cell carcinoma.

Xerosis of Conjunctiva

Characterized by dry, lustreless conjunctiva seen typically in children with vitamin A deficiency.

Bitot's spot: These are defined as collections of foamy material over an area of conjunctival xerosis consisting of desquamated keratinized epithelial cells and saprophytic bacilli. Their presence indicates conjunctival xerosis.

CORNEA

Cornea has to be examined under the following headings (Figs 2.49 and 2.50):

- Size
- Shape
- Surface
- Sheen
- Sensations
- Transparency.

Size: The anterior surface of cornea has a horizontal diameter of 11.7 mm and vertical diameter of 11 mm.

Abnormalities of Size of Cornea

Microcornea

- Anterior horizontal diameter is less than 10 mm
- Inheritance is autosomal dominant or recessive
- Microcornea can be associated with either microphthalmos abnormal small eyeball or nanophthalmos normal small eyeball or it can be isolated anomaly.

It can be associated with other ocular anomalies such as cataract, glaucoma, aniridia. The systemic associations are Ehlers-Danlos syndrome, Weill-Marchesani syndrome and Nance-Horan syndrome (a syndrome characterized by cataract, microcornea,

Contd...

Contd...

dental anomalies and mental retardation), and Turner's syndrome.

Macrocornea (Megalocornea)

Cornea with horizontal diameter of more than 12 mm at birth or more than 13 mm at 2 years of age is called macrocornea. It usually presents as X-linked recessive condition with more than 90% of the affected people being males.

It can present as simple megalocornea not associated with any ocular anomalies or megalocornea in association with anterior megalophthalmos, characterized by enlargement of the structures of the anterior segment of the eye.

It presents as a bilateral condition and it is because of defective growth of the optic cup. It has to be differentiated from buphthalmos—a condition characterized by marked enlargement of the eye ball seen in congenital or infantile glaucoma and keratoglobus—a condition characterized by thinning and protrusion of the cornea.

How to Measure Corneal Size?

Corneal size is measured with callipers. It is not measured routinely unless some abnormality is suspected. Corneal size has to be measured in all cases of congenital glaucomas to differentiate buphthalmos from megalocornea.

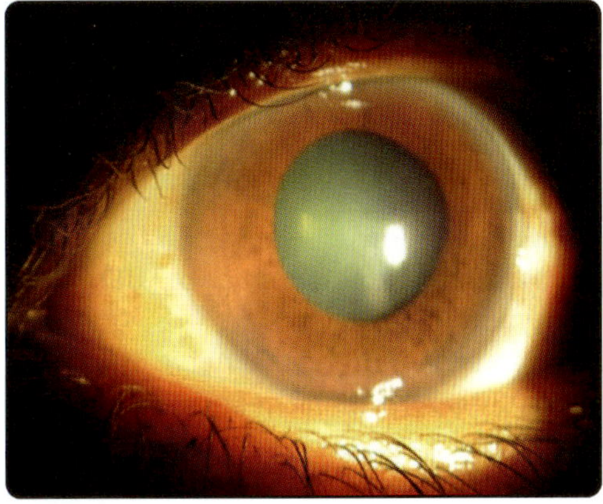

Fig. 2.49: Examination of cornea under diffuse light

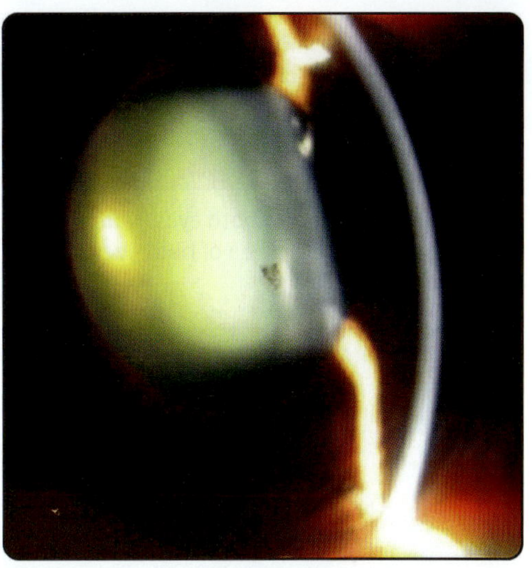

Fig. 2.50: Examination of cornea under slit lamp to study each layer in detail

Shape (Curvature)

Normally cornea is a concavoconvex transparent structure resembling a watch glass with radius of curvature in the optical zone 7.8 mm anteriorly and 7 mm posteriorly. Normal corneal curvature is 44D.

Abnormalities of Corneal Shape (Figs 2.51 to 2.53)

Increased corneal curvature:

- Keratoconus—cone shaped protrusion of cornea
- Keratoglobus—thinning and protrusion of whole of cornea.

  Decreased corneal curvature:
- Cornea plana.

How to Measure Corneal Curvature?

Corneal curvature is measured by:

- Keratometry
- Videokeratography
- Computerized topography
- Orbscan

It is not measured routinely unless some abnormality is suspected.

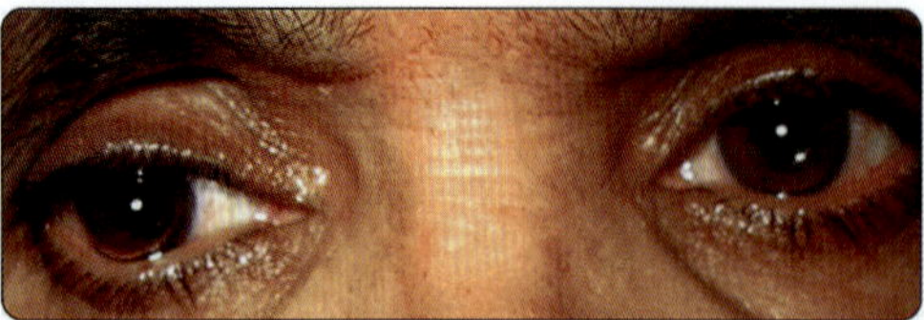

Fig. 2.51: Keratoconus of both eyes (*Note:* Conical protrusion of cornea of both eyes)

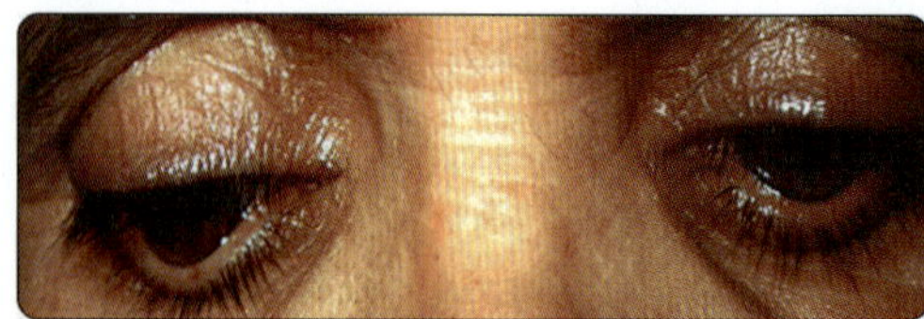

Fig. 2.52: Munson's sign in a patient with severe keratoconus (*Note:* Protrusion of the lower lid margin when the patient looks down).

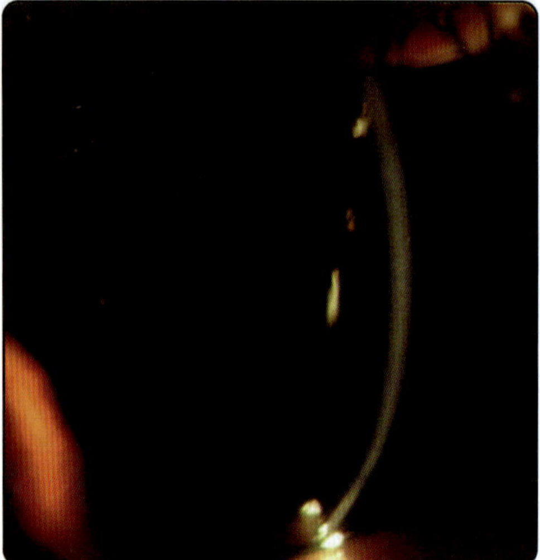

Fig. 2.53: Slit-lamp examination of keratoconus (*Note:* Thinning of cornea inferiorly and conical protrusion of thinned cornea).

Placido's disk test: It consists of alternating black and white circles with a hole in the center, the examiner looks through the hole and looks for the reflection of the alternate white and black circles on the patient's/ subject's cornea. Irregular corneal surface makes the reflected image distorted.

Surface

Normal corneal surface is smooth.

Smoothness of corneal surface is lost in corneal epithelial defects, abrasions, corneal ulcers and corneal opacity.

How to Examine for Corneal Surface?

Window reflex test: Subject is asked to stand in front of a window with bright light from outside; examiner looks for the reflection of the image of the bars of the window. This can also be done by looking for the reflection of the image of the torch light. Irregular corneal surface makes the reflected image distorted.

Sheen

The shining of cornea is called sheen. Normally cornea has a shining surface (Figs 2.54 and 2.55).

Sheen of cornea is lost in dry eye and corneal opacity.

How to Look for Sheen of Cornea?

- Placido's disk or window reflex test is done to look for the sheen of cornea (Fig. 2.56)
- The test is done in the similar way as described above to look for surface
- Sharpness of the image is lost in conditions where sheen of cornea is altered.

Sensation

Normally, cornea is very sensitive.

Diminished Corneal Sensation

- Familial dysautonomia or Riley-Day syndrome
- Paralysis of trigeminal nerve as a result of surgery, trauma, neoplasms

Contd...

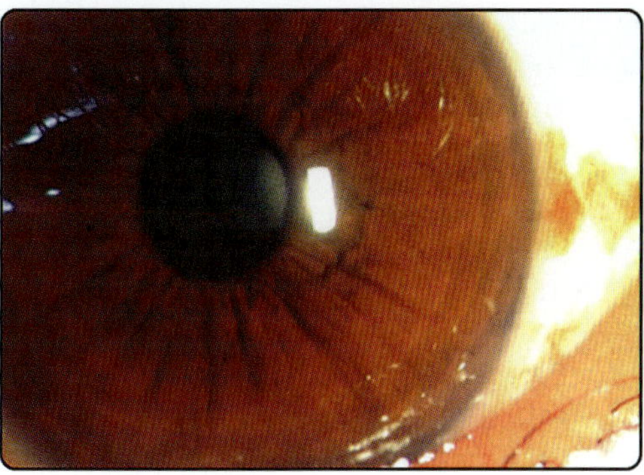

Fig. 2.54: Window reflex for surface and sheen of cornea

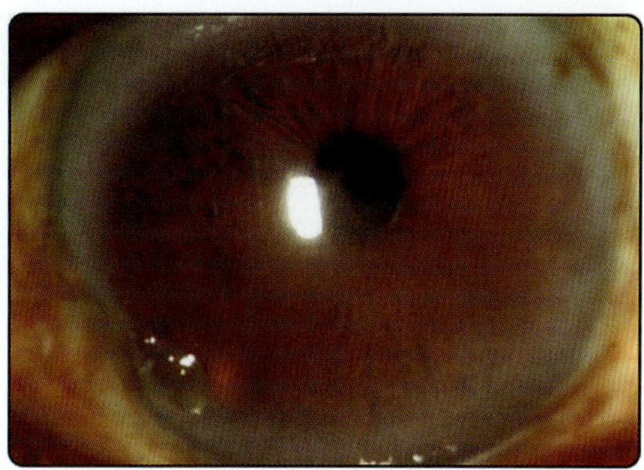

Fig. 2.55: Distorted window reflex sheen of cornea in a patient with corneal edema because of corneal degeneration.

Contd...

- Damage to the sensory nerve endings of cornea as following keratoplasty, refractive corneal surgeries, contact lens wear, herpes simplex keratitis
- Systemic diseases associated with decreased corneal sensation like diabetes mellitus, leprosy
- Drug-induced corneal hypoesthesia as seen with long term use of timolol, betaxolol, ketorolac.

How to Look for Corneal Sensation? (Figs 2.57A and B)

The patient is asked to look straight ahead keeping the eyes wide open; the examiner should touch the corneal surface with dry sterilized cotton and should look for:

- Blinking response
- Ask the patient if he/she can feel the touch of the cotton. The quantitative evaluation of corneal sensitivity can be made from aesthesiometer
- Corneal sensation has to be looked in central and four peripheral quadrants (five in total) and should be compared with the other eye at similar locations (Fig. 2.58).

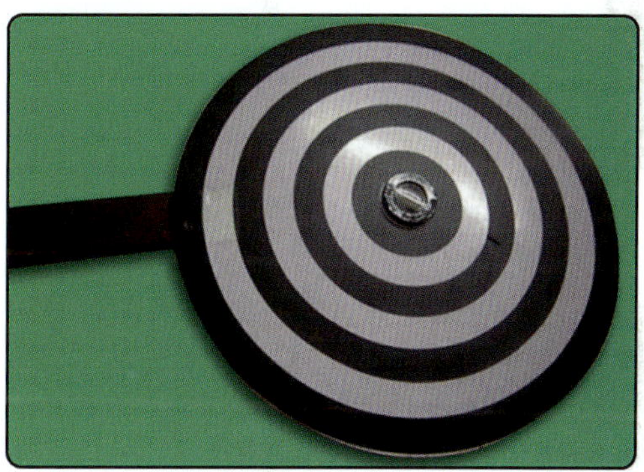

Fig. 2.56: Placido's disk

How to Look for Corneal Sensation in Patients with Reduced/ Absent Blinking Rate?

The test is done in similar way; instead of blinking response Bell's phenomenon is noted.

Transparency: Normally cornea is transparent, i.e. structures inside can be made out clearly.

Why Cornea is Transparent?

Cornea is transparent because of:

- Peculiar arrangement of corneal lamellae (Lattice theory of Maurice)

Contd...

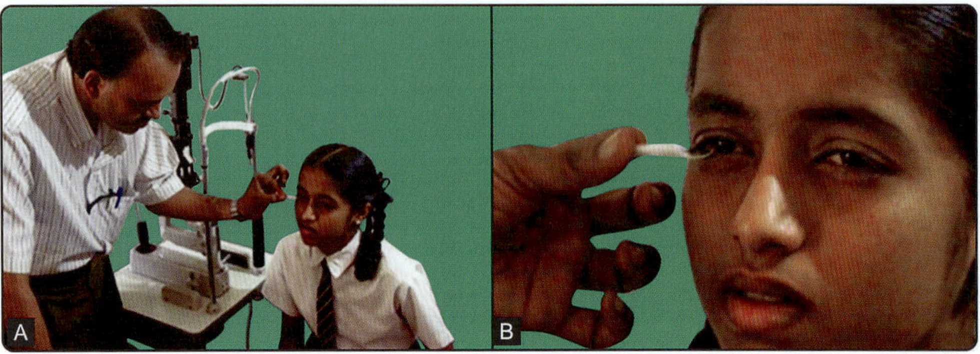

Figs 2.57A and B: Testing for corneal sensation. **A.** The patient/subject is asked to look straight ahead keeping the eyes wide open; **B.** The examiner touches the corneal surface with dry sterilized cotton.

Contd...

- Avascularity
- Relative state of dehydration.

Corneal transparency is lost in corneal edema, corneal ulcer, corneal opacity, corneal degeneration and corneal dystrophies (Figs 2.59 to 2.62).

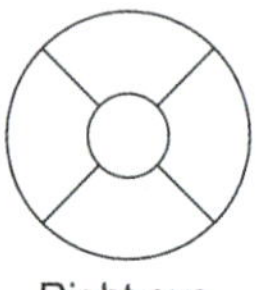

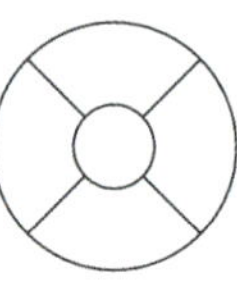

Fig. 2.58: Five quadrants for checking corneal sensation

SCLERA

Normally, sclera is white in color and is covered by the bulbar conjunctiva.

Abnormalities of Sclera

Discoloration

Yellowish discoloration is seen in jaundice and blue sclera due to thinning is seen in:

- Osteogenesis imperfecta
- Marfan's syndrome
- Ehlers-Danlos syndrome
- High myopia
- Buphthalmos.

Staphyloma: Protrusion of thin and weak sclera lined by uveal tissue.

Scleral Inflammation: Characterized by sectoral congestion seen in episcleritis and scleritis.

ANTERIOR CHAMBER

Anterior chamber is examined for:

- Depth
- Contents.

Normally, the anterior chamber is about 2.5 mm deep in center and it contains aqueous humor, which is transparent in nature.

Abnormalities in the Depth of Anterior Chamber

Shallow Anterior Chamber

- Hypermetropia
- Narrow angle glaucoma
- Intumescent cataract
- Phacomorphic glaucoma
- Malignant glaucoma
- Postoperative shallow anterior chamber because of wound leak.

Deep Anterior Chamber

- Keratoconus
- Keratoglobus
- Buphthalmos
- Aphakia
- Myopia.

Irregular Depth Anterior Chamber

- Adherent leucoma
- Annular synechiae leading to iris bombe.

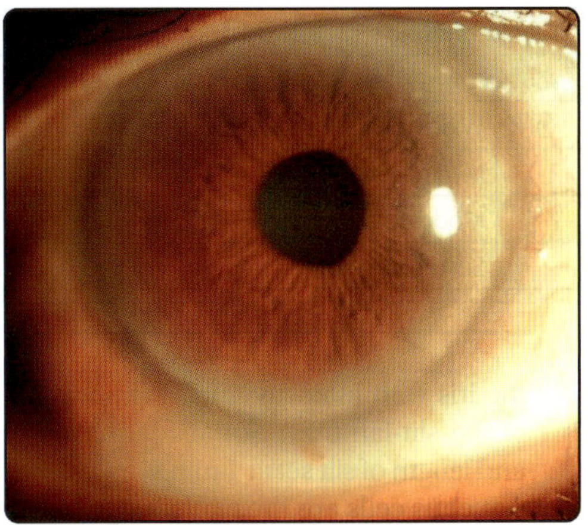

Fig. 2.59: Arcus senilis

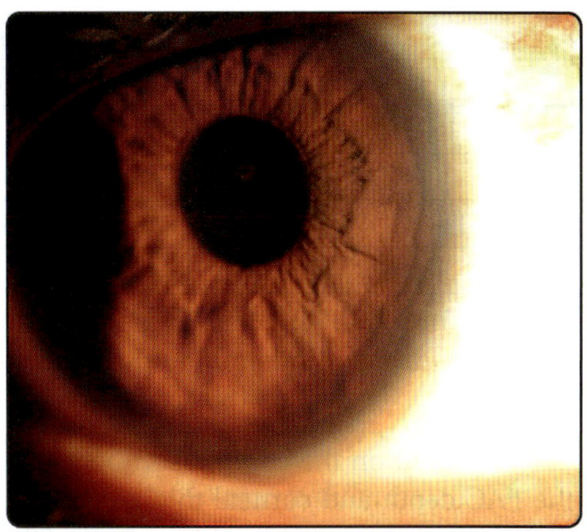

Fig. 2.60: Corneal foreign body

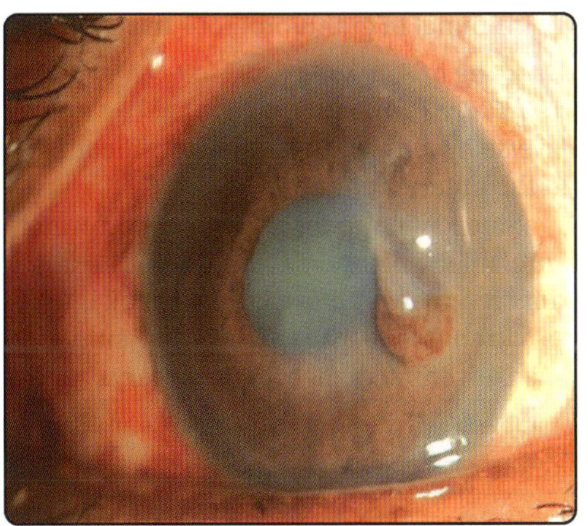

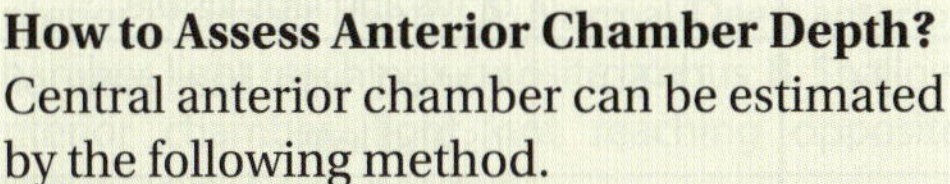

Fig. 2.61: Corneal tear with iris prolapse

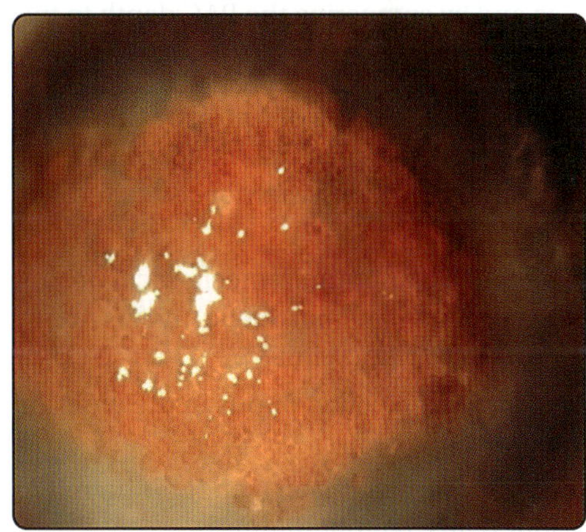

Fig. 2.62: Spheroidal degeneration of cornea (*Note:* The presence of amber colored granules)

How to Assess Anterior Chamber Depth?

Central anterior chamber can be estimated by the following method.

Torch Light Method

Light is thrown from temporal side of limbus, if the illumination is seen at the nasal limbus anterior chamber is said to be normal in depth or not shallow. In case of shallow anterior chamber, illumination will not reach the nasal limbus and nasal half of the iris appears dark as it is not illuminated, this is called eclipse sign.

This method can determine whether depth of anterior chamber is shallow or not, but it cannot determine whether it is normal or deep. Other methods of assessing central anterior chamber depth are:

- Pachymetry by using Haag-Streit optical pachymeter
- Ultrasound pachymetry (A scan)
- Ultrasound biomicroscopy (UBM).

Peripheral anterior chamber (PAC) depth is estimated by slit-lamp method, i.e. Van Herick slit-lamp grading (Table 2.2).

Contd...

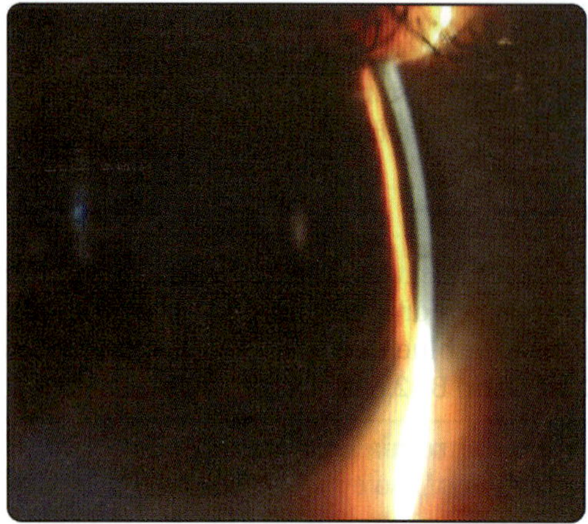

Fig. 2.65: Van Herick slit-lamp grading

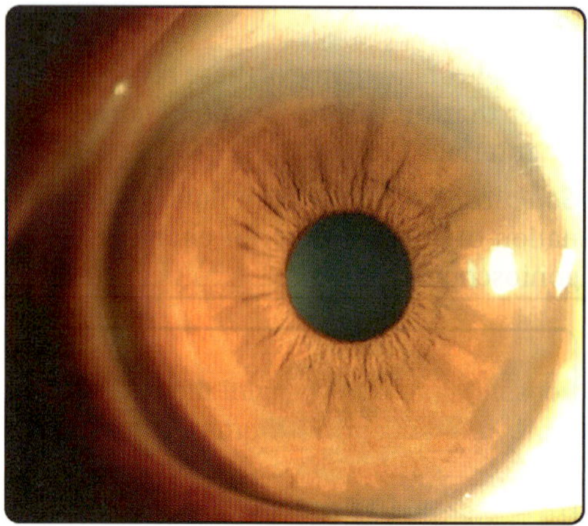

Fig. 2.66: Normal color and pattern of iris (*Note:* The pattern of iris because of presence of collarette, crypts and radial striations on the anterior surface of iris).

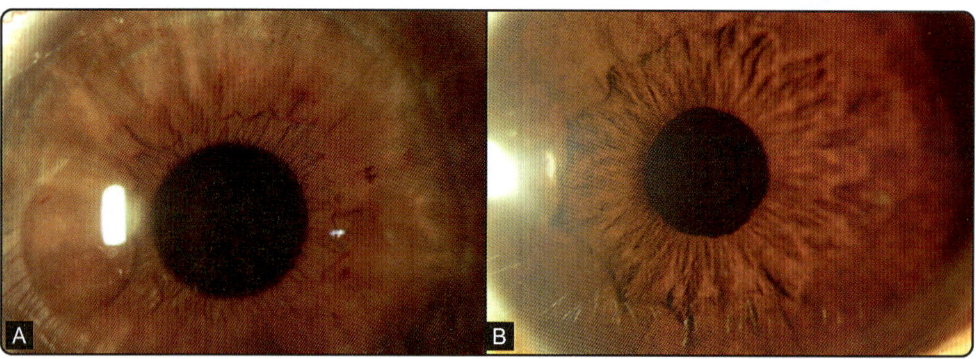

Figs 2.67A and B: Normal variations in color of the iris light brown and dark brown color

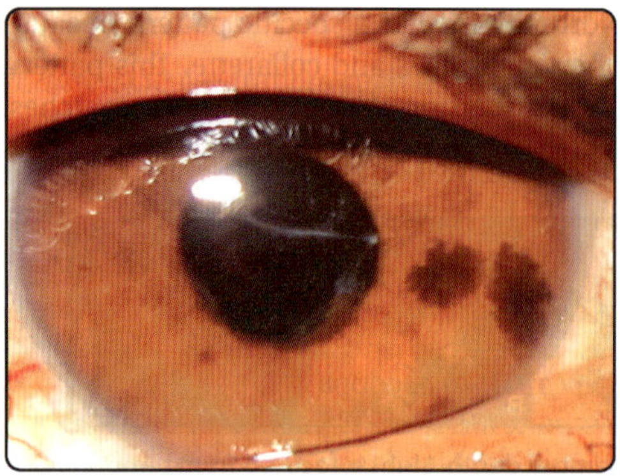

Fig. 2.68: Nevi of iris (*Note:* Dark-pigmented spots on iris, which are relatively common finding)

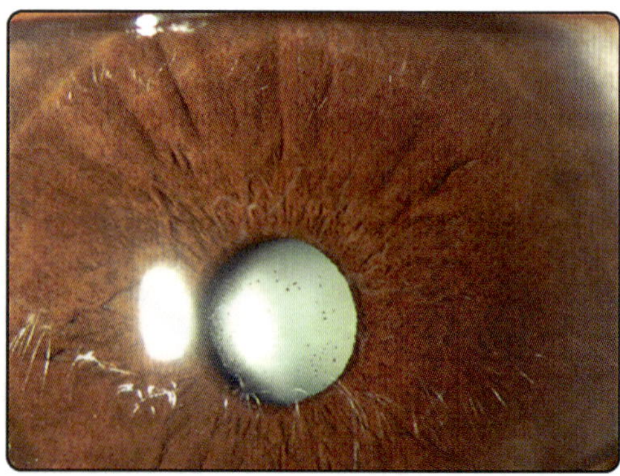

Fig. 2.69: Atrophy of iris (*Note:* Disturbance in the pattern of iris in patient with old healed iridocyclitis)

Abnormalities

1. Iridodonesis: It is tremulousness of iris seen in aphakia due to lack of posterior support, which is normally given by lens.
2. Synechiae: These are adhesions of iris to other intraocular structures:
   a. Anterior synechiae refers to adhesion of iris to structures infront of it like corneal endothelium.
   b. Peripheral anterior synechiae refers to adhesion of iris root to trabecular meshwork. It is made out by gonioscopy and it can result in synechial angle closure.
   c. Posterior synechiae (Figs 2.70 and 2.71) refers to adhesion of iris to structures behind the iris like lens.
3. Pseudoexfoliation: Small flakes seen on the pupillary margin indicate pseudoexfoliation (Fig. 2.72).
4. Pseudoexfoliation syndrome: It is a clinical syndrome characterized by deposition of pseudoexfoliation material on the anterior capsule of the lens, zonules of lens, pupillary margin of the iris, endothelium of cornea, trabecular meshwork and other structures of the anterior segment of the eye. There is a strong relation between glaucoma and pseudoexfoliation. Hence, all patients with pseudoexfoliation should be screened for glaucoma. True exfoliation is seen in glass blowers because of exposure to heat.
5. Persistent pupillary membrane: It is remnant of vascular sheath of lens seen as tags on the surface of iris.
6. Rubeosis iridis: New vessel formation on iris seen in central retinal vein occlusion, diabetes mellitus, Fuchs heterochromic iridocyclitis, anterior segment ischemia, carotid artery occlusive disease, neovascular glaucoma (Figs 2.73 to 2.77).
7. Coloboma of iris: Coloboma means absence of tissue due to failure of closure of embryonic fissure (Fig. 2.78). Coloboma of iris can be typical or atypical, complete or incomplete:
   a. Typical: Seen in inferonasal quadrant.
   b. Atypical: Seen in other position.
   c. Complete: When it extends from iris to optic nerve, i.e. involving iris, lens, retina, choroid and optic disk.
   d. Incomplete: When it fails to extend from iris to optic nerve.

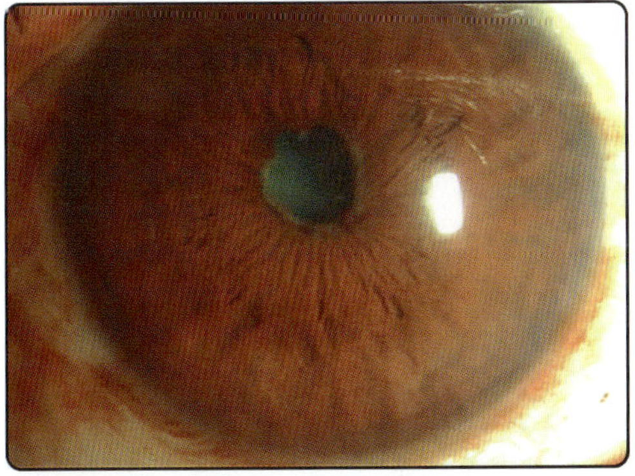

Fig. 2.70: Segmental posterior synechiae (*Note:* The adhesions of iris at some points to underlying lens leading to festooned pupil because of patchy dilatation in response to mydriatic agents).

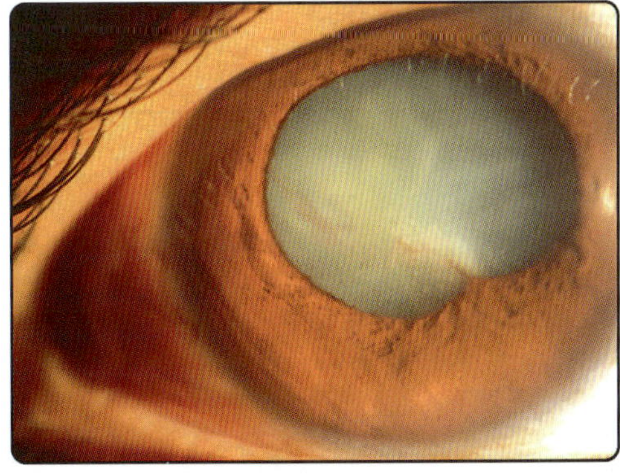

Fig. 2.71: Cataract with posterior synechiae following trauma (*Note:* The adhesion between iris and anterior capsule of lens).

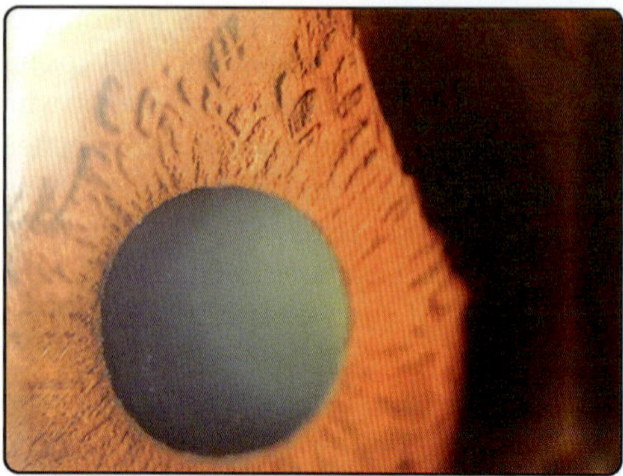

Fig. 2.72: Pseudoexfoliation of iris (*Note:* The presence of white flakes at the pupillary margin of iris)

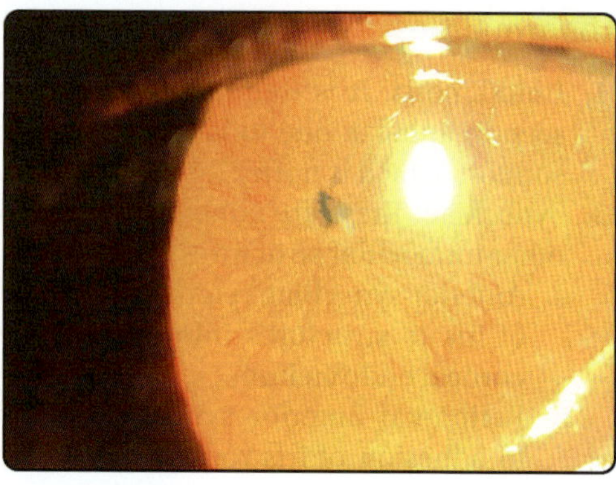

Fig. 2.73: Occlusive pupillae (*Note:* The occlusion of pupil completely due to exudates)

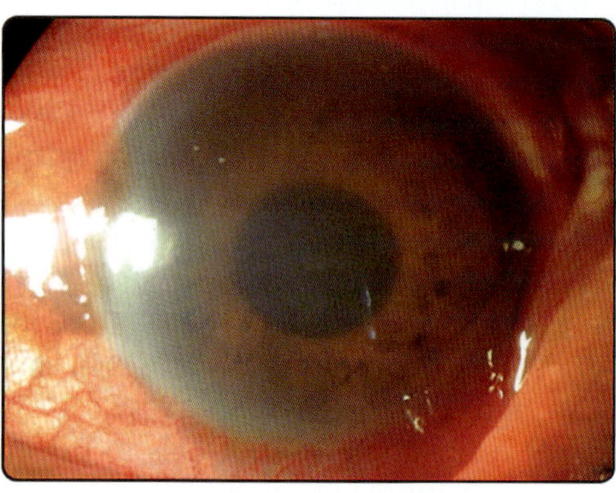

Fig. 2.74: Acute angle closure (Note: Circumcorneal congestion, corneal edema, mid-dilated pupil, shallow anterior chamber).

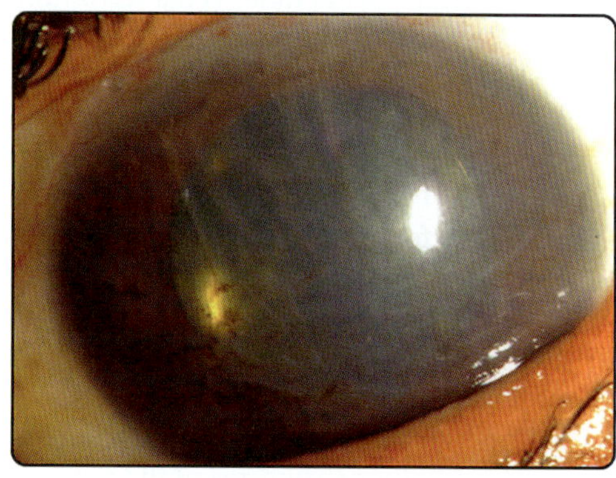

Fig. 2.75: Corneal edema with keratic precipitates over endothelium in a patient with iridocyclitis

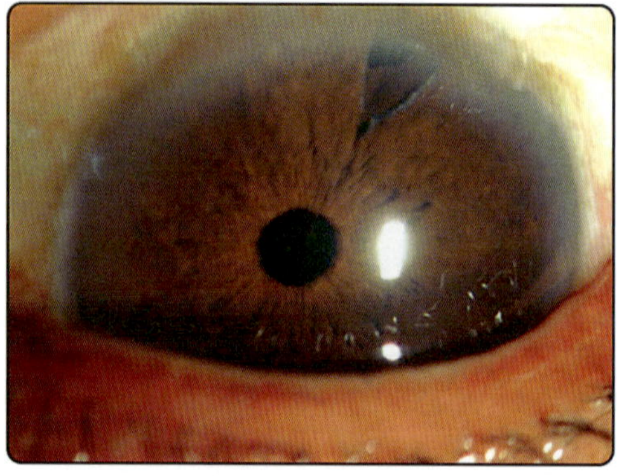

Fig. 2.76: An eye with shallow anterior chamber with prophylactic iridotomy

Fig. 2.77: Slit-lamp photograph demonstrating anterior chamber flare

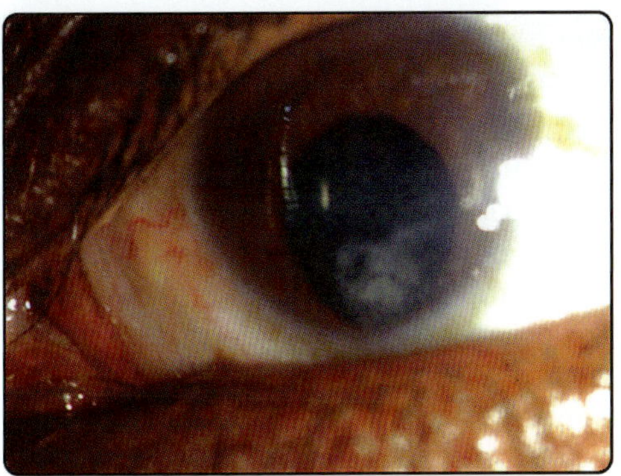

Fig. 2.78: Coloboma of iris (*Note:* The absence of iris tissue in the inferonasal quadrant)

PUPIL

Pupil is an aperture in the center of the iris. Pupil has to be examined under the following headings:

1. Number: Normally there is one pupil. Polycoria congenital presence of more than one pupil.
2. Site: Normally pupil is placed in the center or slightly nasal. Congenital eccentric pupil is called corectopia.
3. Size: Normally, the pupil size is between 3–4 mm.
4. Shape: Normally, pupil is round in shape.
5. Color: It depends on the structures behind the pupil, i.e. lens. Normally pupil is black or grayish black in color.
6. Reflexes/Pupillary reactions: Light reflex and near reflex.

Abnormalities in Pupil Size (Figs 2.79A to C)

The size of the pupil is mainly because of action of two muscles:

1. Sphincter pupillae supplied by parasympathetic fibers.
2. Dilator pupillae supplied by sympathetic fibers:
   a. Abnormally small pupil—miosis.
   b. Abnormally large pupil—mydriasis.

Causes of Miosis

- Physiological: Old age (senile rigid pupil), during sleep, exposure to bright light
- Pharmacological: Effect of parasympathomimetic drugs such as pilocarpine, systemic morphine
- Pathological: Pontine hemorrhage and Horner's syndrome.

Causes of Mydriasis

- Physiological: Exposure to dim light
- Pharmacological: Parasympatholytic drugs such as atropine, homatropine, cyclopentolate, tropicamide and sympathomimetic drugs such as phenylephrine
- Pathological: Optic atrophy, absolute glaucoma, third nerve paralysis and total retinal detachment.

Abnormalities in Pupil Shape

Normally pupil is round in shape. Shape becomes irregular due to synechiae in cases of iridocyclitis.

Festooned pupil: Irregular dilated pupil seen after effect of mydriatics in presence of posterior synechiae (Fig. 2.80).

Abnormalities in Color of Pupil

- Normally color of pupil is black/grayish black
- Grayish white immature cataract
- Pearly white mature cataract
- Milky white hypermature cataract
- Jet black aphakia
- Jet black with shining reflexes pseudophakia
- Yellowish white mid-dilated non-reacting pupil—amaurotic cat's eye (seen in retinoblastoma, retrolental fibroplasias and toxocara endophthalmitis).

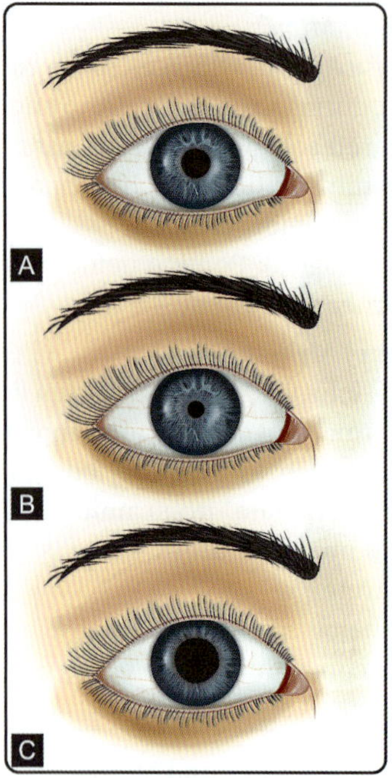

Figs 2.79A to C: Abnormalities in pupil size. **A.** Normal pupil 2–4 mm in diameter; **B.** Miotic pupil < 1 mm in diameter; **C.** Mydriatic pupil > 6 mm in diameter.

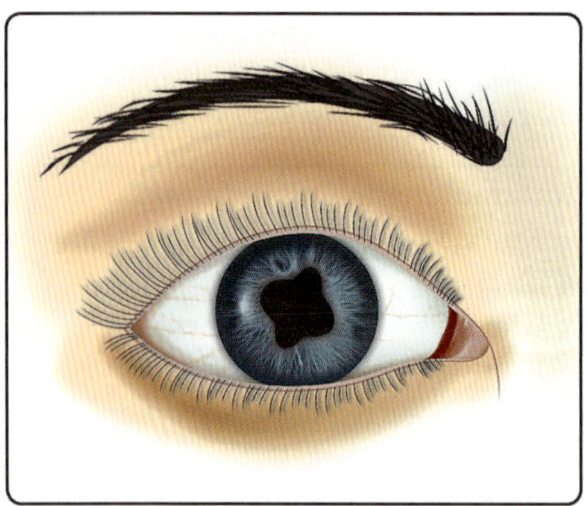

Fig. 2.80: Festooned pupil

How to Look for Pupillary Reactions?

Direct Light Reflex

Subject is seated in dimly illuminated room, two eyes are separated by palm of the hand or a cardboard and light is focused on one eye, while observing for constriction of pupil. Other eye is tested in the same way. Normally pupil constricts on exposure to light.

Indirect Light Reflex/Consensual Light Reflex

Subject is seated in dimly illuminated room, two eyes are separated by palm of the hand or a cardboard and light is thrown on one eye observing for constriction of pupil in the other eye. Other eye is tested in the same way. Normally contralateral pupil also constricts when light is thrown on one eye.

Near Reflex

Subject is asked to look at far object and then asked to see fingertip held at 15 cm from eye observing for constriction of pupil and convergence.

Normally, on looking at nearby objects pupils constrict and eyes converge.

Pathway of Pupillary Reflexes

Light Reflex

Light reflexes are as follows:

- Afferent: Optic nerve
- Center: Edinger-Westphal (EW) nucleus
- Efferent: Oculomotor nerve.

Afferent fibers start from rods and cones in retina, and travel along optic nerve and optic chiasm. In optic chiasm, nasal fibers decussate and travel along the opposite optic tract and temporal fibers travel along the same optic tract to end in pretectal nucleus.

Edinger-Westphal nucleus receives fibers from both pretectal nuclei.

Efferent fibers consists of parasympathetic fibers arising from EW nucleus and travel along the oculomotor nerve to reach the ciliary ganglion. Postganglionic fibers travel along the short ciliary nerves and reach sphincter pupillae.

Near Reflex

Near reflex occurs on looking at a near object. It consists of two components:

1. Convergence reflex:
   a. Afferent: Oculomotor nerve.
   b. Centre: Edinger-Westphal nucleus.
   c. Efferent: Optic nerve.

   Afferent fibres travel along the oculomotor nerve from medial recti to a presumptive convergence center in pretectal region and then to the center, EW nucleus. Efferent fibers arise from EW nucleus and travel along the oculomotor nerve to accessory ciliary ganglion. Postganglionic fibers innervate the sphincter pupillae.
2. Accommodation reflex:
   a. Afferent: Optic nerve.
   b. Center: Edinger-Westphal nucleus.
   c. Efferent: Oculomotor nerve.

   Afferent fibres from retina travel along optic nerve, optic chiasm, optic tract, lateral geniculate body, optic radiations and striate cortex to reach parastriate cortex. From the parastriate cortex, the fibers reach EW nucleus through the occipitomesencephalic tract. Efferent fibers travel along oculomotor nerve to reach the sphincter pupillae and ciliary muscle.

Abnormalities of Pupillary Reflexes

Amaurotic Pupil or Total Afferent Pathway Defect

Amaurotic pupil or total afferent pathway defect is characterized by the absence of direct light reflex on affected side and absence of consensual reflex on normal side. This is seen in complete lesions of optic nerve or retina on the affected side leading to complete blindness.

Marcus Gunn Pupil or Relative Afferent Pathway Defect

Marcus Gunn pupil or relative afferent pathway defect is characterized by the paradoxical response of the pupil to light in the form of dilatation of the pupils both eyes on stimulation of diseased eye and constriction of pupils of both the eyes on stimulation of normal eye. This is seen in incomplete optic nerve lesions. It is tested by swinging flash light test.

Swinging Flash Light Test (Figs 2.81A and B)

A light source is alternatively directed from one eye to the other. First light is directed to normal eye and it results in constriction of both pupils, and then light is directed to affected eye, which results in dilatation of both pupils. This paradoxical dilatation of pupil is called Marcus Gunn pupil.

Wernicke's Hemianopic Pupil

Absence of light reflex when light is focused on the temporal half of retina of the affected side, and nasal half of normal side and vice

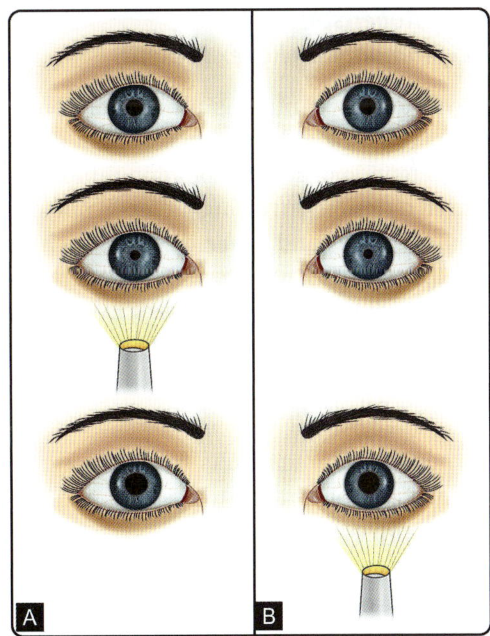

Figs 2.81A and B: Swinging flash light test **A.** On stimulating normal eye (right eye), pupils of both eyes constrict; **B.** On stimulating eye with relative afferent pupillary defect (left eye), pupils of both eyes dilate.

versa, i.e. light reflex is present when light is thrown on the nasal half of the affected side and temporal half of normal side. It is seen in lesions of the optic tract.

Efferent Pupillary Defects

Adie's Tonic Pupil

Adie's tonic pupil is unilateral dilated pupil with absence of poor light reflex, and slow and tonic near reflex. It is seen in parasympathetic denervation as a result of damage to ciliary ganglion. The affected pupil is dilated, but constricts rapidly with 0.125% pilocarpine because of denervation super sensitivity.

Holmes-Adie syndrome

Holmes-Adie syndrome is characterized by the presence of Adie's pupil with decreased deep tendon reflexes and orthostatic hypotension.

Argyll Robertson Pupil (Accommodation Reflex Present)

Argyll Robertson pupil is a bilateral condition characterized by absence of light reflex with retention of accommodation reflex. It is caused by lesions involving pretectal nucleus (neurosyphilis) and other diseases such as multiple sclerosis, tumors of the pretectal region, sarcoidosis and diabetes. The affected pupils are small and irregular in shape.

Horner's Syndrome

Horner's syndrome results from damage to sympathetic innervation to eye.

Features: These are as follows:

- Ptosis because of paralysis of Müller's muscle of upper eyelid
- Inverse ptosis, i.e. elevation of lower eyelid, because of paralysis of Müller's muscle in lower eyelid
- Miosis of pupil due to paralysis of dilator pupillae.

Absences of sweating on the affected side of the face, enophthalmos are the other clinical features. Heterochromia of iris is seen in congenital form.

Causes: The causes for Horner's syndrome are brain stem lesions, multiple sclerosis, syringomyelia result in central Horner's syndrome by affecting the central neurons located in the hypothalamus.

Pancoast's tumor of the lung, apical bronchial carcinoma, malignant cervical lymph nodes and surgeries in the neck result in preganglionic Horner's syndrome by affecting the preganglionic fibers situated between the C8 and T2 of the spinal cord and superior cervical ganglion.

Lesions of the cavernous sinus such as tumors, aneurysms, infections and head injury result in postganglionic Horner's syndrome by affecting the postganglionic fibers.

Central Horner's syndrome is characterized by the presence of sudden onset of vertigo and brainstem signs.

Preganglionic Horner's syndrome is characterized by the presence of anhydrosis of face and neck. Hydroxyamphetamine test differentiates preganglionic Horner's syndrome from postganglionic syndrome. Instillation of hydroxyamphetamine eyedrops cause dilatation of the pupil in case of preganglionic syndrome and pupil will not dilate in postganglionic syndrome as hydroxyamphetamine acts by releasing norepinephrine from the postganglionic nerve endings. The postganglionic nerve endings are normal in preganglionic syndrome, hence hydroxyamphetamine dilates the pupil.

Postganglionic Horner's syndrome can be confirmed by phenylephrine test. Instillation of 10% phenylephrine to both the eyes will result in more dilatation of the pupil with postganglionic syndrome as compared to normal eye because of denervation supersensitivity.

Hutchinson's Pupil

Hutchinson's pupil is characterized by dilated and non-reactive pupil with absence of light reflex. It is seen in head injury or in intracranial mass lesion due to raised intracranial pressure affecting the oculomotor nerve:

- Stage I: Ipsilateral constriction of pupil
- Stage II: Dilatation of pupil with no light reflex
- Stage III: Bilateral dilatation of pupils.

LENS

Lens is a transparent biconvex structure placed in the patellar fossa suspended by the suspensory ligaments of the ciliary processes. Lens has to examine under the headings:

- Position: Normally, lens is biconvex structure with anterior surface less curved than posterior surface
- Shape: Normally, lens is biconvex structure with anterior surface less curved than posterior surface
- Color: Normal color of the lens is grayish black/black
- Transparency: Normal lens is transparent structure.

Abnormalities in Position

Displacement of lens from its normal position. Displacement of lens can be subluxation or dislocation.

Causes

- Congenital simple ectopia lentis
- Ectopia lentis with systemic anomalies such as Marfan's syndrome (typically lens is displaced upwards and outwards), homocystinuria (typically displacement is downwards and inwards), Weill-Marchesani syndrome, Ehlers-Danlos syndrome
- Trauma
- Hypermature cataract.

Subluxation

Partial displacement of the lens from its normal position (Fig. 2.82). Subluxation shows the following:

- Edge of the lens is seen after dilatation of the pupil
- Iridodonesis
- Unilateral diplopia (seen when part of the pupil is phakic and part aphakic).

Dislocation

- Complete displacement of lens from its normal position
- In anterior dislocation, lens is seen in the anterior chamber
- In posterior dislocation, lens is present in vitreous cavity with clinical features of aphakia (Fig. 2.83).

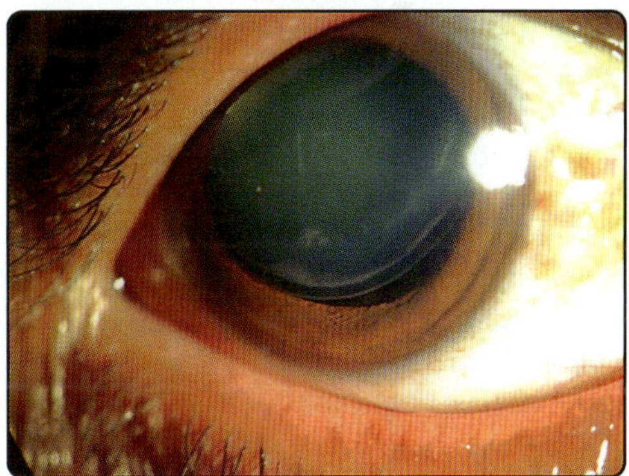

Fig. 2.82: Subluxated lens (*Note:* The inferior lens edge, which is seen after dilatation of pupil)

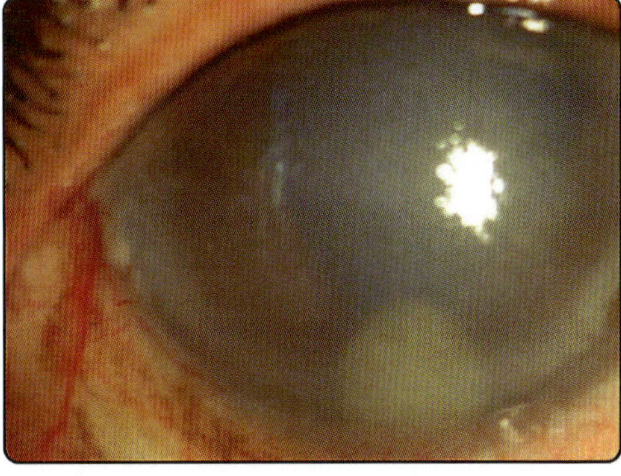

Fig. 2.83: Anterior dislocated lens into anterior chamber (*Note:* The presence of corneal edema with small nucleus of lens in anterior chamber).

Abnormalities in Shape

1. Lenticonus: Cone-shaped bulge seen on anterior or posterior capsule respectively called anterior lenticonus and posterior lenticonus. Anterior lenticonus is seen in Alport's syndrome.
2. Spherophakia (small spherical lens): It is seen in Weill-Marchesani syndrome.

Abnormalities in Transparency

Transparency of lens is lost in cataract.

Abnormalities in Color

Same as abnormalities in color of pupil.

Purkinje's Images Test

Purkinje's images test was described originally to diagnose mature cataract and aphakia. It is not done frequently in clinical practice as by examination of pupillary color mature cataract and aphakia can be easily diagnosed. When light is shown on the eye four Purkinje's images are formed because of four reflecting surfaces, anterior and posterior surfaces of cornea and lens (Figs 2.84 to 2.90A to D):

- Aphakia—both anterior and posterior surfaces of lens are absent, hence both third and fourth images are absent
- Mature cataract—fourth image is absent as light cannot reach posterior surface because of complete opacification of lens.

How to Look for Purkinje's Images?

Torch light is focused on the eye, observing for the reflected image of the torch light on the reflective surfaces of the eye. Of the four reflective surfaces first three, anterior and posterior corneal surfaces, and anterior capsule of lens are convex, i.e. they act like convex mirror, and the fourth reflective surface, posterior lens capsule is concave, i.e. it act like concave mirror. Hence, first three Purkinje's images are virtual and erect (character of image produced by convex mirror), and fourth image is real inverted and minified (character of image produced by concave mirror).

Since, first three images are similar to each other it is difficult to appreciate them separately. The best use of Purkinje's images can be made to differentiate immature and mature cataract. In immature cataract, fourth Purkinje's image is present and in mature cataract, it is absent.

Purkinje's Images

All four present—normal phakic eye, immature cataract, pseudophakia. First three are present and fourth is absent—mature cataract. First two are present, third and fourth are absent—aphakia.

FUNDUS: VITREOUS AND RETINA

Fundus examination is done by:

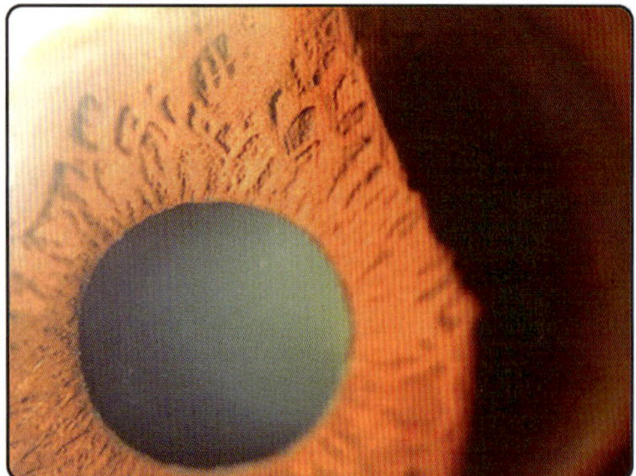

Fig. 2.84: Normal phakic eye (*Note:* The grayish black color of the lens)

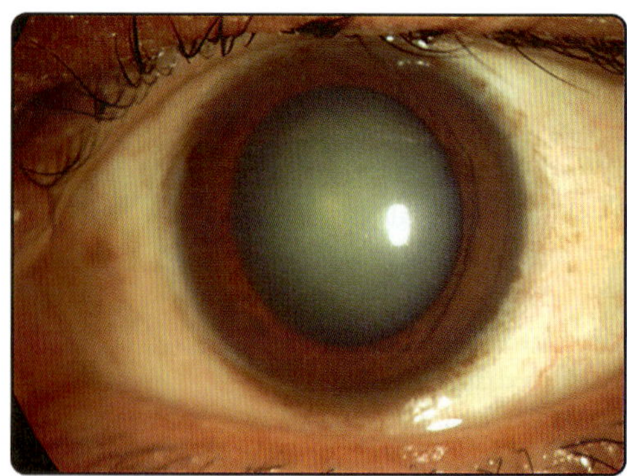

Fig. 2.85: Immature cataract (*Note:* Grayish white color of the lens)

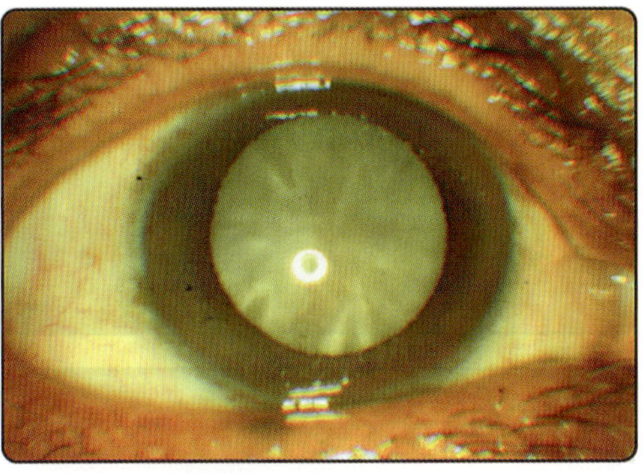
Fig. 2.86: Mature cataract (*Note:* The presence of pearly white color of the lens)

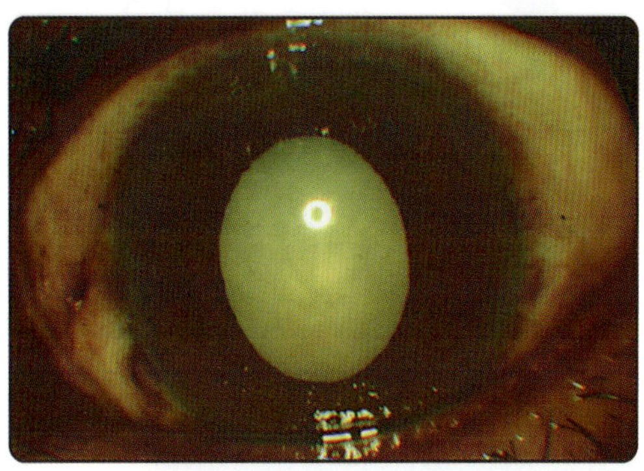
Fig. 2.87: Hypermature cataract (*Note:* The presence of milky white color of the lens)

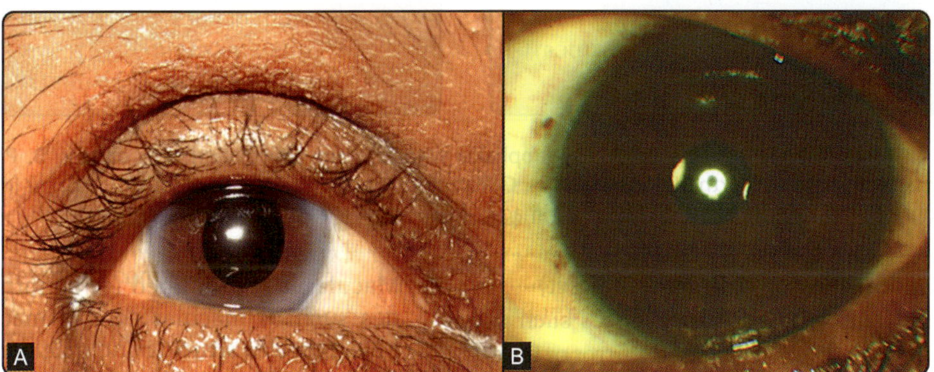
Fig. 2.88A and B: Pseudophakia (*Note:* Jet black color of pupil with shining reflexes)

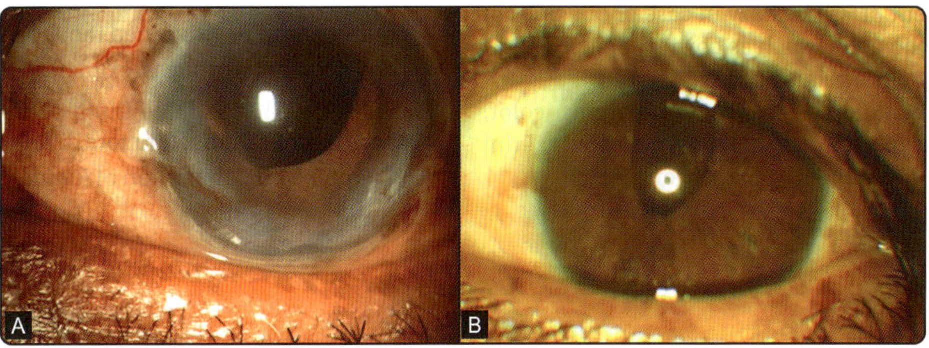
Fig. 2.89A and B: Aphakia (*Note:* Jet black color of pupil)

Eyelids

- Position: ....
- Margins: ....
- Movements: ....
- Palpebral aperture width: ....
- Skin over the eyelids:...........................

Lacrimal apparatus

- Lacrimal puncta:..................................
- Skin over lacrimal sac area: ....
- Regurgitation test: ....

Eyeball

- Size:..
- Position: ....
- Movements of eyeball: ....
- Uniocular movements: ....
- Binocular movements:.........................

Conjunctiva

- Palpebral conjunctiva: ....
- Bulbar conjunctiva: ....
- Conjunctival fornices: ....

Cornea

- Size:..
- Shape:...
- Surface:...
- Sheen:...
- Sensations: ....
- Transparency: ....

Sclera

....

....

Anterior chamber

- Depth:...
- Contents: ....

Iris

- Color: ....
- Pattern:...

Pupil

- Number: ....
- Site: ....
- Size:..
- Shape:...
- Color: ....
- Pupillary reactions: ....
- Direct light reflex: ....
- Indirect light reflex: ....
- Near reflex:..

Lens

- Position: ....
- Shape:...
- Color: ....
- Transparency: ....

Fundus

....

....

Intraocular pressure

....

....

DIFFERENTIAL DIAGNOSIS

....

....

....

PROVISIONAL DIAGNOSIS

....

....

....

INVESTIGATIONS

....

....

....

TREATMENT

....

....

....

Chapter 4

Case Presentation

Chapter Outline

- Cataract
- Pseudophakia
- Aphakia
- Corneal Opacity
- Adult Dacryocystitis
- Chalazion
- Pterygium
- Corneal Ulcer
- Ptosis

CATARACT

Cataract is the most common cause for blindness in India accounting for 62.6% of the blindness.

Refractive error 19.7%, corneal opacity 0.9%, glaucoma 5.8% are the other leading causes in India.

Cataract is defined as opacification of lens and/or its capsule, congenital or acquired, progressive or stationary, partial or complete, with or without visual impairment.

The word cataract literally means waterfalls. The word cataract is derived from a Latin word 'cataracta' meaning waterfalls. It implies that vision of a patient with cataract is foggy as if he/she is seeing through a glass covered with water droplets and it also indicates the color of the lens in total cataract (mature cataract) is white as that of waterfalls.

Cataract is the commonest cause for avoidable blindness worldwide and in India. Cataract is responsible for 51% of worldwide blindness.

CASE PROFORMA (Box 4.1)

Box 4.1: Proforma for cataract

Biodata

Here is a male/female patient aged about..............years,..............by occupation, hailing from..............

Important Facts

Age

- Congenital cataract onset at birth
- Developmental cataract onset after birth to puberty

Contd...

Contd...

- Presenile cataract onset after puberty before 50 years of age
- Senile cataract onset after 50 years of age.

Occupation

Total amount of annual exposure to sunlight has a direct relation to high incidence of senile cataract seen in the hot and dry areas of the world. Cataract is more common in people of rural origin.

Presenting Complaints

His presenting complaints are:

- Diminution of vision in right eye (RE)/left eye (LE)/both eyes (BE) since..............months/years
- ....

History of Presenting Illness

He/She was apparently normal.................months/years back. He/She noticed diminution of vision insidious in onset, gradually progressive in nature. Initially he/she was able to see things at..............meters, now he/she can see things at..............meters.

- Diminution of vision is (choose one among three):
  - Same for both near and distance vision
  - More for near vision
  - More for distance vision.
- Diminution of vision is (choose one among three):
  - Same in dim light and bright light
  - More in dim light
  - More in bright light.
- Diminution of vision is associated with:
  - Glare
  - Pain
  - Redness
  - Watering
  - Discharge
  - Brow ache
  - Headache.

Important Facts

Cuneiform cataract: As the cataract starts at periphery, visual disturbances are noted at a comparatively late stage. As the pupil dilates (Fig. 4.1) in dim light these patients experience more diminution of vision in dim light.

Cupuliform cataract: As the cataract starts in the center, visual disturbances are noticed at early stage. As the pupil is constricted (Fig. 4.2) in bright light, these patients experience more diminution of vision in bright or day light.

Nuclear cataract: In nuclear sclerosis, distant vision decreases and near vision improves due to index myopia. Hence such persons will be able to read without presbyopic glasses. This improvement in near vision is called second sight.

Symptoms: Glare is one of the earliest symptoms of cataract and is due to diffraction of light by lenticular opacity. Other earliest symptoms of cataract are colored halos and uniocular polyopia. Pain, redness, watering, discharge are seen in:

- Complications associated with cataract such as phacoanaphylactic uveitis, phacomorphic glaucoma and phacolytic glaucoma, etc.
- Other ocular diseases such as acute dacryocystitis and conjunctivitis, etc. when present along with cataract.

Contd...

Contd...

Ocular History

- He/She is/was wearing spectacles for (choose one among three):
  - Near vision
  - Distance vision
  - Both.
- He/She give history of surgery/no history of surgery to RE/LE/BE
- He/She give history of trauma/no history of trauma to RE/LE/BE
- He/She history of using eyedrops for long duration/no history of using eyedrops to RE/LE/BE.

Important Facts

- Posterior subcapsular cataracts are associated with prolonged use of steroids
- Anterior subcapsular cataracts are associated with long-term use of miotics such as echothiophate and demecarium chloride
- Amiodarone, chlorpromazine and busulfan are some other drugs associated with development of cataract.

Trauma is associated with:

- Vossius ring
- Conclusion cataract
- Rosette cataract (Fig. 4.3)
- Subluxation of lens
- Dislocation of the lens.

Past History

- He/She is a known diabetic on treatment/not a known diabetic
- He/She is a known hypertensive on treatment/not a known hypertensive
- He/She is a known patient of chronic obstructive pulmonary disease (COPD), asthma, ischemic heart disease on treatment/not a known patient of COPD, asthma, ischemic heart disease
- He/She give past history of tuberculosis/no past history of tuberculosis.

Important Facts

Diabetes and Cataract

Diabetes is associated with early onset of senile cataract or with true diabetic cataract. True diabetic cataract is called snow flake cataract or snow storm cataract. When blood sugar levels are elevated above 200 mg/mL, the enzyme hexokinase is saturated and remaining glucose is converted by aldose reductase to sorbitol, which accumulates in the lens fibers and causes cataract by osmotic stress.

Other Ocular Signs in Diabetes

- Transient variation in refraction as hyperglycemia causes increased refractive index of the lens causing myopic shift and hypoglycemia causes decreased refractive index of the lens causing hypermetropic shift
- Increased incidence of:
  - Extraocular muscle paresis/paralysis
  - Stye and internal hordeolum
  - Infective keratitis
  - Vitreous hemorrhage, central retinal vein occlusion, primary open angle glaucoma and neovascular glaucoma.
- Diabetic retinopathy
- Delayed epithelial healing due to abnormality in epithelial basement membrane.

Family History

- Significant/Not significant
- His/Her father/mother/both had history of cataract/cataract surgery
- His/Her brothers/sisters had history of cataract/cataract surgery.

Contd...

Contd...

Important Facts

- Heredity plays an important role in age of onset and maturation of senile cataract.

Personal History

- Diet
- Appetite
- Habits.

Important Facts

Deficiency of proteins, calcium, essential elements such as copper, selenium and zinc has been postulated in the development of cataract. Vitamins E and C, and riboflavin are involved in lens metabolism, by acting as antioxidants they prevent cataract formation.

Socioeconomic History

He/She belongs to:

- Upper class
- Middle class
- Lower class.

Important Facts

Cataract is more common in people of poor socioeconomic status. For management socioeconomic status plays an important role in advising the type of surgery and type of intraocular lens (IOL) considering the affordability of the patient. Surgeries in camp set-up are done free of cost. Cataract surgeries with multifocal IOL cost around ₹50,000.

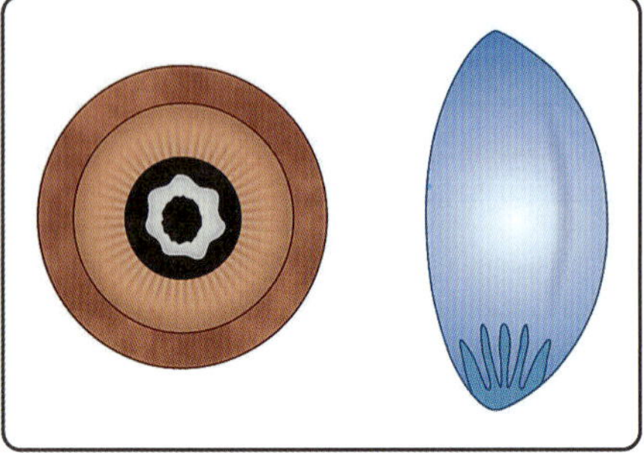

Fig. 4.1: Cuneiform cataract

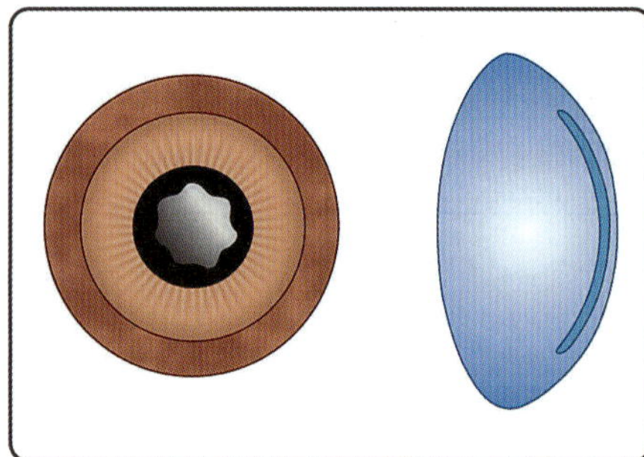

Fig. 4.2: Cupuliform cataract

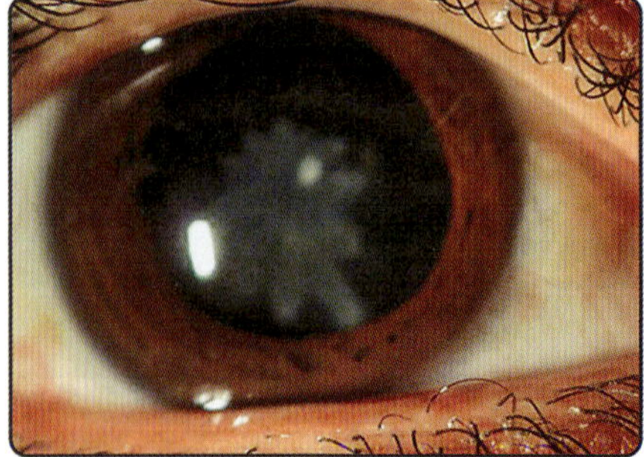

Fig. 4.3: Rosette cataract seen after blunt trauma

CASE DISCUSSION

1. How the cataract is diagnosed?

History: Painless diminution of vision insidious in onset and gradually progressive.

On examination: Visual acuity decreased.

Immature cataract: 6/6p (p indicates person can read only a part of the 6/6) to counting fingers close to face.

Mature cataract: Hand movements, perception of light and projection of rays present.

Hypermature cataract: Perception of light and projection of rays present.

2. What are the significant features of lens in cataract?

Lens opacity

Immature cataract

- Grayish white color of the lens (Fig. 4.4)
- Iris shadow present (Fig. 4.5)
- Purkinje images—all 4 are present.

Mature cataract

- Pearly white color of the lens (Figs 4.6A and B)
- Iris shadow absent
- Purkinje images—first 3 are present.

Hypermature cataract

- Milky white color of the lens
- Iris shadow absent
- Purkinje images—first 3 are present.

Complete loss of vision, i.e. perception of light (PL) negative can never be caused by cataract. Diseases of lens or cornea can never cause PL negative unless there is a problem in retina and/or in optic nerve.

Lens anatomy

- Transparent biconvex crystalline structure
- Anterior surface—radius of curvature is 10 mm
- Posterior surface—radius of curvature is 6 mm
- Refractive index—1.39
- Total power—16 D
- Accommodation:
  - 14–16 D (at birth)
  - 7–8 D (at 25 year)
  - 1–2 D (at 50 year).

Lens transparency

Lens is transparent due to:

- Regular arrangement of lens fibers
- Presence of protective factors such as glutathione in high concentration, which protect the lens against oxidative damage
- Avascularity of lens
- Pump mechanism of lens, which maintains it in a state of relative dehydration.

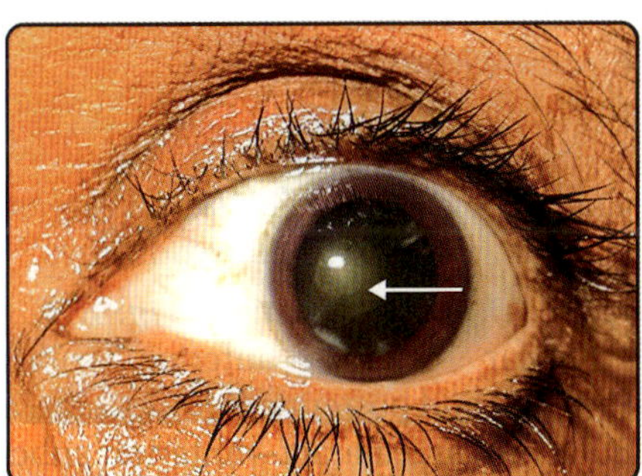

Fig. 4.4: Immature cataract (subtype—posterior subcapsular cataract, e.g. cupuliform cataract) (*Note:* Grayish white color of the lens).

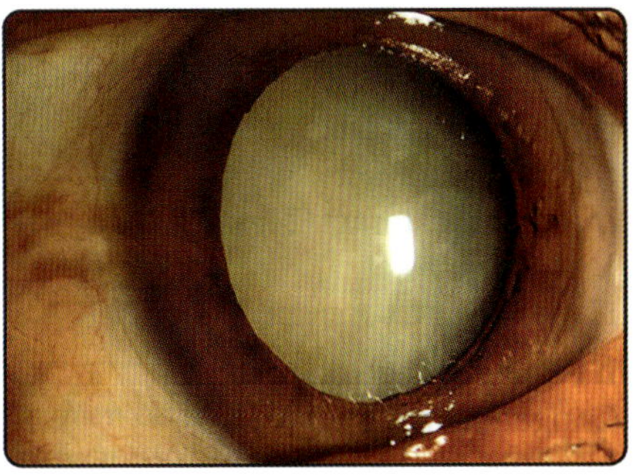

Fig. 4.5: Immature cataract (*Note:* Presence of iris shadow)

a. Inflammatory conditions of the eye such as uveitis including iridocyclitis, intermediate uveitis, choroiditis, endophthalmitis and keratitis.
b. Diseases of the retina such as long-standing retinal detachment, retinitis pigmentosa, gyrate atrophy, Leber's congenital amaurosis.
c. Glaucoma, including primary and secondary glaucomas.
d. Pathological myopia.
e. Intraocular tumors including primary tumors such as retinoblastoma, malignant melanoma and metastatic tumors.

10. What are the characteristic features of complicated cataract?

a. Complicated cataract usually begins in the posterior cortex as posterior subcapsular opacity (Fig. 4.12).
b. Breadcrumb appearance and polychromatic luster are the characteristic features of complicated cataract (Figs 4.13A and B).

11. Classify congenital cataract.

- Lamellar cataract
- Cataracta centralis pulverulenta
- Sutural cataract
- Blue dot cataract
- Anterior polar cataract
- Posterior polar cataract
- Total congenital cataract.

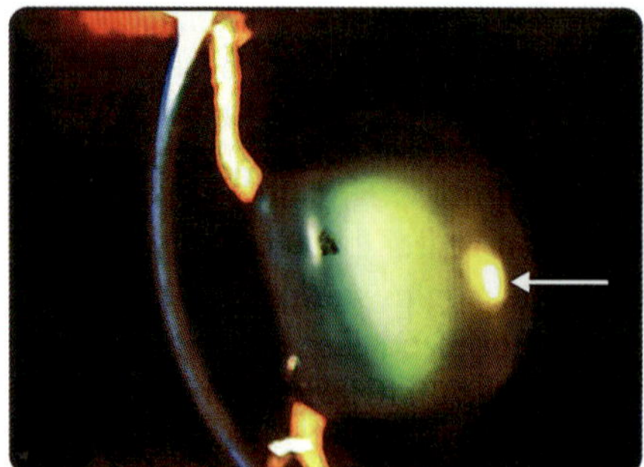

Fig. 4.12: Complicated cataract (*Note:* Presence of opacity in the center of the posterior cortex as shown in the slit-lamp section of lens.

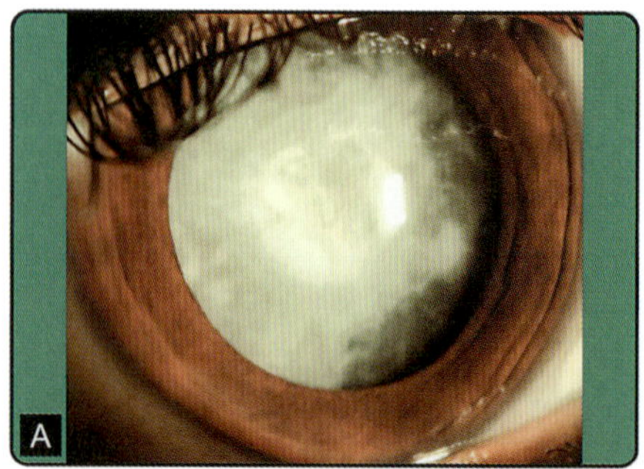

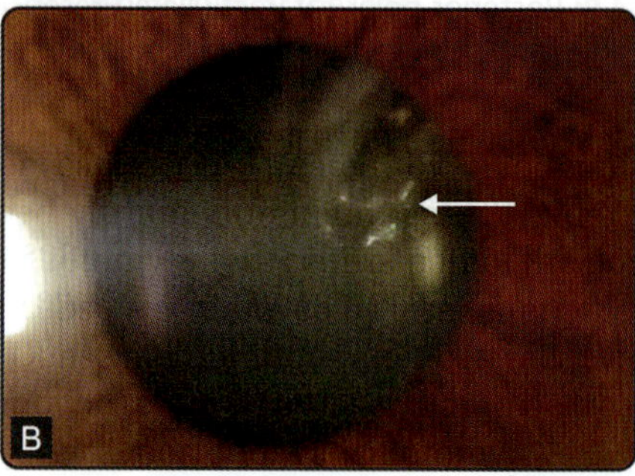

Figs 4.13A and B: Complicated cataract. **A.** Presence of yellowish, dirty, chalky white color of the lens; **B.** Polychromatic luster in a patient with complicated cataract.

12. What is the mechanism of formation of cataract?

Cortical cataract: Decreased level of proteins and amino acids with increasing age leading to increase in the permeability of lens capsule resulting in increased levels of sodium causing increased hydration. Increased hydration of the lens leads to opacification of lens fibers. The cortical cataract is because of overhydration and the cortical cataract is called soft cataract.

Nuclear cataract: Nuclear cataract is because of dehydration and it is called hard cataract. The mechanism of formation of nuclear cataract is from dehydration leading to increase in water-insoluble proteins and compaction of nucleus. Nuclear cataract may be associated with deposition of urochrome or melanin derived from the amino acids.

13. What is nuclear cataract?

Cataract, which occurs as a result of age-related sclerosis is called nuclear cataract. Nuclear cataract can be:

- Cataracta brunescens (brown cataract)
- Cataracta rubra (red cataract)
- Cataracta nigra (black cataract).

14. What is nuclear sclerosis?

Nuclear sclerosis is the hardness of the nucleus. It is found in both cortical and nuclear cataracts and in immature or mature cataract. Nuclear sclerosis can be graded by examining the color and size of the lens after dilatation of the pupil.

15. How do you grade nuclear sclerosis (Figs 4.14A to C)?

- Grade I—grayish yellow
- Grade II—grayish orange
- Grade III—grayish brown
- Grade IV—black.

16. What is second sight?

Improvement in near vision in patients with nuclear sclerosis due to progressive index myopia is called second sight. This is because of neutralization of the 'plus' power of presbyopia by the 'minus' power of myopia, which is because of index myopia as a result of increase in the refractive index of the lens caused by nuclear sclerosis.

17. What is Iris shadow?

Crescenteric shadow of pupillary margin of iris formed on the grayish opacity of the lens when an oblique beam of light is thrown on the pupil is called iris shadow. When lens is completely transparent or opaque, no iris shadow is formed. Hence, iris shadow is a sign of immature cataract (Figs 4.15A and B).

18. Why Iris shadow is seen?

For shadow to form this requirement is the transparent media, which allows light and opaque media, which acts as a screen on which the image is formed. This requirement is fulfilled only in immature cataract.

In immature cataract, there is a clear lens between the iris and the lens opacity, thus iris shadow is formed in immature cataract.

Normally, lens is completely transparent in mature and the hypermature cataract lens is completely opaque. Hence, iris shadow is not seen in these two conditions and seen only in immature cataract in which lens is partly transparent and partly opaque.

19. Name retinal and macular function tests.

Retinal function tests

Projection of rays

The patient is asked to identify the direction of light from which light is coming while projecting light from various directions. Each

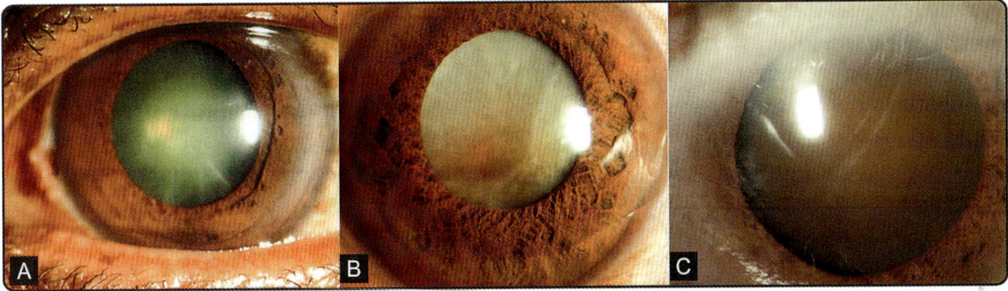

Figs 4.14A to C: Grading of nuclear sclerosis. **A.** Yellowish color in the center (in nucleus)—grade I nuclear sclerosis; **B.** Orange color in the center (in nucleus)—grade II nuclear sclerosis; **C.** Brown color in the center (in nucleus)—grade III nuclear sclerosis (cataracta brunescens).

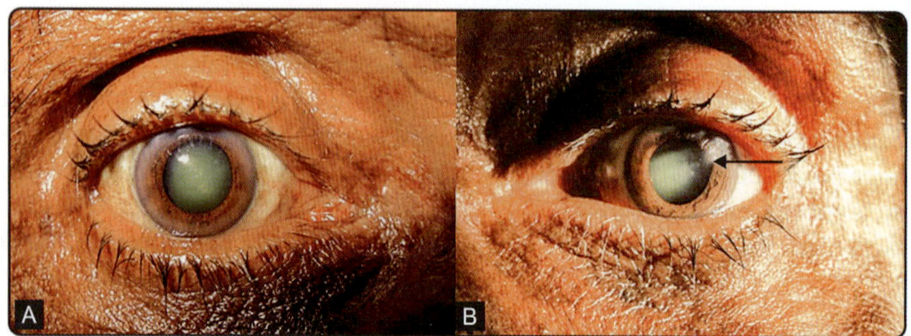

Figs 4.15A and B: Demonstration of iris shadow. **A.** Front view; **B.** Presence of crescentic shadow of the iris on the temporal side when light is directed on the eye from temporal side.

eye is tested separately with the other eye being closed. If the patient can identify the direction from which the light is coming, it indicates good retinal function. Usually projection of rays is tested in the four quadrants to check for the retinal function in the four quadrants of retina:

a. Entoptic visualization: It is done by placing a point source of light against the closed eyelids and asking the patient if he/she can perceive the retinal vascular pattern. The presence of entoptic visualization indicates good retinal function.
b. Test for Marcus Gunn pupillary response, presence of Marcus Gunn pupil indicates afferent pathway defect.
c. B-scan: To detect anatomical state of retina and vitreous.
d. Electroretinogram.
e. Electrooculogram.
f. Visual evoked potential.

Macular function tests

a. Cardboard test (two point discrimination test): Patient is asked to see through a cardboard with two holes close to each other with light behind the holes if two lights are appreciated. It indicates good macular function.
b. Maddox rod test: Patient is asked to look through a maddox rod at a bright light. If the patient sees continuous, unbroken and undistorted red line it indicates that the macula is normal; if the line is broken, it indicates diseases of macula.
c. Amsler grid test: It can be used in eyes with better vision. Patient is asked to close one eye and to see at Amsler chart with the other eye holding at normal reading distance. Patient is asked to look for any distortion in the grid while looking at the central fixing dot; when present, distortion indicates macular pathology. The test is repeated with the other eye.
d. Laser interferometry: It is done by laser interferometer—an instrument used to detect visual acuity in the presence of opaque media.
e. Potential acuity meter: It is done by projecting a slit-lamp miniature Snellen's chart into the eye and the macular function can be judged by lines read by the patient.

20. How do you calculate IOL power?

Calculation of IOL power

Without biometry

a. Using standard power +19 D.
b. Based on basic refraction (refractive error present prior to the onset of cataract):

$$P = +19\ D + (1.25\ R)$$

where,

P = Implant power

R = Basic refractive error.

Contd...

Contd...

With biometry

a. Using regression formulae:
   - SRK-I, SRK-II, SRK-T, modified SRK-II, holladay, etc. [*Note:* SRK formulae are most commonly used (SRK stands for 'Sanders-Retzlaff-Kraff')]:

     $P = A - 2.5L - 0.9K$

   where,

     P = Implant power
     A = Constant
     L = axial length
     K = corneal power in diopters (D).
   - Value of A:
     - For posterior chamber IOL: 118.2 (value of constant varies with the type of lens)
     - For anterior chamber IOL: 114.

21. What is presenile cataract?

Cataract formation because of age-related changes in people aged less than 50 years is called presenile cataract. In all cases of presenile cataract, other causes for cataract have to be ruled out, i.e. trauma, metabolic diseases such as diabetes, intraocular diseases causing complicated cataract, drug intake such as corticosteroids and other drugs causing cataract and skin diseases causing cataract (Table 4.1).

Table 4.1: Some specific type of cataracts and their causes

Types	Causes
Snowflake cataract	Diabetic cataract
Oil droplet cataract	Galactosemic cataract
Sunflower cataract	Inborn errors of copper metabolism, e.g. Wilson's disease
Glass-blower's cataract	Prolonged exposure to heat
Toxic cataract	Long-term use of steroids and miotics such as echothiophate and demecarium bromide
Syndermatotic cataract	Cataract with skin diseases

22. What is the work up for a patient with cataract posted for cataract surgery?

Diagnosis of cataract

History: Diminution of vision insidious in onset and gradually progressive.

On examination

Decrease in visual acuity varying according to the stage of cataract:

a. In immature cataract—6/6 parts to counting fingers close to face (6/6 parts—cannot read complete letters in 6/6, can read only a part of it.
b. In mature cataract—hand movements, perception of light and projection of rays.
c. In hypermature cataract—perception of light and projection of rays.

Presence of lens opacity

a. Grayish white opacity and iris shadow present—immature cataract.
b. Pearly white opacity—mature cataract.
c. Milky white opacity—hypermature cataract.

Eye has got two refractive structures—cornea and lens, which project light rays onto the retina, which travel via optic nerve to the visual sensory area in the occipital lobe.

Diminution of vision should have problem in one of these structures or there can be a problem in all three or two structures at the same time.

Confirm diagnosis and exclude other associated causes for diminution of vision. Slit-lamp examination/anterior segment examination to rule out corneal disorders such as dystrophies and degenerations; pterygium encroaching the pupillary area.

Retinoscopy to rule out refractive error

Ophthalmoscopic examination of retina (fundoscopy), to look for retinal pathologies such as age-related macular degeneration, chorioretinal degeneration and optic atrophy.

Systemic investigations to confirm fitness of the patient for surgery

a. Urine sugar/random blood sugar (RBS) to rule out diabetes mellitus. If the patient is known diabetic, fasting and postprandial blood sugar (FBS and PPBS) has to be done.
b. Blood pressure measurement to rule out hypertension.
c. Electrocardiography (ECG) to know the cardiac status.
d. If the patient is known to have chronic disorders such as COPD and IHD, they have to be controlled before posting the patient for surgery.
e. HIV and HBsAg to take safety precautions if the patient is seropositive.
f. Rule out any potential source of infection such as infected abscess and open infected wound, which may act as a foci for development of endophthalmitis.

Ocular investigations

a. Rule out any ocular infections/inflammatory diseases such as conjunctivitis, stye, chronic dacryocystitis/active uveitis.
b. Lacrimal syringing to rule out chronic dacryocystitis.
c. Retinal and macular function tests to know visual prognosis.
d. Biometry for calculation of IOL power, which includes keratometry and A-scan.
e. Xylocaine test dose to rule out hypersensitivity to xylocaine.

To summarize

Systemic

- Urine sugar/RBS
- Blood pressure
- Electrocardiography
- Human immunodeficiency virus
- Hepatitis B surface antigen
- Evaluation of any chronic disorder and treating it appropriately
- Rule out any septic foci of infection anywhere in the body.

Ocular

- Measurement of intraocular tension
- Lacrimal syringing
- Retinal and macular function tests
- Biometry.

23. What are the differential diagnoses for immature cataract?

Immature cataract has to be differentiated from nuclear sclerosis (Table 4.2).

24. What are the differential diagnoses of mature cataract and hypermature cataract?

Mature and hypermature cataracts have to be differentiated by pseudoglioma (Table 4.3).

Table 4.2: Differences between immature cataract and nuclear sclerosis

Clinical features	Immature cataract	Nuclear sclerosis
Vision	Diminution of vision, painless and progressive in nature No improvement with pinhole	Diminution of vision, painless and progressive in nature Improvement with pinhole
Anterior segment examination	Grayish white color of the lens, iris shadow present	Grayish color of the lens (color varies according to the grade of nuclear sclerosis), iris shadow absent
Distant direct ophthalmoscopy	Black spots against red background	Only red glow is seen

Table 4.3: Differences between mature/hypermature cataract and pseudoglioma

Clinical features	Mature cataract and hypermature cataract	Pseudoglioma
Vision	Decreased, painless and progressive in nature	Decreased, nature of diminution of vision depends on the cause
Pupil	White color	White color and usually semi-dilated pupil
Anterior segment examination	Cataractous lens, fourth Purkinje image absent	Clear lens, opacity behind the lens, fourth Purkinje image present
B-scan	Normal	Vitreous/Retinal pathology is seen

Pseudoglioma

Pseudoglioma includes conditions, which present as leukocoria other than retinoblastoma (glioma). Common conditions included in this list are:

- Retinopathy of prematurity
- Persistent hyperplastic primary vitreous
- Toxocara endophthalmitis
- Coat's exudative retinopathy.

25. What is intracapsular cataract extraction?

Intracapsular cataract extraction (ICCE) is a surgical procedure for cataract, where entire cataractous lens is removed along with intact capsule. It was practiced till 1980, now it is not performed because of increased rate of complications and availability of better surgical techniques. The only indication for ICCE now is dislocated lens into anterior chamber.

26. What is extracapsular cataract extraction?

Extracapsular cataract extraction (ECCE) is a surgical procedure for cataract, where cataractous lens is removed leaving behind intact posterior capsule. It is of three types:

- Conventional ECCE
- Small incision cataract surgery (SICS)
- Phacoemulsification.

27. What are the steps of SICS?

a. Anesthesia: Local anesthesia in the form of peribulbar block or sub-Tenon's anesthesia. Peribulbar block is the preferred one.
b. Preparation of the eyeball by painting the eye with povidone-iodine draping the eye with eye towel.
c. Insertion of the wire speculum.
d. Superior rectus stitch or bridle suture for fixation of the globe.
e. Conjunctival peritomy and cauterization of the bleeding vessels.
f. Scleral groove and sclerocorneal tunnel construction using crescent blade.
g. Paracentesis or side port entry into anterior chamber: It is made by using a paracentesis needle and it is self-sealing, as the dimension is less than 1 mm. This is made at 90° to the main incision. The main purpose of side port incision is to remove the subincisional cortical matter. This can also be used to do capsulotomy/capsulorhexis and injection of viscoelastic because of easy maneuverability.
h. Injection of viscoelastic into the anterior chamber.
i. Capsulotomy or capsulorhexis.
j. Entry into anterior chamber with keratome and enlargement of the wound up to 5.5–6.5 mm.
k. Hydrodissection and hydrodelineation.
l. Removal of nucleus.
m. Removal of cortical matter and epinucleus by irrigation and aspiration.
n. Posterior chamber (PC) IOL insertion.
o. Formation of anterior chamber and closure of conjunctiva.
p. Subconjunctival injection of antibiotic with steroid.
q. Pad and bandage.

28. What are the methods of nucleus delivery in SICS?

a. Phacosandwich method: Nucleus is removed by sandwiching between lens loop and spatula.
b. Phacofracture: Nucleus is removed by cutting it into two or more pieces.
c. Phacofragmentation: Nucleus is removed by fragmenting the nucleus into multiple small pieces by nucleus fragmentor.
d. Fishhook technique: Nucleus is removed by hooking it with a hook mounted on a 1 mL syringe.
e. Blumenthal technique: Nucleus is removed by using a anterior chamber maintainer and a lens glide.
f. Irrigating vectis: Nucleus is removed by inserting a irrigating vectis.

29. What is the relation between corneal astigmatism and scleral incision?

Corneal astigmatism is directly related to the cube of length of the incision and it is inversely related to the distance of incision from the limbus. Hence, shorter incisions close to the limbus and longer incisions away from limbus have the same effect on corneal astigmatism. The preferred incisions are straight and frown-shaped incision, which produces less astigmatism when compared to smile incision or incision along the limbus (C shaped).

30. What is hydrodissection and hydrodelineation?

Injection of fluid under the anterior capsule to separate the cortex and nucleus from capsule is called hydrodissection.

Injection of fluid into the cortical layer of the lens to separate the outer soft epinucleus from inner compact nucleus is called hydrodelineation.

31. What is the anesthesia used for cataract surgery?

General anesthesia: It is used in children, mentally retarded and non-cooperative patients.

Local anesthesia: It is used in rest all. This is in the form of:

- Retrobulbar anesthesia
- Peribulbar anesthesia
- Sub-Tenon's anesthesia
- Topical anesthesia.

Peribulbar anesthesia is the preferred and most commonly used for small incision cataract surgery, as the risk of complications associated with peribulbar block is low, while retaining all the advantages of retrobulbar block.

Lignocaine 2% with duration of action 45 minutes to 2 hours and bupivacaine 0.75% with duration of action 5–8 hours are the most commonly used anesthetic agents for infiltration anesthesia. Lignocaine 4% and proparacaine are used for topical anesthesia.

32. What are the complications of cataract surgery?

During anesthesia (Figs 4.16A and B)

- Globe perforation
- Intravascular injection
- Damage to optic nerve
- Brainstem anesthesia
- Oculocardiac reflex (sinus bradycardia)
- Retrobulbar hemorrhage.

During surgery (operative)

- Damage to cornea:
  - Detachment of Descemet's membrane
  - Damage to endothelium.
- Damage to iris and ciliary zonules:
  - Iridodialysis
  - Zonular dialysis.

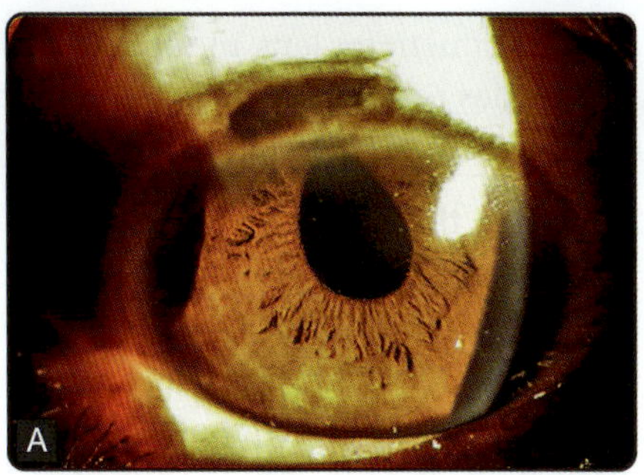

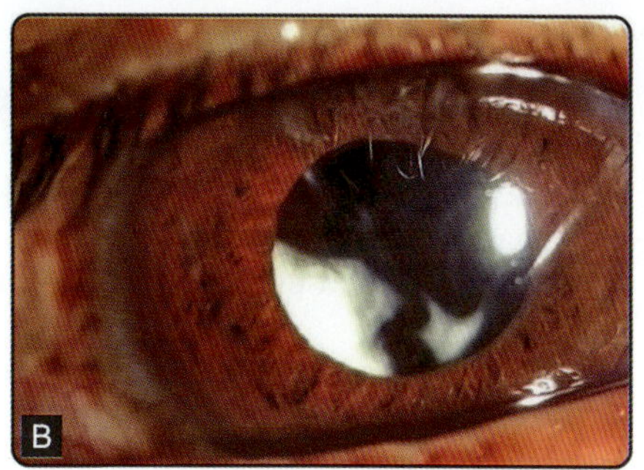

Figs 4.16A and B: Complications of cataract surgery. **A.** Iris prolapse (*Note:* Pear-shaped pupil with iris in the scleral wound); **B.** Retained cortical matter (*Note*: White lens matter in the inferonasal quadrant with pseudophakia).

- Damage to posterior capsule:
  - Posterior capsular tear
  - Vitreous loss
  - Posterior dislocation of lens fragments.
- Expulsive choroidal hemorrhage.

Early postoperative (within 3 week)

- Iris prolapse
- Shallow anterior chamber either because of wound leak or pupillary block glaucoma
- Residual lens matter
- Severe postoperative inflammation (iridocyclitis, phacotoxic uveitis, etc.)
- Endophthalmitis
- Hyphema
- Striate keratopathy.

Late postoperative

- Cystoid macular edema
- Posterior capsular calcification (after cataract)
- Anterior capsular contracture (phimosis)
- Retinal detachment
- Corneal endothelial decompensation—Bullous keratopathy
- Vitreous touch syndrome (Irvine-Gass syndrome)—vitreous touch, bullous keratopathy and cystoid macular edema
- Epithelial ingrowth
- Fibrous downgrowth.

33. What are the IOL-related complications?

IOL-related complications are described under 'Pseudophakia'.

34. What is the postoperative management after cataract surgery?

a. Postoperatively, dressing is removed after 6 hours of surgery.
b. Antibiotic-steroid eyedrops, e.g. ofloxacin-prednisolone acetate, ciprofloxacin-dexamethasone are prescribed for 6 weeks in tapering dosage:
   - 10 times per day in 1st week
   - 8 times per day in 2nd week
   - 6 times per day in 3rd week
   - 4 times per day in 4th week
   - 3 times per day in 5th week
   - 2 times per day in 6th week.
c. Non-steroidal eyedrops such as flurbiprofen, ketorolac are prescribed four times per day for 6 weeks.
d. Patient is seen on the 1st postoperative day, after 2 weeks and after 6 weeks.
e. Visual rehabilitation in the form of spectacles is prescribed after 6 weeks.

Visual rehabilitation

Final spectacle correction is given after:

- 4 weeks after phacoemulsification
- 6 weeks after SICS
- 8 weeks after suture removal in ECCE conventional.

Postoperative instructions

- Not to rub the operated eye

Contd...

Contd...

- Avoid exposure of the operated eye to dust and smoke
- To use protective eye goggles for 2 weeks
- No head bath for 2 weeks
- To use prescribed eyedrops as per the advice
- To report immediately, if the patient notices pain, redness and diminution of vision.

The treatment for lens-induced glaucomas includes reduction of IOP followed by lens extraction.

35. What are the complications of cataract if it is not operated even after its maturation?

Lens-induced glaucomas:
- Lens-induced uveitis
- Subluxation or dislocation of lens because of degeneration of ciliary zonules.

Lens-induced glaucomas

Phacomorphic glaucoma: It is a type of angle closure lens-induced glaucoma caused by swollen or intumescent lens resulting in mechanical closure of the angle of the anterior chamber (AC).

Phacolytic glaucoma: It is a type of open-angle lens-induced glaucoma caused by obstruction of aqueous outflow in the trabecular meshwork by high-molecular weight lens proteins, which leak from microscopic defects in the intact capsule of mature or hypermature cataract.

Lens particle glaucoma: It is a type of open angle lens-induced glaucoma caused by obstruction of aqueous outflow in the trabecular meshwork by lens particles liberated into the anterior chamber following disruption of the lens capsule after cataract surgery or following trauma.

Phacoanaphylactic glaucoma: It is a type of open angle lens-induced glaucoma caused by obstruction of aqueous outflow in the trabecular meshwork by lens particles liberated into the anterior chamber following disruption of the lens capsule and inflammatory cells in response to inflammatory reaction elicited by lens antigen.

36. What are the retinal function tests/investigations to be done before operating on mature and hypermature cataract?

- Test for Marcus Gunn pupillary response, which indicates afferent pathway defect
- Projection of rays—crude, but easy test for assessing the status of peripheral retina
- B-scan—to detect anatomical state of retina and vitreous.

37. Describe the management of cases when cataract is associated with other ocular and systemic diseases.

Cataract with glaucoma

Senile cataract may be associated with glaucoma, as both are seen in elderly age people. The treatment options are surgery for cataract and medical treatment/laser trabeculoplasty or trabeculectomy (surgical treatment of glaucoma).

Cataract surgery along with medical treatment for glaucoma is the preferred treatment for cases in which glaucoma is well controlled with low-dose medical regimen with little or no glaucomatous damage.

Simultaneous cataract and glaucoma surgery (trabeculectomy) is indicated in cases with:
- Uncontrolled glaucoma with maximal medical treatment
- Intolerance to medical treatment or noncompliance to medical treatment
- Advanced glaucoma.

Before operating on patients with cataract and glaucoma together, proper evaluation of the glaucoma should be done by measurement of IOP, visual field examination, assessing optic disk changes due to glaucoma.

Cataract with pterygium

Cataract and pterygium are more frequently seen in association. Cataract and pterygium excision can be done together or separately depending on the surgeon's preferences. Cataract with atrophic pterygium—requires treatment for only cataract in the form of cataract surgery, as atrophic pterygium is usually asymptomatic and would not require surgical intervention.

Cataract surgery with pterygium excision together

Advantages

Operating for both pterygium and cataract during same setting will cure both at once and hence would not require second surgery. Cataract with progressive pterygium not crossing pupillary area—combined surgery, cataract surgery first followed by pterygium excision during the same setting. In cases with progressive pterygium crossing pupillary area and obscuring the view of the lens making the cataract surgery difficult, pterygium excision can be done first followed by cataract surgery during the same setting.

Disadvantage

Pterygium excision will lead to epithelial defect of the cornea and it is not wise to use potent steroids (required postoperatively following cataract surgery) with corneal epithelial defect, as it may get infected.

Cataract surgery with pterygium excision separately

Advantages: It avoids the risks associated with using steroids with corneal epithelial defect. Depending on the cause for visual impairment, cataract or pterygium is operated first followed by the other one.

Disadvantage: Patient requires two surgeries

Cataract with corneal opacity

If the corneal opacity is leukomatous, requiring full thickness keratoplasty, both cataract surgery and keratoplasty can be done together. After removing diseased recipient's cornea and entering anterior chamber, open-sky extracapsular cataract extraction and IOL implantation is done and keratoplasty is completed by suturing donor cornea to recipient's corneal rim. This is called triple procedure—Cataract extraction + IOL implantation + Keratoplasty.

Cataract when associated with infective conditions

Ocular infective diseases such as conjunctivitis, acute dacryocystitis, external hordeolum, internal hordeolum, orbital cellulitis, infective keratitis. Systemic infective conditions such as abscess anywhere in the body and infective ulcer are the contraindications for cataract surgery because of risk of endophthalmitis; hence the infective condition has to be treated appropriately before posting the patient for cataract surgery.

Cataract with chronic dacryocystitis

Cataract surgery is contraindicated in patients with chronic dacryocystitis because of risk of endophthalmitis. Chronic dacryocystitis has to be treated first either by dacryocystectomy (to make the eye safe by removing lacrimal sac, which may be reservoir/source of infection) or dacryocystorhinostomy (to re-establish the patency of lacrimal drainage system).

Treatment protocol

a. In patients with cataract and chronic dacryocystitis, first either DCT or DCR has to be done.
b. Removal of skin sutures after 2 weeks.
c. Conjunctival swab for culture and sensitivity to confirm the sterile ocular surface a prerequisite for cataract surgery.
d. Cataract surgery if conjunctival swab shows no growth of infective organisms (if there is any growth, appropriate antibiotics depending on the culture andsensitivity report have to be used to make the eye sterile before proceeding to cataract surgery).

Cataract with ocular inflammatory conditions

In cases where cataract is associated with non-infective inflammatory conditions such as acute iridocyclitis, cataract surgery should only be done once the active inflammation is treated with appropriate treatment by use of steroids because of the risk of increased postoperative ocular inflammation.

Cataract with chalazion

Though chalazion is non-infective, performing cataract surgery in the presence of chalazion is contraindicated as:

- Chalazion is granulomatous inflammatory condition
- Chalazion may get secondarily infected leading to internal hordeolum
- Hence cataract surgery is performed after treating chalazion.

Medical management of cataract

It is indicated in early stages of cataract where visual impairment is not significant. Medical management of cataract involves:

a. Use of drugs to delay progression of cataract:
   - Antioxidants such as glutathione, beta-carotene, vitamin C, N-acetyl carnosine, etc.
   - Aldose reductase inhibitors such as sulindac to delay the progression of diabetic cataract.
b. Treatment of cause of cataract such as adequate control of diabetes in case of diabetic cataract, withdrawal of steroids in steroid-induced cataract.
c. Improving vision by refraction and correction, using drugs such as mydriatics in small central cataract.

Cataract with diabetes mellitus

All patients with diabetes mellitus must be screened for diabetic retinopathy by detailed fundus examination (Fig. 4.17).

If there is no diabetic retinopathy, cataract surgery should be performed and patient should be followed as per the screening protocol (as described later).

General instructions for cataract surgery in diabetic patients

a. Preferably, IOL of large diameter, i.e. 6.5 mm, which facilitates subsequent panretinal photocoagulation or vitrectomy, if required later, should be used.
b. Polymethyl methacrylate (PMMA) IOL is preferred over silicone IOL, as patients may require silicone oil insertion after vitrectomy, if needed.
c. Anterior chamber IOL should be avoided, as this may prevent pupillary dilatation thereby making it difficult to do panretinal photocoagulation or vitrectomy, if required later.

If there is diabetic retinopathy, cataract surgery may worsen the diabetic retinopathy leading to poor vision; hence it has to be treated before performing surgery.

Diabetic macular edema requires treatment by focal laser for focal diabetic maculopathy and grid laser for diffuse diabetic maculopathy before cataract surgery. Proliferative diabetic retinopathy (PDR) should be treated by panretinal photocoagulation (PRP) before cataract surgery.

If the dense cataract precludes laser treatment, IVTA injection should be injected during cataract surgery for diabetic macular edema to prevent worsening of the edema; PDR requires treatment by immediate PRP by indirect ophthalmoscope either during surgery or after extraction of cataractous lens or in the early postoperative period.

If the cataract is mature and no view of the retina is possible before cataract surgery,

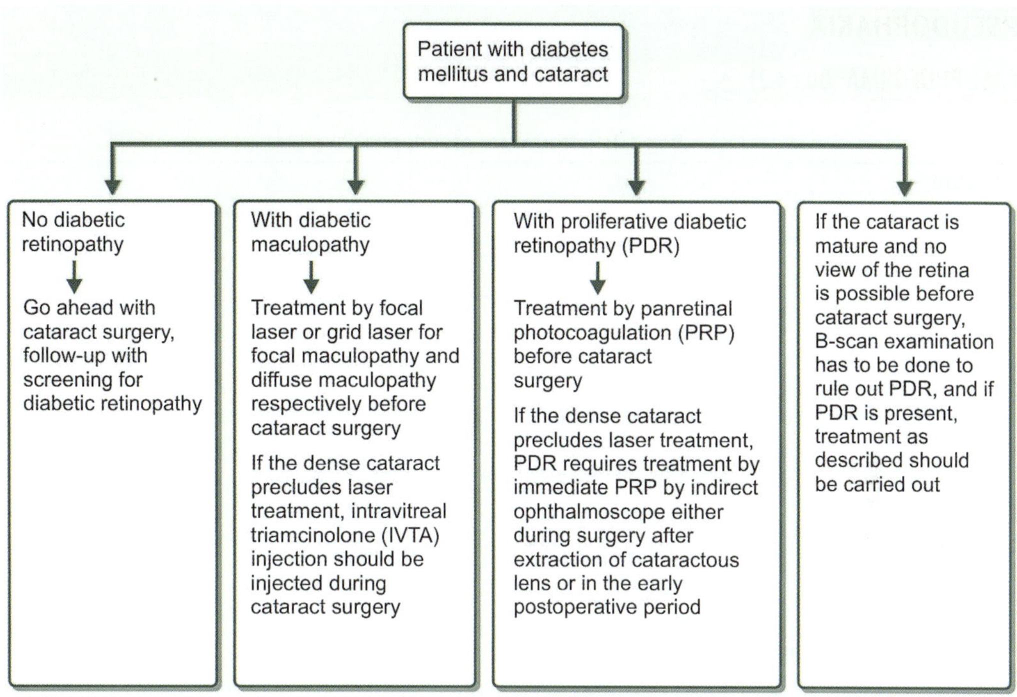

Fig. 4.17: Management of cataract associated with diabetes

B-scan examination has to be done to rule out PDR and if PDR is present, then treatment as described, should be carried out.

Screening for diabetic retinopathy

a. Type 2 diabetes mellitus:
   - First screening is done as soon as the diagnosis is made and then once in a year till no diabetic retinopathy or mild non-proliferative diabetic retinopathy (NPDR)
   - Moderate NPDR—once in 6 months
   - Severe NPDR—once in 3 months
   - PDR with no high-risk characteristics—once in 2 months.

b. Type 1 diabetes mellitus:
   - Since the diabetic retinopathy is rare before puberty, first screening is done at puberty and rest is same as for type 2 diabetic individuals
   - Screening involves measurement of visual acuity and fundus examination following pupillary dilatation.

Cataract with ischemic heart disease

Cataract surgery should be performed after cardiac evaluation by a physician or a cardiologist. If the patient is on aspirin, it should be stopped 5–7 days prior to surgery, as this may cause increased bleeding during surgery or hyphema following surgery.

Cataract with chronic pulmonary disease

Cataract surgery should be performed after COPD is well controlled because uncontrolled COPD may cause repeated iris prolapse during surgery or postoperative iris prolapse because of violent coughing.

Cataract with abscess or infected wound anywhere in the body

Cataract surgery should be performed after treating the abscess or infected wound because of the risk of endogenous endophthalmitis if performed in the presence of infection.

PSEUDOPHAKIA

CASE PROFORMA (Box 4.2)

Box 4.2: Proforma for pseudophakia

Biodata

Here is a male/female patient aged about....... years,...... by occupation, hailing from...........

Presenting Complaints

- Pseudophakia will not have any complaints as it is the treatment done for the complaint, i.e. cataract
- All pseudophakics require spectacles to have normal distant and near vision
- All people with pseudophakia will not have near vision as accommodation is completely lost after surgery until unless accommodative intraocular lens (IOL) or multifocal IOL has been put. The distant vision depends on the final astigmatism induced by surgery.

Causes for Diminution of Vision in Pseudophakia

- Astigmatism induced by surgery
- Wrong power IOL implanted causing consecutive myopia or hypermetropia
- After cataract
- Cystoid macular edema
- Retinal detachment
- Pseudophakic glaucoma
- IOL-related complications.

History of Presenting Illness

He/She was apparently normal........... months/years back. He/She noticed diminution of vision in right eye (RE)/left eye (LE)/both eyes (BE) for which he/she was operated at...........,........... months/years back. Before surgery he/she was able to see........... meters, after surgery he/she was able to see.......... meters. He/She is wearing spectacles/not wearing spectacles.

If he/she complains of diminution of vision the same should be evaluated below the headings of onset, duration, associated features.

Ocular History

He/She is/was wearing spectacles for (choose one among three):

- Near vision
- Distance vision
- Both.

Past History

- He/She is/was a known diabetic on treatment/not a known diabetic
- He/She is/was a known hypertensive on treatment/not a known hypertensive
- He/She is/was a known patient of chronic obstructive pulmonary disease (COPD), asthma, ischemic heart disease on treatment/not a known patient of COPD, asthma, ischemic heart disease
- He/She give past history of tuberculosis/ no past history of tuberculosis.

Family History

- Significant/Not significant
- His/Her father/mother/both had history of cataract/cataract surgery
- His/Her brothers/sisters had history of cataract/cataract surgery.

Personal History

- Diet
- Appetite
- Habits.

Contd...

Contd...

Socioeconomic History

....

....

- The word pseudophakia literally means false lens
- Pseudophakia is a condition where the natural lens is replaced by artificial lens
- Pseudophakia can be:
  - Posterior chamber IOL (most common)
  - Anterior chamber IOL
  - Iris-fixated IOL.

CASE DISCUSSION

1. How pseudophakia is diagnosed?

Pseudophakia is diagnosed as follows:

- History of cataract surgery
- Limbal scar may be seen (except in clear corneal phacoemulsification)
- Jet black pupil with shining reflexes (Fig. 4.18)
- Posterior chamber IOL—IOL will be behind iris in posterior chamber (Fig. 4.19)
- Anterior chamber IOL—IOL will be in front of the iris in anterior chamber (Fig. 4.20).

2. What is the refractive status of a pseudophakic eye?

- Emmetropia—the power of the IOL implanted is correct
- Consecutive myopia—the power of the IOL is more than required
- Consecutive hypermetropia—the power of the IOL is less than required.

3. What is the status of near vision of a pseudophakic eye?

All pseudophakic eyes require near vision correction unless multifocal IOL or accommodative IOL is placed or consecutive myopia is done by over correction, i.e. by implanting higher power IOL than required (myopia—short-sightedness, person can see near things clearly).

4. Name the various generations of IOLs.

- First generation: Posterior chamber IOL (Ridley's posterior chamber IOL)
- Second generation: Anterior chamber angle-fixated lenses
- Third generation: Iris supported lenses
- Fourth generation: Modified one piece anterior chamber lenses
- Fifth generation: Modified posterior chamber lenses

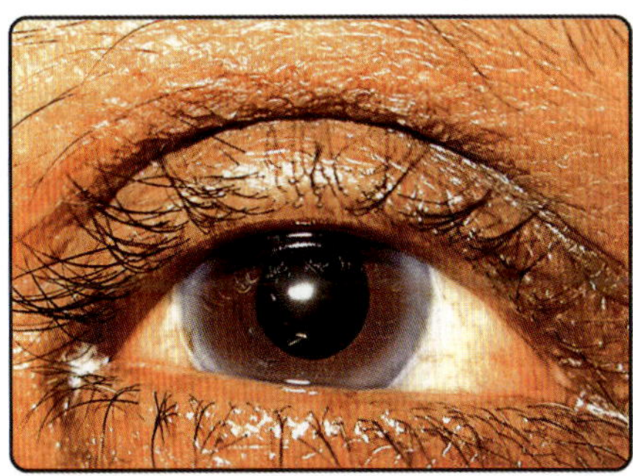

Fig. 4.18: Pseudophakia with posterior chamber intraocular lens look for jet black pupil with shining reflexes

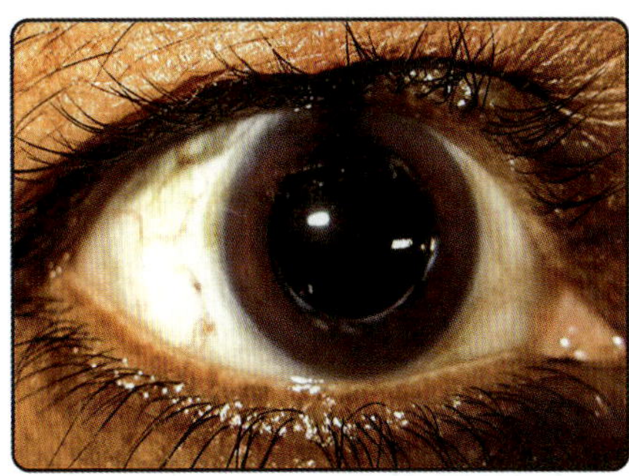

Fig. 4.19: Pseudophakia with posterior chamber intraocular lens after dilatation of pupil (*Note:* Presence of fourth Purkinje image, which is absent in aphakia).

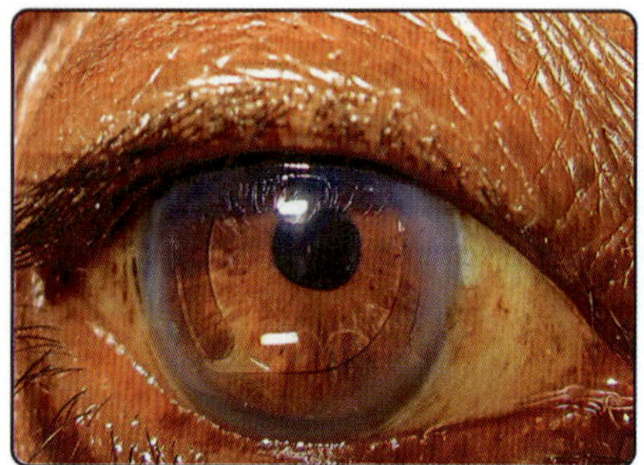

Fig. 4.20: Pseudophakia with anterior chamber intraocular lens

- Sixth generation: Modern capsular posterior chamber IOL and modern anterior chamber IOL.

> Sir Harold Ridley, a British Ophthalmologist was the first to use IOLs in cataract surgery in the year 1949.

5. What are the recent advances in IOLs?

- Multifocal IOLs
- Foldable IOLs.

6. What are the materials by which IOLs made of?

- Polymethyl methacrylate (PMMA)
- Silicone
- Acrylic
- Hydrogels.

7. What are the parts of IOL?

The IOL has got two parts, i.e. optic and haptic.

8. What are the types of IOLs?

- Depending on the site where they are placed (Fig. 4.21):
  - Anterior chamber IOL
  - Iris-fixated IOL
  - Posterior chamber IOL.
- Depending on the nature:
  - Rigid IOL
  - Foldable IOL.
- Depending on the components:
  - Three-piece IOL: Optic and haptic, made of different material or same material (optic and haptic are made separately later joined)
  - Single-piece IOL: Optic and haptic made of same material.

9. How IOLs are sterilized?

- Chemical sterilization: It is done by soaking the lens in 10% sodium hydroxide solution
- Gas sterilization: It is done by exposing the lens to ethylene oxide
- Radiation sterilization: It is done by exposing to gamma rays up to 2.5 M rad.

10. What are the IOL-related complications?

Malposition of IOLs (Fig. 4.22)

- Decenteration
- Subluxation: Sunset syndrome, i.e. inferior subluxation, sunrise syndrome, i.e. superior subluxation
- Dislocation: Lost lens syndrome, i.e. dislocation of IOL into vitreous chamber
- Wind shield wiper syndrome: Movement of the IOL with movements of the eye as a result of small IOL placed in the ciliary sulcus.

Pupillary capture (Fig. 4.23)

Formation of synechiae between the posterior surface of the optic and the underlying iris.

Iris tuck

Entrapment of peripheral iris within the haptic of IOL:

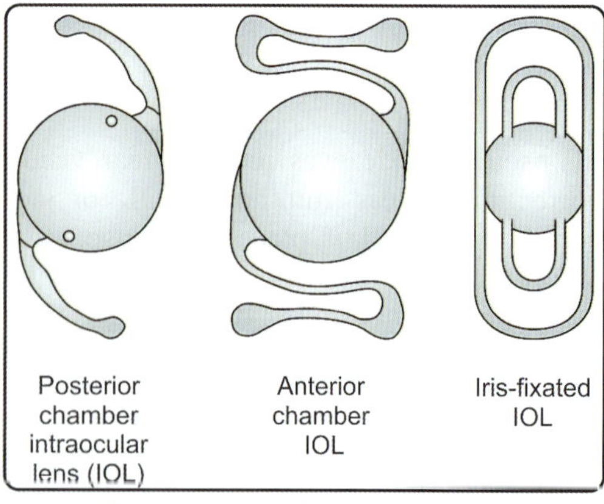

Fig. 4.21: Types of intraocular lenses

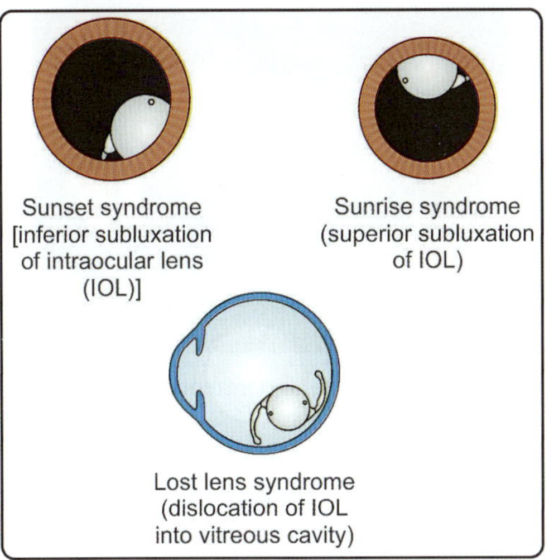

Fig. 4.22: Malposition of intraocular lenses

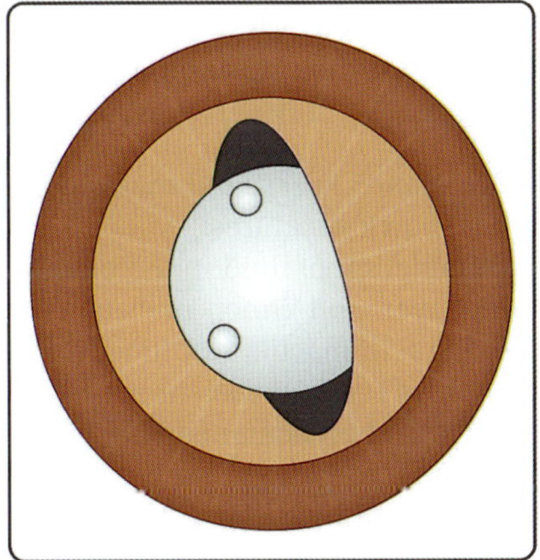

Fig. 4.23: Pupillary capture (*Note:* Optic of the intraocular lens partly on the iris and rest behind the iris).

- Uveitis-glaucoma-hyphema (UGH) syndrome: UGH because of mechanical rubbing of the iris on a sharp edge due to improper finishing quality of the IOL
- Corneal retinal inflammatory syndrome (CRIS): Constant IOL uveal contact and toxic material of the IOL leads to chronic inflammation
- Persistent corneal edema and corneal decompensation.

Other complications of IOLs

- Cystoid macular edema
- Posterior capsular opacification
- Toxic lens syndrome: Uveitis caused by toxins associated with lens such as ethylene gas used for sterilizing lens.

11. What are the causes for diminution of vision in a pseudophakic eye?

After cataract and cystoid macular edema are the two most common causes for diminution of vision in pseudophakic eyes.

Preoperative causes

Failure to identify pre-existing causes before surgery:

- Pre-existing glaucoma
- Retinal diseases such as diabetic maculopathy, age-related macular degeneration and retinal detachment.
- Pre-existing amblyopia
- Early postoperative complications
- Corneal edema
- Pseudophakic pupillary block glaucoma
- Endophthalmitis.

Late postoperative complications

- After cataract
- Cystoid macular edema (CME)
- Retinal detachment.

12. What is after cataract?

- It is also called posterior capsule opacification (PCO) (Figs 4.24A and B, 4.25)
- After cataract is opacification of posterior capsule of the lens following ECCE
- Incidence is 10–50% following ECCE.

After cataract can never be seen in ICCE as lens is removed along with both anterior and posterior capsule.

13. What are the types of after cataracts (Fig. 4.26)?

- Membranous after cataract: Cells proliferate such as membrane
- Elschnig's pearl: Cells proliferate and distend to form spherical cells

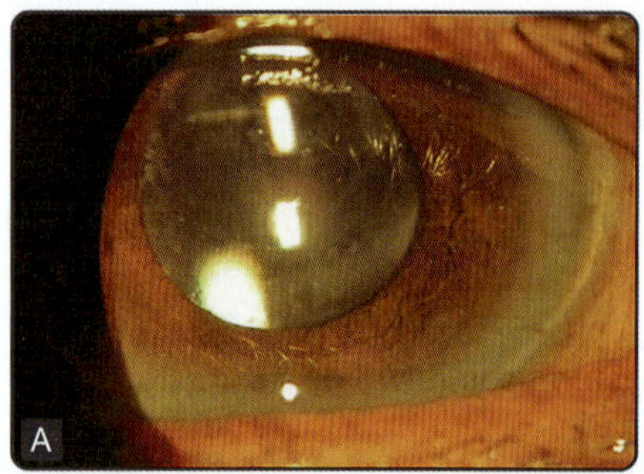

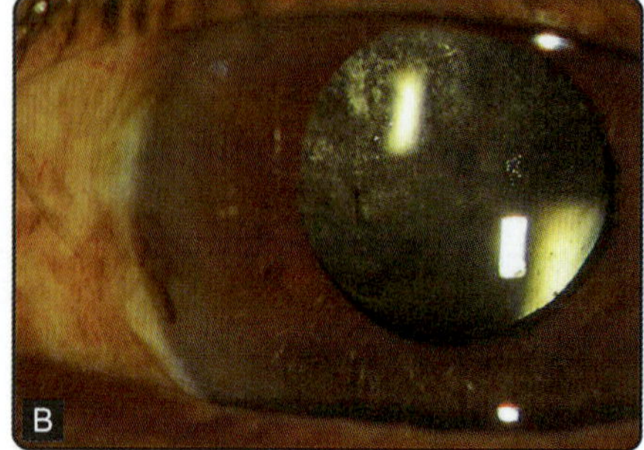

Figs 4.24A and B: Posterior capsule opacification (*Note*: Membrane behind intraocular lens)

- Soemmering's ring: Cells proliferate and get enclosed between two layers lens capsule and appear as a ring, hence seen at the periphery.

14. What is the mechanism of after cataract?

The equatorial epithelium, which remains active throughout life is the primary source of after cataract especially for Elschnig's pearl and Soemmering's ring. The membranous type is because of posterior proliferation of anterior epithelium cells.

15. How after cataract can be prevented?

a. Reducing the source for after cataract by:
   - Complete removal of cortical matter
   - Polishing of the posterior capsule
   - Polishing of the under surface of the remaining anterior capsule to remove the anterior and equatorial epithelial cells
   - Reduce the stimulus for after cataract by using biocompatible IOL to reduce stimulation of cellular proliferation.

b. Prevent the after cataract from reaching posterior capsule by:
   - Using IOL with square truncated edges, which prevent migration of anterior epithelial cells posteriorly
   - Using biconvex IOL or planoconvex IOL with convexity towards the posterior capsule and placing it in the capsular bag, so that it obliterates the space between IOL and posterior capsule.

16. How after cataract is treated?

After cataract is treated by neodymium-doped yttrium aluminium garnet (Nd-YAG) capsulotomy where central part of the posterior capsule is removed by laser energy.

Dense membranous after cataract, which cannot be removed by laser, has to be treated by surgical posterior capsulotomy.

17. What is CME?

The CME stands for cystoid macular edema with the following features:

- Accumulation of fluid in the outer plexiform layer and inner nuclear layer of the retina in macula resulting in the formation of cystic spaces in the macula is called cystoid macular edema
- On fundoscopy, it gives typical honeycomb appearance (Fig. 4.27)
- On fundus fluorescein angiography, it gives flower petal appearance.

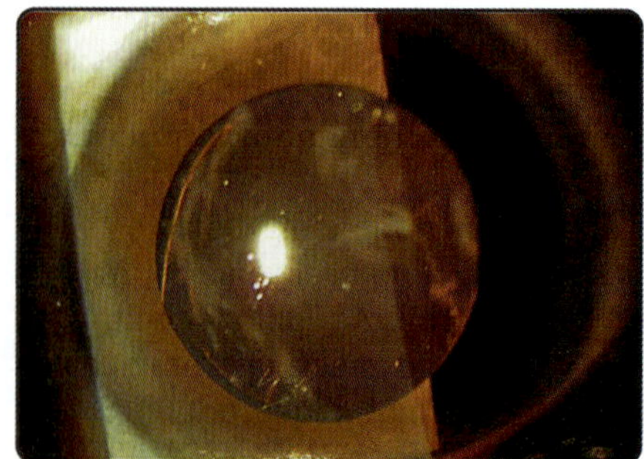

Fig. 4.25: Posterior capsule opacification as seen in retroillumination

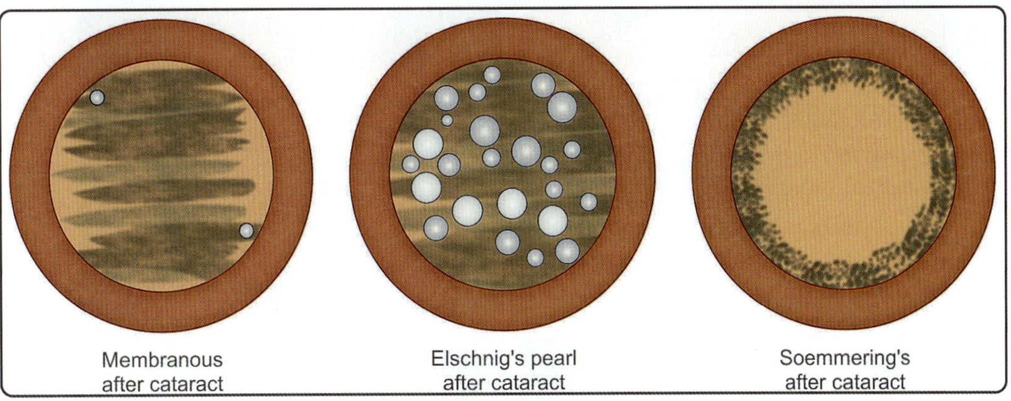

Fig. 4.26: Types of after cataracts

Anatomy of macula

In the macular region, which surrounds the fovea centralis, the outer plexiform layer is thicker than elsewhere in the retina and it is called Henle's layer.

In fovea centralis, rods are absent, cones are tightly packed and other layers of retina are absent. It consists of cones and their nuclei covered by a thin internal limiting membrane.

The thinness of fovea centralis (provides little protection against inflammatory exudates that pass through vitreous) and the thickness of Henle's layer (because of its thickness can absorb large quantities of fluid) are responsible for accumulation of inflammatory exudates at macular region.

18. What is the mechanism of CME?

Release of inflammatory mediators, i.e. prostaglandins result in edema at macula. Inflammatory mediators are released due to:

- Postoperative inflammation because of iridocyclitis
- Systemic factors such as uncontrolled diabetes and hypertension
- Vitreous disturbances such as vitreous loss and vitreous incarceration in the wound.

19. How CME is treated?

- Topical antiprostaglandins such as ketorolac, indomethacin are used as initial treatment or as prophylactic treatment before cataract surgery to prevent development of cystoid macular edema.
- Topical steroids, periocular steroids and systemic steroids are helpful in established cases.

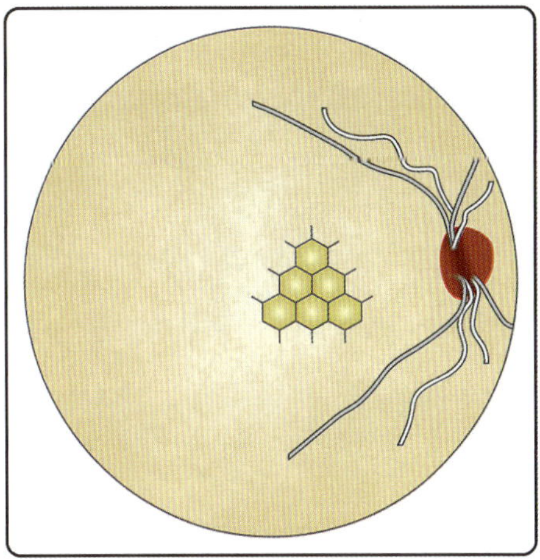

Fig. 4.27: Cystoid macular edema (honeycomb appearance)

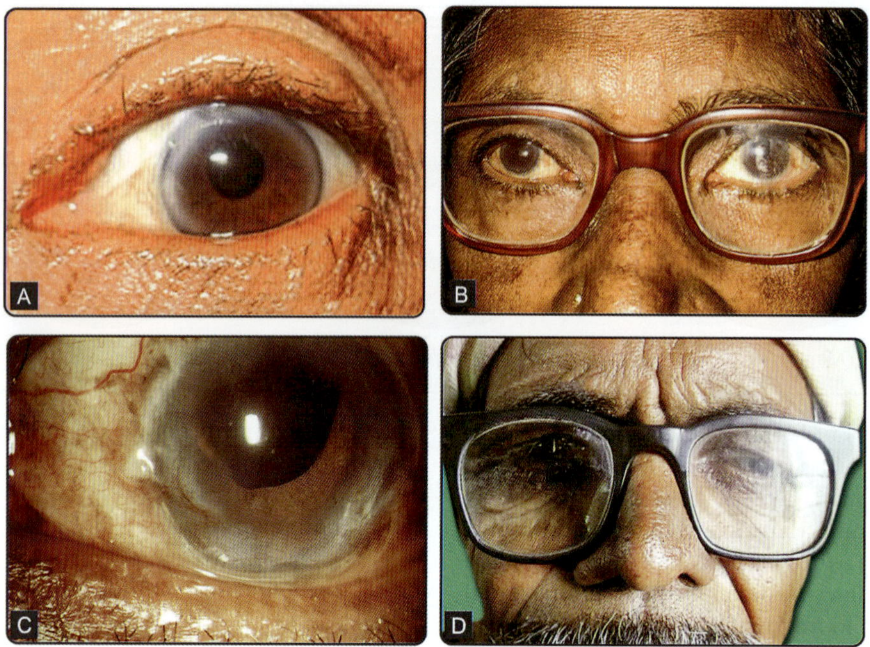

Figs 4.28A to D: Aphakia. **A.** Jet black pupil and absence of shining reflexes; **B.** Aphakic patient wearing aphakic glasses for her left eye (*Note:* Aphakic glass is thick in the center and produces magnification of the image); **C.** U-shaped pupil commonly due to sectoral iridectomy; **D.** Aphakic patient wearing aphakic glasses for his left eye.

APHAKIA

Aphakia is a defined as a condition in which lens is absent from its normal position, i.e. from pupillary area (patellar fossa).

Aphakia literally means absence of lens from the eye (Figs 4.28A to D).

- Phakia means lens
- Aphakia means absence of lens from its normal position
- Pseudophakia means presence of artificial lens in the eye.

CASE PROFORMA (Box 4.3)

Box 4.3: Proforma for aphakia

Biodata

Here is a male/female patient aged about........years,........ by occupation, from........

Presenting Complaints

Diminution of vision in right eye (RE)/left eye (LE)/both eye (BE) for far and near, which improves with spectacles with history of cataract surgery to RE/LE/BE.

Reasons for Poor Vision in Aphakia

Since in aphakia lens is removed, the power of the eye is reduced by +16 D [diopters (D)] (from +60 D in normal eye to +44 D in aphakic eye), hence the eye becomes highly hypermetropic causing diminution of vision for far and near. Vision in aphakia without correction by spectacles is approximately about 3/60 (counting fingers 3 m).

History of Presenting Illness

He/She give history of cataract surgery............. months/years back. He/She noticed diminution of vision in RE/LE/BE after surgery for distance and near, which improved with spectacles.

History regarding trauma and spontaneous dislocation has to be enquired, if there is no history of cataract surgery. Spontaneous dislocation of lens, which may occur in hypermature cataract may cause improvement in vision spontaneously from hand movements + (vision in hypermature cataract) to counting fingers up to 3 m (vision in aphakia without spectacles) without history of cataract surgery.

Causes for Aphakia

Surgical: After cataract surgery.

Trauma: Traumatic extrusion of lens.

Dislocation: Posterior dislocation of lens spontaneously or following trauma.

Congenital: Absence of lens very rarely.

Surgical aphakia is the most common cause of aphakia.

Causes for Diminution of Vision in Aphakia with Spectacles

- Cystoid macular edema
- Retinal detachment
- Aphakic glaucoma
- Astigmatism induced by surgery
- Aphakic bullous keratopathy.

Ocular History

- He/She is/was wearing spectacles for (choose one among three):
- Near vision
- Distance vision
- Both.

He/She give history of cataract surgery.

Contd...

Contd...

Past History
- He/She is a known diabetic on treatment/not a known diabetic
- He/She is a known hypertensive on treatment/not a known hypertensive.

Family History
Significant/Not significant.

Personal History
- Diet
- Appetite
- Habits.

Socioeconomic History

....

....

CASE DISCUSSION

1. How aphakia is diagnosed?

History

History of cataract surgery or trauma or spontaneous dislocation.

Visual acuity

- Vision without spectacles up to counting fingers 3 m
- Vision with spectacles (with +10 D) improvement in vision
- Retinoscopy shows hypermetropic refractive error.

Ocular examination

- Limbal scar (scar of previous cataract surgery seen in surgical aphakia)
- Anterior chamber is deep and iridodonesis is present, i.e. tremulousness of iris because of lack of posterior support
- Jet black color of the pupil
- Purkinje's images: Only two are present. (Third and fourth images are absent because anterior capsule and posterior capsule both are absent).

2. Describe the optics of aphakia.

- If the eye was emmetropic earlier, it becomes highly hypermetropic as the total power of the eye is reduced from +60 D to +44 D
- The anterior focal distance is 23 mm (normally 15 mm) and posterior focal distance is 31 mm (normally 24 mm)
- Accommodation is totally lost due to absence of lens.

3. Describe the treatment of aphakia.

Aphakia is corrected by convex lenses of appropriate power to correct hypermetropia:

- Spectacles
- Contact lenses
- Intraocular lens implantation
- Refractive corneal surgery such as hypermetropic LASIK.

Spectacles for aphakia

- Approximately +10 D spherical convex lens
- Cylindrical lenses for correction of surgically induced astigmatism +3 D of convex spherical lens addition for near vision
- The above mentioned condition is for previously emmetropic eyes. In patients with ammetropia, refractive power has to be calculated by doing refraction.

4. What are the advantages and disadvantages of aphakic glasses?

Advantages

Cheap and easy method of correcting aphakia.

Disadvantages

- The glasses are very thick and heavy; hence cause cosmetic disfigurement and inconvenience to use them
- Image magnification is of about 30%

- Prismatic aberration producing roving ring scotoma, also called jack in the box phenomenon
- Spherical aberration producing pincushion distortion
- Reduced field of vision
- Anisometropia, if the other eye is normal or pseudophakic.

Roving ring scotoma

A ring scotoma produced by the prismatic effect at the periphery of the thick convex lens, which moves against the movement of the eye.

Since this scotoma shifts with the movement of the eyes, the scotoma appears and disappears with the changing position of the eyes from object to object. This is called jack in the box phenomenon.

5. What are the advantages and disadvantages of correction of aphakia with contact lenses?

Advantages

- Cosmetically gives better acceptance
- Image magnification is less, it is about 8%
- Spherical and prismatic aberrations are not present
- Wider field of vision.

Disadvantages

- Costlier than spectacles
- Requires care and maintenance of contact lenses
- Contact lens intolerance
- Contact lens complications such as giant papillary conjunctivitis, corneal abrasion, microbial keratitis, corneal warping and superficial punctate keratitis.

6. What are the advantages and disadvantages of correction of aphakia with intraocular lens?

Advantages

- Best method to correct aphakia
- Will not have disadvantages associated with aphakic glasses
- Anisometropia is not seen if the other eye is normal or pseudophakic.

Disadvantages

Requires one more surgery, hence complications associated with cataract surgery can be seen.

Case 1: A patient with aphakia in one eye and the other eye being pseudophakia or normal. What is the preferred modality of correction of aphakia?

Spectacles are not preferred, because it will cause anisometropia. Anisometropia is a refractive condition in which the refraction of the two eyes is unequal. A difference of more than 2.5 D is not tolerated causing diplopia. Contact lens correction is possible. Intraocular lens correction is the best and preferred method.

Case 2: A patient with aphakia in right eye and immature/mature cataract in left eye. What is the preferred treatment?

Treatment options are:

a. Cataract surgery in left eye without IOL implantation, i.e. making the eye aphakic and later giving aphakic correction to both eyes so that anisometropia is avoided. Though bilateral aphakia will not cause anisometropia this treatment is not preferred because of disadvantages associated with aphakic spectacles, not cause anisometropia this treatment is not preferred because of disadvantages associated with aphakic spectacles.
b. Cataract surgery in the left eye with posterior chamber IOL implantation followed by secondary IOL implantation in right eye. This is the preferred treatment.

7. What is secondary IOL implantation?

Secondary IOL implantation is defined as insertion of IOL into an eye, which is rendered aphakic by prior cataract surgery.

Secondary IOL implantation

After ICCE

- Anterior chamber IOL implantation
- Iris fixated IOL implantation
- Scleral fixated IOL.

After ECCE

With intact posterior capsule

- Posterior chamber IOL.

Without posterior capsule support

- Anterior chamber IOL implantation
- Iris fixated IOL implantation
- Scleral fixated IOL.

8. What are the causes for surgical aphakia?

- Intracapsular cataract extraction
- Intraoperative complications during extracapsular cataract extraction such as posterior capsule tear and zonular dehiscence.

9. What are the complications of aphakia?

- Cystoid macular edema
- Retinal detachment incidence is higher in aphakics because of associated vitreous loss and vitreous traction
- Vitreous touch syndrome—vitreous touch, bullous keratopathy and cystoid macular edema (Irvine-Gass syndrome)
- Aphakic bullous keratopathy
- Aphakic glaucoma.

CORNEAL OPACITY

CASE PROFORMA (Box 4.4)

Box 4.4: Proforma for corneal opacity

Biodata

Here is a male/female patient aged about..........years,.......... by occupation, from...........

Presenting Complaints

His presenting complaints are:

- White opacity in right eye (RE)/left eye (LE)/both eye (BE) since.........,.......... months/years
- Diminution of vision in RE/LE/BE since.........,.......... months/years.

History of Presenting Illness

He/She was apparently normal from.........,.......... months/years back. He/She noticed white opacity in RE/LE/BE insidious/sudden in onset gradually progressive/stationary in nature after trauma/corneal ulcer/congenital.

Causes of Corneal Opacity

Tears in the endothelium and Descemet's membrane (STUMPED) corneal ulcers and inflammation (STUMPED).

Congenital

- **S**: Sclerocornea
- **T**: Tears in Descemet's membrane
- **U**: Ulcer
- **M**: Metabolic conditions such as mucolipidosis, mucopolysaccharidosis
- **P**: Posterior corneal defect such as Peter's anomaly
- **E**: Endothelial dystrophy such as congenital hereditary endothelial dystrophy
- **D**: Dermoid.

Acquired

- Post-trauma following chemical injuries, mechanical injuries
- Corneal degenerations
- Postinfection or inflammation of cornea following infective or non-infective keratitis.

Corneal opacity is associated/not associated with:

- Diminution of vision
- Glare
- Pain
- Redness
- Watering.

- Corneal opacity in the periphery will not cause any visual problems
- Corneal opacity in the visual axis will cause diminution of vision
- Nebular and macular grade corneal opacity cause diminution of vision by causing glare and irregular astigmatism
- Leukomatous grade corneal opacity causes diminution of vision by completely obstructing the light rays
- Corneal opacity is the end result of any form of insult/disease of cornea. Since corneal opacity is not an active disease, it is not associated with symptoms such as pain and redness.

Ocular History

He/She is/was wearing spectacles for (choose one among three):

- Near vision
- Distance vision
- Both.

He/She gives history of surgery/no history of surgery to RE/LE/BE.

Contd...

Contd...

Past History
- He/She is a known diabetic on treatment/not a known diabetic
- He/She is a known hypertensive on treatment/not a known hypertensive
- He/She is a known patient of chronic obstructive pulmonary disease (COPD), asthma, ischemic heart disease on treatment/not a known patient of COPD, asthma, ischemic heart disease
- He/She give past history of tuberculosis/no past history of tuberculosis.

Family History
Significant/not significant.

Personal History
- Diet
- Appetite
- Habits.

Socioeconomic History
He/She belongs to:
- Upper class
- Middle class
- Lower class.

Corneal opacity is more common in low socioeconomic status:
- Because of more incidence of trauma
- Particularly in children because of deficiency of vitamins, e.g. vitamin A deficiency causing keratomalacia.

CASE DISCUSSION

1. How corneal opacity is diagnosed based on ocular examination?

Corneal opacity is examined under the following headings:
- Position of corneal opacity in relation to the limbus and pupil
- Number: Can be single or multiple
- Shape: It varies according to cause of corneal opacity
- Size: It varies according to cause of corneal opacity
- Depth and grading of opacity
- Staining of opacity: Corneal opacity will not stain with dyes such as fluorescein since epithelium is intact in corneal opacity
- Vascularization of pacity
- Iris incarceration in opacity
- Corneal sensation: It will be absent in corneal opacity.

- Normal cornea is avascular except for peripheral 1 mm
- Vascularization of cornea is always pathological. It can be superficial or deep vascularization.

Superficial corneal vascularization
It is seen in conditions causing keratocon. junctivitis such as trachoma, phlyctenular keratoconjunctivitis and in contact lens wearers. It is usually subepithelial in location and the vessels can be traced onto the conjunctival vessels. The vessels in superficial vascularization show multiple branching arborizing patterns, with source being conjunctival vessel.

Deep corneal vascularization
It is seen in diseases of corneal stroma such as interstitial keratitis, disciform keratitis, sclerosing keratitis. It is usually located in the stroma and the vessels are derived from anterior ciliary vessels, hence they are not

Contd...

Contd...

continuous with conjunctival vessels. The vessels in deep vascularization are straighter with minimal branching.

Diminished corneal sensation

- Congenital: Trigeminal anesthesia and corneal hypoesthesia of congenital type
- Pharmacological: Local anesthetics, e.g. xylocaine
- Pathological:
  - Ocular: Viral infections of cornea such as herpes simplex, corneal degenerations and dystrophies
  - Systemic: Leprosy, diabetes, etc.
  - Post-trauma/surgical: Corneal scars, keratoplasty, corneal refractive surgeries.

2. Define corneal opacity.

Corneal opacity is defined as presence of opaque cornea replacing the transparent cornea as a result of loss of transparency. Corneal opacity is one of the leading causes of blindness globally and it accounts for about 4% of all cases of blindness.

3. Mention the histological layers of cornea.

Histologically cornea is made up of five layers; recently a new layer is added to it making it six layers:

1. Epithelium of cornea: It is 5–7 layers thick and it is of stratified squamous subtype.
2. Bowman's membrane: It is not a true membrane, but it is condensation of collagen of superficial stroma. It is about 12–14 µm thick and it is tough layer.
3. Stroma: It is about 500 µm thick accounting for 90% of thickness of cornea. It is composed of collagen fibrils arranged in lamellar form.
4. Dua's layer: It is about 15 µm thick present between stroma and Descemet's layer. It is named after Harminder S Dua who first proved its presence in the year 2013. It can be used as plane to separate the cornea for posterior lamellar keratoplasty.
5. Descemet's membrane: It is a true membrane and it is the basement membrane of endothelial cells. It is about 12 µm in thickness and it is a tough layer.
6. Endothelium: It is the innermost layer of the cornea consisting of single layer of cells. The endothelial cells cannot regenerate and the number of endothelial cells decreases as the age increases. The endothelial cell count in children is about 4,000 cells per mm^2 and it will decrease to 2,500 cells per mm^2 mm by 70 years of age.

4. Name the factors responsible for transparency of cornea.

1. Avascularity of cornea: Cornea is avascular in nature except for periphery of cornea and this helps to keep cornea transparent.
2. State of relative dehydration: The hydration of cornea is about 80% thus making it relatively dehydrated compared to tear film, which lies anterior to cornea and aqueous humor, which lies posterior to cornea. Cornea is kept in this relatively dehydrated state by epithelium, which acts as a barrier anteriorly and by endothelium with its metabolic pump mechanism.
3. Absence of myelinated nerve fibers: Though cornea is densely innervated by nerve supply, the nerves in the cornea are not myelinated, which helps to keep cornea transparent.
4. Arrangement of the collagen fibrils in corneal stroma: It contributes significantly to the transparency of cornea as explained by the following theories.
5. Maurice's theory of Lattice: This was proposed by David Maurice. It states that cornea is transparent because of regular

lattice arrangement of the collagen fibrils, which leads to destruction of scattered light by destructive interference or mutual interference.

6. Goldman theory of minimal separation of collagen fibrils: This was proposed by Goldman and Benedek. It states that cornea is transparent because of presence of small diameter collage fibrils with small separation, which will not cause scattering of light. The collagen fibrils are separated by less than one third of wavelength of light and to cause scattering of light because of interference with transmission of light the separation has to be more than one third of wavelength of light.

5. What is the mechanism of loss of corneal transparency?

The common pathogenic pathways involved in loss of corneal transparency are:

- Corneal edema
- Corneal vascularization
- Corneal opacity.

6. What are the causes for corneal opacity?

Congenital (STUMPED)

- **S**clerocornea
- **T**ears in Descemet's membrane
- **U**lcer
- **M**etabolic conditions such as mucolipidosis, mucopolysaccharidosis
- **P**osterior corneal defect, e.g. as in Peter's anomaly
- **E**ndothelial dystrophy such as congenital hereditary endothelial dystrophy
- **D**ermoid.

Acquired

- Post-trauma following chemical injuries, mechanical injuries
- Corneal degenerations
- Postinfection or inflammation of cornea following infective or noninfective keratitis.

7. What are the grades of corneal opacity (Fig. 4.29)?

Nebular grade corneal opacity: Corneal opacity involving less than one third of corneal thickness involving the epithelium and Bowman's membrane.

Macular grade corneal opacity: Corneal opacity involving one third to half of corneal thickness (Fig. 4.30).

Leukomatous grade corneal opacity: Corneal opacity involving more than half of corneal thickness (Figs 4.31A and B, 4.32A and B).

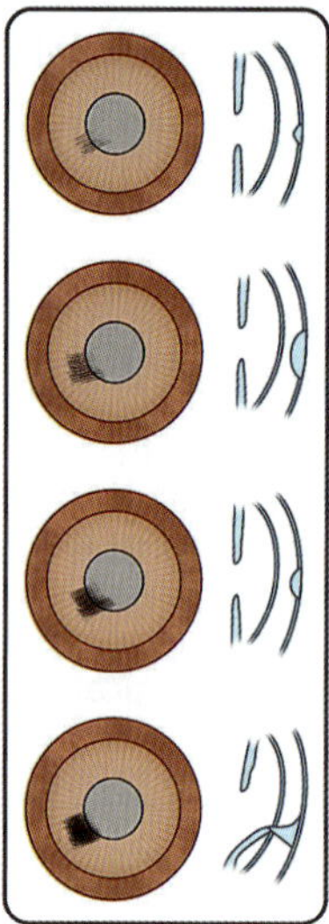

Fig. 4.29: Grades of corneal opacity

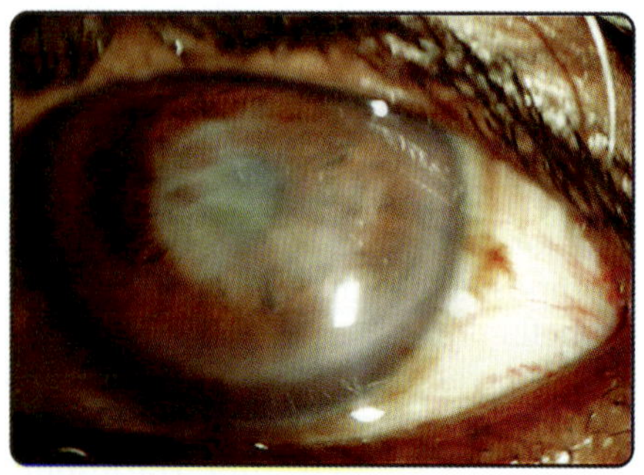

Fig. 4.30: Macular grade corneal opacity

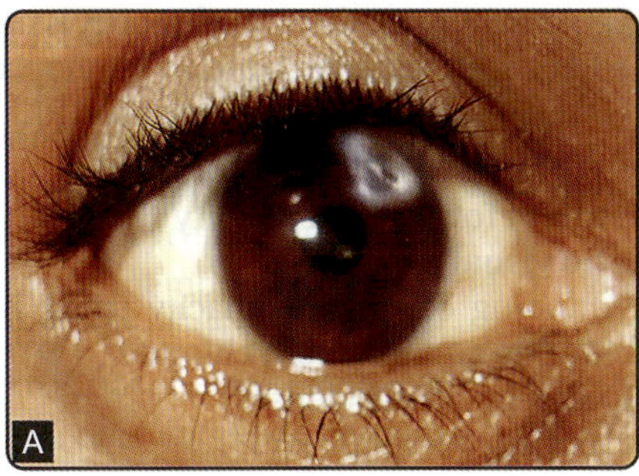

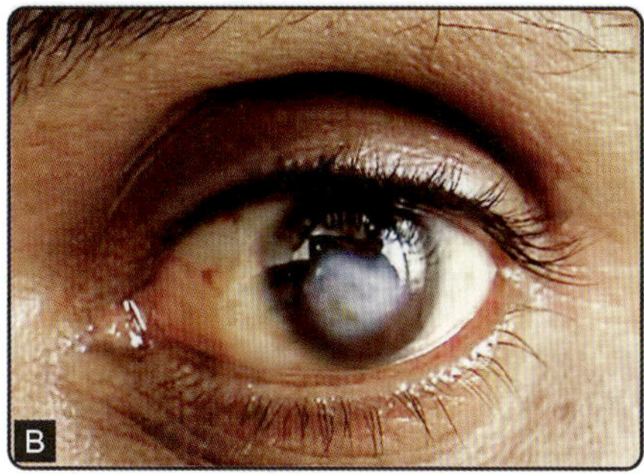

Figs 4.31A and B: Leukomatous grade corneal opacity. **A.** Peripheral; **B.** Central.

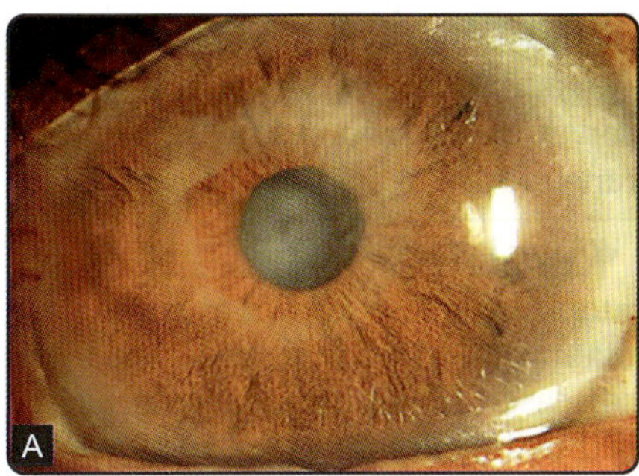

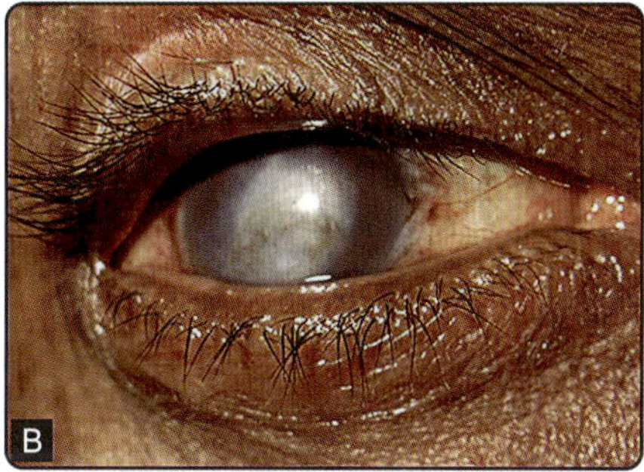

Figs 4.32A and B: Leukomatous grade corneal opacity

Adherent leukoma (Fig. 4.33)

Leukomatous corneal opacity with incarceration of iris into the opacity. A small nebular grade corneal opacity in the visual axis will cause more visual discomfort than a small leukomatous opacity because nebular corneal opacity causes diffraction of light resulting in glare where as leukomatous opacity just obstructs all the light in its path.

8. What is staphyloma?

The word 'staphyloma' means bunch of grapes. The abnormal protrusion of uveal tissue through weak outer coat of the eyeball is called staphyloma.

9. What are the types of staphyloma?

a. Anterior staphyloma: It is abnormal protrusion of iris through weak and thinned out cornea. It usually follows perforated corneal ulcer or perforating corneal injury (Fig. 4.34).
b. Intercalary staphyloma: It is abnormal protrusion of root of the iris through weak and thinned out limbus. It usually follows perforated peripheral corneal ulcer or perforating injury involving limbus.
c. Ciliary staphyloma: It is abnormal protrusion of ciliary body through weak and thinned out sclera in the ciliary zone, which lies 3 mm away from limbus. It usually follows scleritis or perforating injury involving the ciliary zone.

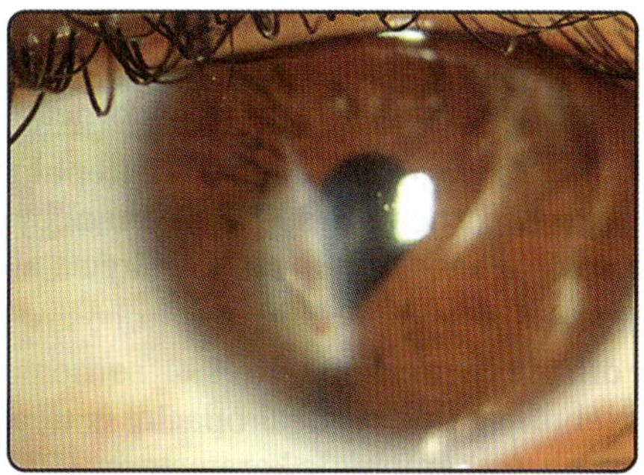

Fig. 4.33: Adherent leukoma

18. Mention contraindications for use of donor eye.

Ocular: Intrinsic eye diseases such as intraocular tumors, intraocular inflammations, corneal degenerations, corneal dystrophies, corneal opacity, etc.

Systemic: AIDS or HIV seropositivity, rabies, Creutzfeldt-Jakob disease, viral hepatitis:

- Death from unknown cause
- Septicemia
- Malignancies such as leukemia, lymphoma, etc.

ADULT DACRYOCYSTITIS

CASE PROFORMA (Box 4.5)

Box 4.5: Proforma for adult dacryocystitis

Biodata

Here is a male/female patient aged about............. years,............. by occupation, hailing from.............

Important Facts

Age: Adult dacryocystitis is more common between 40 and 60 years.
Sex: It is more common in females due to comparatively narrow lumen of the bony canal (nasolacrimal duct).

Presenting Complaints

- His/Her presenting complaints are:..
- Watering in right eye (RE)/left eye (LE)/both eyes (BE) since,............. months/years.

- If swelling is present, it should be included in presenting complaints
- If watering is associated with pain and redness of eye as in acute dacryocystitis, they have to be included in presenting complaints and the same has to be described in history of presenting illness.

History of Presenting Illness

- He/She was apparently normal............. months/years back.

He/She noticed:

- Watering in RE/LE/BE since............. months/years
- Associated with swelling in the lacrimal sac region, i.e. medial to medial canthus
- Associated with discharge (mucoid/mucopurulent/purulent)
- Associated with/without recurrent episodes of pain, redness (to rule out episodes of inflammation).

Ocular History

- He/She give history of surgery/no history of surgery to RE/LE/BE for complaints of watering
- He/She give history of trauma/no history of trauma to RE/LE/BE.

After dacryocystectomy (DCT), patient will have watering as lacrimal sac is totally removed and no longer tears can be drained via nasolacrimal duct. Trauma involving lacrimal drainage system such as canalicular tear, eversion of punctum because of cicatricial ectropion can result in watering as tears are no longer drained by lacrimal drainage system.

Past History

History of similar complaints may be present in past in case chronic dacryocystitis and in cases of recurrent dacryocystitis due to failure of treatment, i.e. following failed dacryocystorhinostomy (DCR):

- He/She is a known diabetic on treatment/not a known diabetic
- He/She is a known hypertensive on treatment/not a known hypertensive.

Family History

Significant/Not significant.

Personal History

....

....

Socioeconomic History

He/She belongs to:

- Upper class
- Middle class
- Lower class.

It is more common in low socioeconomic group because of poor personal hygiene, which may act as predisposing factor.

CASE DISCUSSION

1. How to diagnose adult dacryocystitis?

Ocular examination

Inspection

a. Look for watering of the eye.
b. The eye appears wet with accumulation of tears at the medial canthus. There may be discharge at the medial canthus. The conjunctiva may show congestion indicating chronic dacryocystitis.
c. Look for any swelling over lacrimal sac area, if there is a swelling, the swelling has to be described under:
    - Site
    - Size
    - Shape
    - Surface
    - Skin over the swelling.
d. Look for any surgical scar seen in cases of DCT or DCR.
e. Look for any evidence of trauma in the form of irregular scar over the lacrimal drainage system or cicatricial ectropion.
f. Look for any fistula over the lacrimal sac area.

Palpation

a. Presence of tenderness, which indicates whether the swelling is acute or chronic.
b. Regurgitation test (Figs 4.36A and B).

Diagnosis

Acute dacryocystitis: History of watering and discharge associated with a painful swelling in the lacrimal sac area (Figs 4.37A and B).

Chronic dacryocystitis: History of watering with or without mucoid discharge. It may or may not be associated with painless swelling in lacrimal sac area (Fig. 4.38).

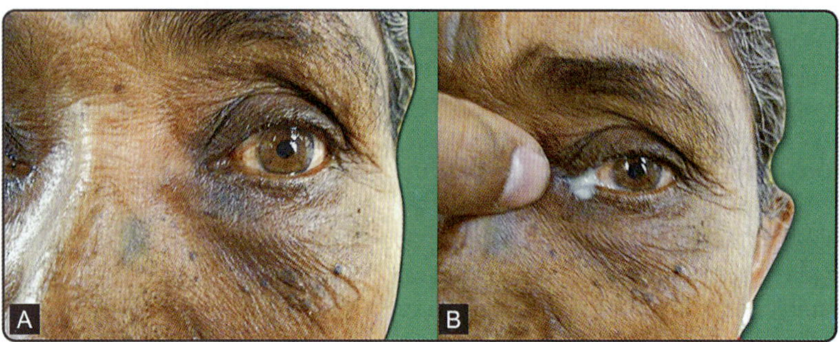

Figs 4.36A and B: Regurgitation test (*Note:* Regurgitation of mucoid fluid on applying pressure over lacrimal sac area with thumb of the examiner)

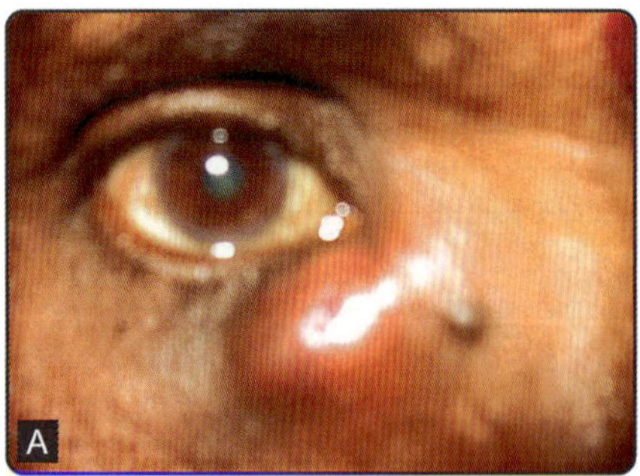

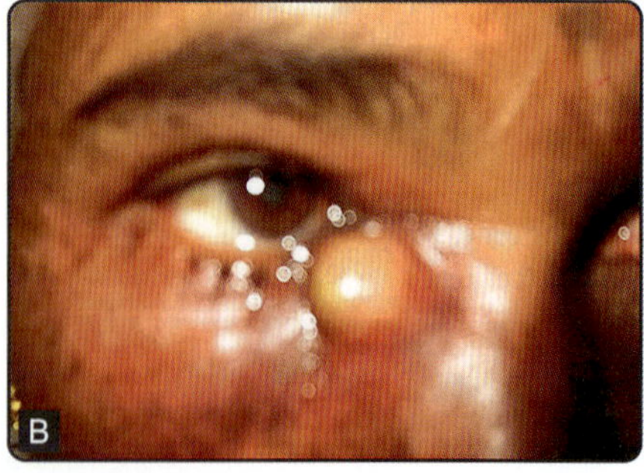

Figs 4.37A and B: Acute dacryocystitis. **A.** Presence of inflammatory signs, i.e. redness over lacrimal sac area; **B.** Acute dacryocystitis with pyocele.

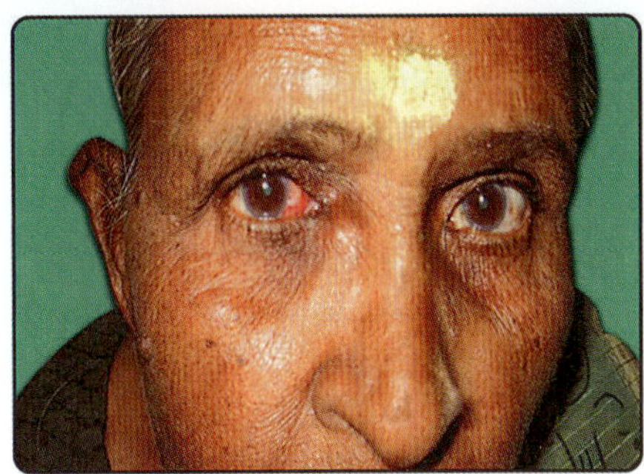

Fig. 4.38: Chronic dacryocystitis

Differential diagnosis

a. Hyperlacrimation caused by reflex lacrimal hypersecretion secondary to ocular inflammations such as conjunctivitis and keratitis, etc.
b. Epiphora due to obstruction of lacrimal drainage system. Chronic dacryocystitis is the most common cause for epiphora.

2. What are the causes for hyperlacrimation?

Reflex hyperlacrimation, which occurs due to stimulation of the sensory nerve endings of trigeminal nerve is the commonest cause of hyperlacrimation. It occurs in inflammatory diseases of the eye such as conjunctivitis, keratitis, episcleritis, scleritis, iridocyclitis, etc. in eyelid conditions such as trichiasis, entropion and conjunctival/corneal foreign body, etc. Reflex lacrimation is because of reflex between the sensory trigeminal nerve and motor facial nerve.

Primary oversecretion of tears from the lacrimal glands is seen in inflammatory conditions of lacrimal gland, tumors of the lacrimal glands and cholinergic drugs because of stimulation of parasympathetic fibers.

Central hyperlacrimation is seen in supranuclear causes such as emotional stress and infranuclear causes such as aberrant regeneration of facial nerve.

3. What are the causes for epiphora?

The cause for epiphora may lie in punctum, canaliculi, lacrimal sac, nasolacrimal duct or lacrimal pump:

- Causes in punctum:
  - Punctal obstruction because of congenital atresia or acquired stenosis following trauma, chronic use of drugs such as pilocarpine
  - Punctal ectropion.
- Causes in canaliculi:
  - Congenital stenosis or acquired stenosis following the trauma and inflammation.
- Causes in lacrimal sac:
  - Congenital anomalies of lacrimal sac such as dacryocystocele and acquired causes, e.g. dacryocystitis, lacrimal sac tumors, dacryolith.
- Causes in nasolacrimal duct:
  - Congenital nasolacrimal duct obstruction and acquired causes such as inflammations, involutional stenosis, tumors.
- Causes in lacrimal pump:
  - Lacrimal pump weakness because of laxity of eyelids or weakness of orbicularis oculi.
- Causes in eyelids:
  - Abnormalities in the eyelids such as ectropion, lagophthalmos.

4. What is dacryocystitis?

The inflammation of lacrimal sac is called dacryocystitis.

5. What are the causative organisms for chronic dacryocystitis?

Bacteria are the most common causative agents; common bacteria causing dacryocystitis are *Staphylococcus epidermidis, Staphylococcus aureus, Pseudomonas, Pneumococcus, Propionibacterium* and *Escherichia coil.* Granulomatous inflammations such as tuberculosis, syphilis and fungi such as *Aspergillus, Candida* are rare cause of dacryocystitis.

6. Mention the predisposing/risk factors for chronic dacryocystitis.

a. Chronic dacryocystitis of adults is commonly seen in middle age group in the fourth decade.

b. It is more common in females probably because of narrow nasolacrimal duct.
c. It is more common on left side with less commonly affecting the right side probably because the tears are drained with more ease on right side compared to left side as the nasolacrimal duct and lacrimal fossa form a greater angle on the right side.
d. It is more common in white races and rare in black races because of presence of shorter, straighter and wider nasolacrimal duct in blacks.
e. It is more common in individuals with narrow facial configuration compared to those with broad face because of presence of narrow bony nasolacrimal canal in individuals with narrow face.
f. It is more common in people with nasal tumors, nasal polyps, deviated nasal septum, hypertrophied inferior nasal turbinate, etc. because of obstruction to nasolacrimal outflow.

7. Mention the pathogenesis for chronic dacryocystitis.

a. Stagnation and stasis of tears in lacrimal sac because of slowing or obstruction to lacrimal outflow.
b. Infection of the stagnant secretions leading to inflammation of the lacrimal sac.
c. Inflammatory edema and fibrosis further reduces the lacrimal outflow, leading to increased stagnation and stasis, which further leads to increased inflammation and the vicious cycle sets in.

8. What are the stages of chronic dacryocystitis?

- Stage of catarrhal dacryocystitis
- Stage of lacrimal mucocele
- Stage of chronic suppurative dacryocystitis with or without acute exacerbations
- Stage of fibrosis.

9. What are the stages of acute dacryocystitis?

- Stage of cellulitis
- Stage of lacrimal abscess
- Stage of fistula formation.

10. What is dacryoadenitis?

Dacryoadenitis is the inflammation of lacrimal gland.

Acute dacryoadenitis

It is caused by viral infections such as mumps, measles, influenza, mononucleosis, herpes and cytomegalovirus. Viral infections are responsible for dacryoadenitis in children. In adults, bacteria such as *Staphylococcus aureus, Neisseria gonorrhea, Haemophilus influenzae* and *Chlamydia trachomatis* are the usual causative agents. It presents as acute and painful swelling involving the upper and outer part of the orbit. On examination typical S-shaped swelling of the lid is seen because of swelling of the lateral one third of the upper eyelid.

Chronic dacryoadenitis

It is caused by chronic granulomatous inflammations such as tuberculosis, syphilis and autoimmune diseases such as sarcoidosis, Wegener's granulomatosis, Grave's disease, Sjögren's syndrome.

11. What are the differential diagnoses for swelling in the lacrimal sac region?

The differential diagnoses for swelling in the lacrimal sac region are:

- Lacrimal mucocele
- Lacrimal abscess
- Dermoid cyst
- Lacrimal sac tumors.

12. What are the complications of chronic dacryocystitis?

- Acute exacerbations resulting in acute dacryocystitis

- Intractable conjunctivitis
- Increased risk of hypopyon corneal ulcer following corneal abrasion
- Increased incidence of postoperative endophthalmitis.

13. What is regurgitation test?

Regurgitation test is done by applying pressure over the lacrimal sac area with either thumb or index finger. In cases with nasolacrimal duct obstruction such as chronic dacryocystitis, the contents of the sac regurgitate through the punctum.

Interpretation

- In chronic dacryocystitis the contents of the sac shall regurgitate through the lower, or lower and upper punctum
- In chronic dacryocystitis with functional block, i.e. pump failure, the contents of the sac shall empty in the nose
- In chronic dacryocystitis with encysted mucocele there is no regurgitation of the contents.

14. What is lacrimal syringing test?

Lacrimal syringing test is done by injecting saline into lacrimal drainage system with a lacrimal cannula fixed to a syringe filled with saline. It is done to know the patency of lacrimal drainage system. It can also localize the site of obstruction in the lacrimal drainage system.

Procedure

It is done under topical anesthesia by injecting normal saline into the lacrimal sac from lower or upper punctum with a lacrimal cannula fixed to syringe filled with saline. It is interpreted as follows:

- Saline is passing freely into throat as seen by swallowing reflex and appreciation of salt taste by patient indicates normal patent lacrimal passage
- Fast regurgitation of clear fluid from same punctum indicates obstruction in same canaliculi.
- Fast regurgitation of clear fluid from opposite punctum indicates obstruction at common canaliculi.
- Slow regurgitation of mucoid/mucopurulent fluid from same and opposite punctum indicates obstruction in lacrimal sac or nasolacrimal duct.
- Partial regurgitation of saline from punctum and partial saline going into throat indicates partial obstruction in the lacrimal passage.

15. What is hard stop and soft stop?

a. It is the type of resistance seen during lacrimal syringing by the lacrimal cannula or during probing by a lacrimal probe.
b. If cannula/probe enters the sac, it comes to a stop at medial wall of the sac and the lacrimal bone is felt hard—hard stop.
c. Hard stop excludes obstruction of canaliculi and common canalicular junction (Fig. 4.39A).
d. But if the cannula/probe stops proximal to the junction of common canaliculus and lacrimal sac, i.e. at lateral wall of the sac, there will be spongy feeling because cannula/probe presses the soft tissue of common canaliculus, lateral wall and the medial wall of the sac before touching the bone behind—soft stop.
e. Soft stop indicates that the block is at the level of common canalicular junction (Fig. 4.39B).

16. What is fluorescein dye disappearance test?

Fluorescein dye is instilled into conjunctival sac and tear meniscus is observed for disappearance of dye. Normally no dye is seen in conjunctival sac after 5 minutes. Prolonged retention of the dye for more than 5 minutes indicates epiphora.

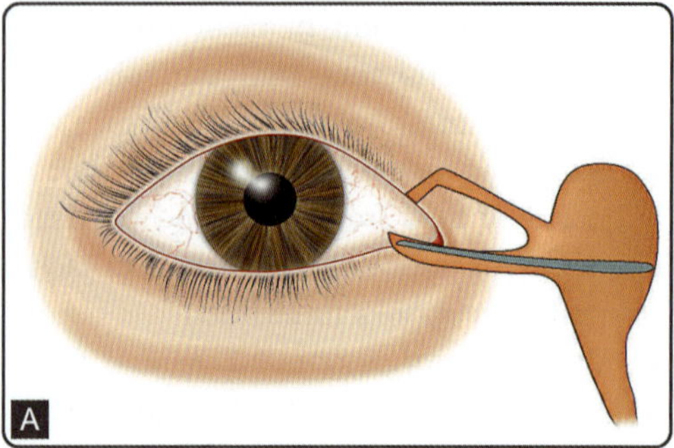

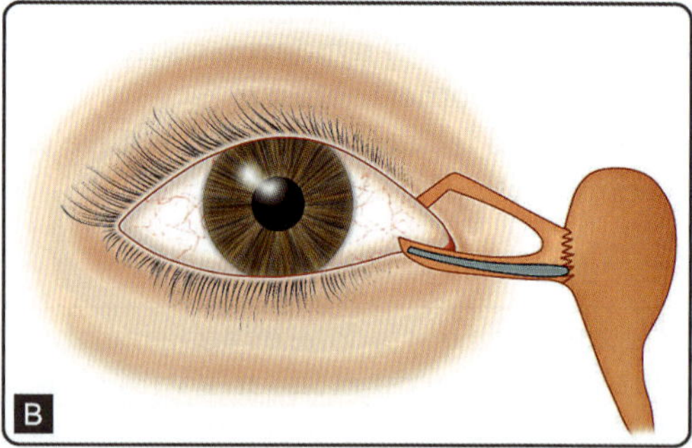

Figs 4.39A and B: Resistance to lacrimal probing. **A.** Hard stop (probe stopping at the medial wall of lacrimal sac and lacrimal bone); **B.** Soft stop (probe stopping proximal to common canalicular junction due to common canalicular block).

17. Describe Jones dye tests.

Jones dyes tests are done in cases of suspected partial obstruction of lacrimal passage. Jones test I differentiates partial obstruction from hyperlacrimation. Jones test II differentiates partial obstruction from lacrimal pump failure.

Jones test I

It is done by instilling 2% fluorescein dye into conjunctival sac and placing a cotton bud in the inferior meatus. After 5 minutes the cotton bud is inspected for staining with dye. Cotton bud stained with dye indicates that lacrimal passage is patent and the cause of watering is hyperlacrimation. A negative test indicates partial of the lacrimal passage or lacrimal pump failure.

Jones test II

It is done in cases of negative Jones test I. Lacrimal syringing is done following negative Jones test I. Cotton bud stained with dye after lacrimal syringing indicates partial obstruction of lacrimal passage. A negative Jones test II indicates lacrimal pump failure.

18. What is dacryocystography?

Dacryocystography is performed by injecting radiopaque dye such as lipiodol into lacrimal passage and taking X-ray to visualize the passage of the dye. Dacryocystography localizes the site of obstruction in the lacrimal passage. This test determines the site, nature and extent of block.

19. Describe the treatment for acute dacryocystitis.

Treatment is mainly by conservative methods and surgical treatment in the form of DCT/DCR should be avoided till the acute inflammation subsides. Treatment is by topical antibiotic eyedrops, oral antibiotics and anti-inflammatory drugs. Intravenous antibiotics are indicated in patients with severe inflammation or with complications (e.g. orbital cellulitis).

Lacrimal abscess if seen in cases not responding to treatment is treated by incision and drainage.

20. Describe the treatment for chronic dacryocystitis.

Surgery is the main treatment of chronic dacryocystitis. Medical management in the form of antibiotic eyedrops is advised to prevent acute exacerbation till surgery is done. Dacryocystorhinostomy (DCR) is the treatment of choice. Dacryocystectomy (DCT) is done in cases where DCR cannot be done or DCR is contraindicated.

Type of surgery depends on the site of obstruction in the lacrimal outflow tract:

- Chronic dacryocystitis with NLD block or block in the lacrimal sac—dacryocystorhinostomy (DCR)
- Chronic dacryocystitis with common canalicular block—canaliculocystorhinostomy
- Chronic dacryocystitis with block in the canaliculi—conjunctivo-canaliculocystorhinostomy—insertion of Lister's Jones tube
- Chronic dacryocystitis with external fistula—fistulectomy with dacryocystorhinostomy.

Dacryocystectomy

Dacryocystectomy (DCT) is a surgical procedure where the lacrimal sac is removed completely.

Indications

- Elderly, debilitated patient with shrunken and fibrosed sac
- Tumors or chronic granulomatous inflammations of sac such as tuberculosis, where sac has to be removed
- Nasal contraindications, e.g. atrophic rhinitis.

Dacryocystectomy leaves the patient with watering for the rest of his/her life as the entire sac is removed, but it prevents recurrent infections thus making the eye safe for any intraocular surgeries.

Dacryocystorhinostomy

Dacryocystorhinostomy (DCR) is a surgical procedure, which re-establishes the lacrimal drainage by connecting lacrimal sac to middle meatus of nose by making an ostium between lacrimal sac and nose (made by removing the lacrimal bone).

Work up/Investigations before dacryocystorhinostomy (DCR)

- Lacrimal syringing test
- ENT examination to rule out nasal contraindications
- Systemic investigations such as blood pressure measurement, blood sugar examination, bleeding time, clotting time, HIV, HBsAg, ECG.

Indications

DCR is the surgery of choice except for the indications mentioned in DCT.

Types of DCR

Lacrimal sac can be approached by three routes:

- Through canaliculi—canalicular DCR (LASER DCR)
- Through skin over lacrimal sac area—external DCR
- Through nose—nasal DCR (endonasal DCR).

Anesthesia for DCR

Usually it is done under local anesthesia. Local anesthesia is given by:

- Infiltration of the anesthetic agent along the skin incision over the lacrimal sac area
- Infratrochlear nerve block by inserting needle below trochlea
- Infraorbital nerve block by inserting the needle at the junction of inferior orbital margin with anterior lacrimal crest
- Anesthesia of nasal mucosa by packing nose with a gauze piece moistened with 4% lignocaine.

Steps of DCR

a. Nasal package: Nose is packed with sterile gauze soaked in 4% lignocaine and adrenaline.
b. A straight vertical or curved incision is made within 3 mm or more than 8 mm medial to the inner canthus to avoid damage to angular vessels.
c. Skin and fibers of orbicularis oculi are dissected to expose medial palpebral ligament. Below the medial palpebral ligament lies the lacrimal sac. Lacrimal sac is separated from medial wall and floor to expose the lacrimal fossa. The anterior lacrimal crest and the bone from the lacrimal fossa are removed.
d. Bowman's probe is introduced into the lacrimal sac and the sac is incised in an H-shaped manner to create two flaps.
e. A vertical incision is made in the nasal mucosa to create anterior and posterior flaps.
f. The posterior flaps and anterior flaps are sutured respectively.
g. The medial canthal tendon is resutured to periosteum and the skin incision closed with interruptured sutures.

Complications of DCR

a. Hemorrhage from injury to angular vein or nasal mucosa is the most common intraoperative complication.
b. Blockage of anastomosis resulting in failure of the surgery is the most common late postoperative complication.

21. How do you treat failed DCR?

- Failed DCR is treated by: Repeat DCR
- DCR with artificial implants such as Pawar implant to prevent the closure of the ostium
- Lester Jones tube insertion.

22. What is a lacrimal sac tumor?

Lacrimal sac tumors usually masquerade as chronic dacryocystitis; hence high index of suspicion is required for early diagnosis of lacrimal sac tumors.

Malignancy should be suspected in patients presenting with:

- Firm and non-compressible mass above the medial palpebral ligament
- Presence of epistaxis or blood-stained tears
- Cervical lymphadenopathy
- Presence of ulceration over the lacrimal sac mass.

CHALAZION

Subacute or chronic non-suppurative inflammation of meibomian gland is called chalazion. It is also called tarsal cyst or meibomian cyst.

Chalazion is more common in people with poor facial hygiene with habits of rubbing of eyes with dirty fingers.

CASE PROFORMA (Box 4.6)

Box 4.6: Proforma for chalazion

Biodata
Here is a male/female patient aged about.............. years,.............. by occupation, hailing from..............

Presenting Complaints
His/Her presenting complaints are swelling in eyelid since.............. months/years.

Chalazion is the most common nodular swelling of the eyelids.

History of Presenting Illness
He/She was apparently normal.............. months/years back. He/She noticed painless swelling in upper/lower eyelid of right eye (RE)/left eye (LE)/both eyes (BE) insidious in onset, gradually progressive/stationary in nature. Initially it was of the size of about.............. mm, now it has progressed to the present size.

Associated Features
- Pain
- Redness
- Watering
- Discharge
- Diminution of vision.

Pain, redness, watering are features of inflammation seen in internal hordeolum and external hordeolum, which have to be differentiated from chalazion, which is painless in nature (Table 4.4).
Secondary infection of a chalazion leads to formation of internal hordeolum which presents with pain, redness. Discharge is seen when external/internal hordeolum ruptures or when associated with lid abscess. Diminution of vision is rarely seen in chalazion when seen it is either because of mechanical ptosis or due to astigmatism because of upper lid chalazion pressing on the cornea.

Ocular History
He/She is/was wearing spectacles for (choose one among three):
- Near vision
- Distance vision
- Both.

He/She give history of similar complaints/no history of similar complaints.

Chalazion is more common in people with refractive errors, diabetes. It can recur after incision and curettage if the contents are not completely removed.

Past History
- He/She is a known diabetic on treatment/not a known diabetic
- He/She is a known hypertensive on treatment/not a known hypertensive.

Chalazion is more common in diabetics, immunocompromised individuals.

Family History
Not significant.

Personal History and Socioeconomic History
....
....

c. Incision and curettage of the chalazion is required for large chalazion. After local infiltration of the lignocaine vertical incision is put on the conjunctival side and the cheesy material is scooped out. The incision has to be put vertically to avoid damage to the ducts of the neighboring glands.

Work up of patient with chalazion

a. Look for refractive error and chronic blepharitis, correct it if present.
b. Urine sugar/RBS to screen for diabetes.
c. Bleeding time and clotting time since incision and curettage for chalazion involves incision on the conjunctiva.

Incision and curettage

Anesthesia: Topical 4% xylocaine eyedrops are instilled to the conjunctival sac, skin above the swelling is infiltrated with 2% xylocaine and chalazion clamp is applied.

Vertical incision is made on the conjunctival side to avoid injury to the neighboring meibomian ducts (incision has to be made on the conjunctival side as chalazion usually presents toward conjunctival side and conjunctival incision prevents scar, which may be seen in skin incision).

The contents of the chalazion (cheesy material) are curetted out with a chalazion scoop. Antibiotic eye ointment is applied and a pressure bandage is applied for about 3 hours for hemostasis.

8. What is the treatment of internal hordeolum?

Treatment is mainly conservative including hot fomentation, topical antibiotics, oral antibiotics and anti-inflammatory drugs.

9. What is recurrent chalazion/multiple chalazion?

They are common in patients with posterior blepharitis or meibomianitis or in patients with poor lid hygiene.

In elderly patients it may be masquerade syndrome of sebaceous gland carcinoma. Uncontrolled diabetics and those with immunodeficiency can have recurrent chalazion or multiple chalazia.

Meibomian gland carcinoma

It is third most common malignant tumor of the eyelid accounting for 1–5% of all malignant lid tumors. It is a highly aggressive tumor seen in elderly females and it is characterized by high rate of local recurrence, regional and distant metastases. More incidences are seen in individuals with prior radiation therapy.

The diagnosis of meibomian gland carcinoma is usually missed in the initial stages as it simulates chalazion or chronic blepharitis. SGC should be suspected in elderly patients diagnosed with chalazion, when chalazion is associated with features such as madarosis and destruction of meibomian gland orifices and recurrence after incision and curettage for more than three times.

PTERYGIUM

The word Pterygium is derived from Greek word pterygos meaning wing. Pterygium is a degenerative condition of the conjunctiva characterized by proliferation of subconjunctival tissue as a triangular fleshy mass to invade the cornea involving the Bowman's membrane and the superficial stroma.

CASE PROFORMA (Box 4.7)

Box 4.7: Proforma for pterygium

Biodata

Here is a male/female patient aged about........... years,........... by occupation, hailing from...........

Pterygium is a common degenerative condition of conjunctiva seen in middle aged and elderly people. It is most common in people living in hot climates.

Presenting Complaints

His/Her presenting complaints are:

- Growth in right eye (RE)/left eye (LE)/both eyes (BE) since........... months/years.

Most of the times patient may not come to hospital because of pterygium as it is asymptomatic except for cosmetic intolerance, unless it causes one of the symptoms:

- Inflamed pterygium causing pain, redness and watering
- Diminution of vision due to:
  - Astigmatism because of encroachment to cornea
  - Encroachment of pupillary area.

History of Presenting Illness

He/She was apparently normal........... months/years back. He/She noticed growth in RE/LE/BE insidious in onset gradually progressive/stationary in nature on nasal side/temporal side.

History has to be asked to rule out complications of pterygium such as inflammation of pterygium and visual disturbances to assess the growth of pterygium to know whether it is progressive or atrophic.

Ocular history

He/She is/was wearing spectacles for (choose one among three):

- Near vision
- Distance vision
- Both.

He/She gives history of surgery/no history of surgery to RE/LE/BE for similar complaints.

- Recurrence of pterygium is the most common complication after pterygium excision
- Recurrence rate is 30–50%.

Past history

- He/She is a known diabetic on treatment/not a known diabetic
- He/She is a known hypertensive on treatment/not a known hypertensive.

Family History

Not significant.

Personal History and Socioeconomic History

....

....

CASE DISCUSSION

1. How to diagnose pterygium?

Ocular examination

Pterygium has to be addressed as growth during examination and should be examined under:

- Site
- Size
- Shape
- Extent
- Vascularization
- Fibrous/Fleshy.
- Encroachment of cornea:
  - Crossing limbus
  - Midway between limbus and pupillary margin
  - Up to pupillary margin
  - Crossing pupillary margin.

Differential diagnosis (Table 4.5)

a. Pterygium has to be differentiated from pinguecula, pseudopterygium, papilloma and ocular surface squamous neoplasia (OSSN) (Figs 4.42A and B). Pinguecula appears as a yellowish nodule near the limbus with apex away from the cornea (Fig. 4.43). Papilloma and OSSN have lobulated appearance with sentinel vessel (Fig. 4.44).

b. Inflamed pterygium has to be differentiated from episcleritis, scleritis and phlyctenular conjunctivitis. All three present as nodular inflammation whereas pterygium will have characteristic wing shaped or triangular appearance (Figs 4.45A and B).

2. What is the etiology of pterygium?

Definite etiology is not known. Pterygium is known to be because of damage to limbal stem cells because of cumulative effect of exposure to ultraviolet radiation and dry, dusty and sandy weather.

Altered limbal epithelial cells results in the increased production of matrix metalloproteinase's resulting in elastotic degeneration of the collagen fibers of the substantia propria and destruction of Bowman's membrane. Activation of fibroblasts and angiogenesis results in proliferation of the vascularized granulation tissue (refer Table 4.5).

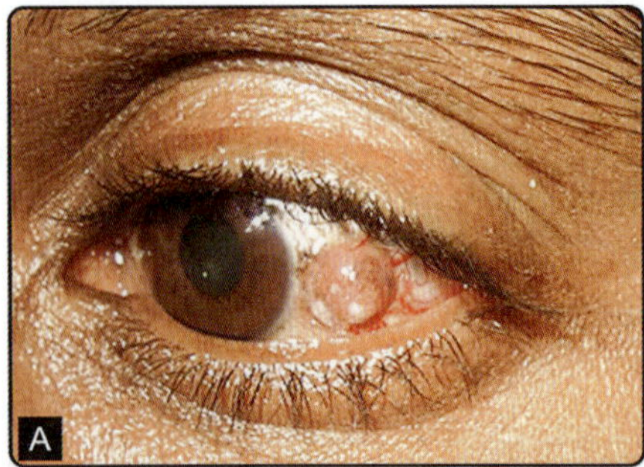

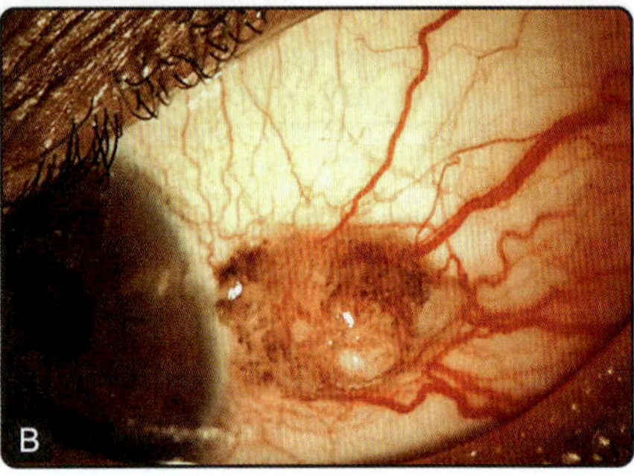

Figs 4.42A and B: Ocular surface squamous neoplasia

3. What is the pathology of pterygium?

Pathology of pterygium is characterized by elastotic degeneration of the collagen fibers of the substantia propria of conjunctiva with fibrovascular proliferation of granulation tissue under the epithelium.

4. What are the parts of pterygium?

- Apex or head—apical part present on the cornea
- Neck—limbal part
- Body—scleral part
- Cap—infiltrates infront of the apex.

5. What is pseudopterygium?

Adhesion of a fold of scarred conjunctiva to part of peripheral cornea or sclera following inflammation (refer Table 4.5).

Table 4.5: Difference between pterygium and pseudopterygium		
Features	**Pterygium**	**Pseudopterygium**
Definition	Degenerative condition	Inflammatory condition
Etiology	Ultraviolet radiation, dry, dusty, sandy weather	Chemical burns, trauma
Age	Middle age and elderly people	Seen at any age
Clinical course	Progressive or stationary	Stationary
Site	Nasal or temporal bulbar conjunctiva in the horizontal meridian	Seen at any meridian
Probe test	Probe cannot be passed under the neck of the pterygium	Probe can be passed under the neck of the pterygium as it is attached only at the apex
Treatment	Treatment is by surgical excision; recurrence following is surgery is seen and the incidence varies according to the method of surgical excision	Treatment is by surgical excision and recurrence is not seen

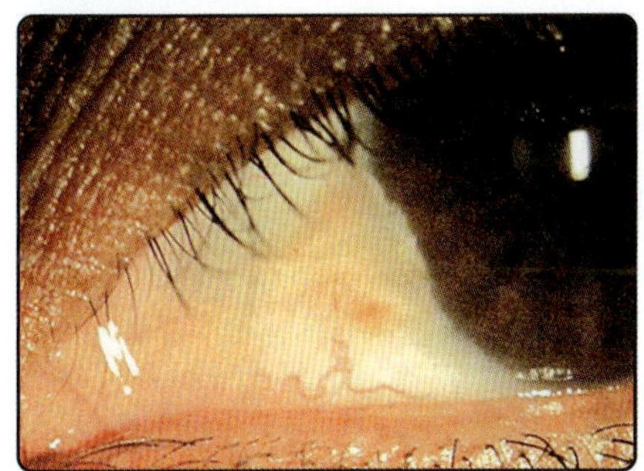

Fig. 4.43: Pinguecula (*Note:* Yellowish white triangular patch near limbus with apex away from cornea)

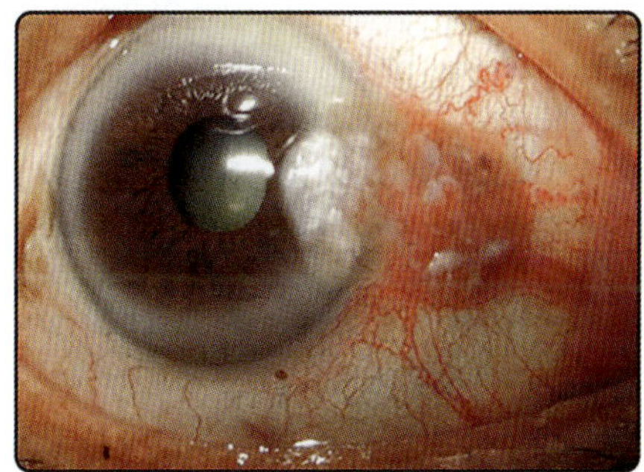

Fig. 4.44: Papilloma (*Note:* Lobulated mass with dilated vessels surrounding the mass)

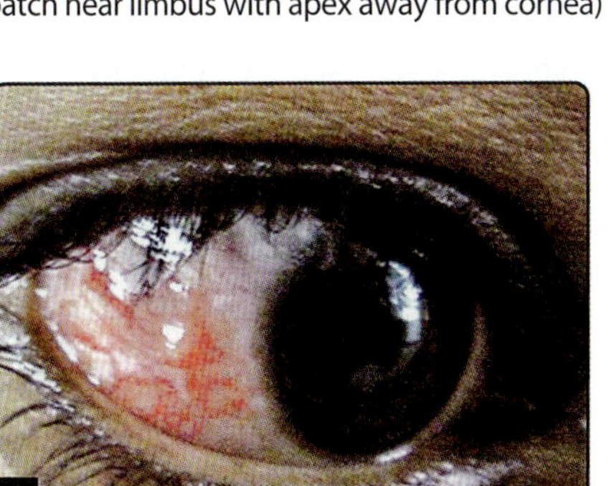

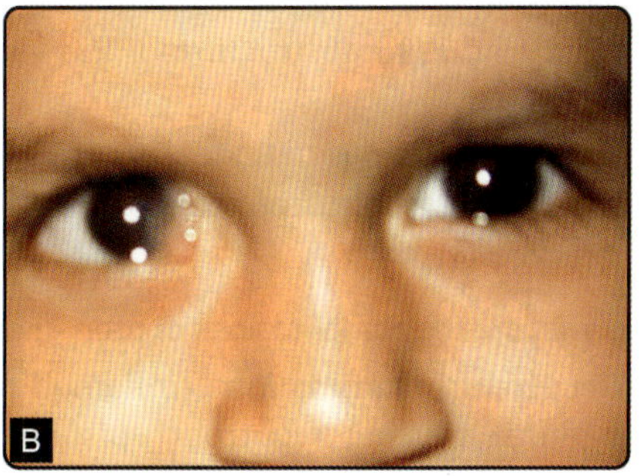

Figs 4.45A and B: **A.** Episcleritis (*Note:* Nodular lesion away from limbus and the congestion is deep to conjunctiva); **B.** Limbal dermoid of right eye.

6. What is Stocker-Busaca's line?

Deposition of iron infront of the apex of the pterygium is called Stocker-Busaca's line.

7. Name other conditions of deposition of iron in cornea.

a. Fleischer's ring: Iron deposition seen at the base of the keratoconus.
b. Hudson-Stahli's line: Iron deposition seen as horizontal line in cornea at the junction of meeting of upper and lower eyelids.
c. Ferry's line: Iron deposition seen in front of filtering bleb.
d. Coat's ring: Iron deposition seen in rust ring, left after removing corneal foreign body.

8. What are the stages or types of pterygium?

a. Progressive pterygium: It presents as thick fleshy vascular with infiltrations in front of the head of the pterygium (cap of the pterygium) (Figs 4.46A to C).
b. Atrophic pterygium: It presents as thin, attenuated fold with little vascularization and infiltrations in front of the head of the pterygium (cap) is absent.

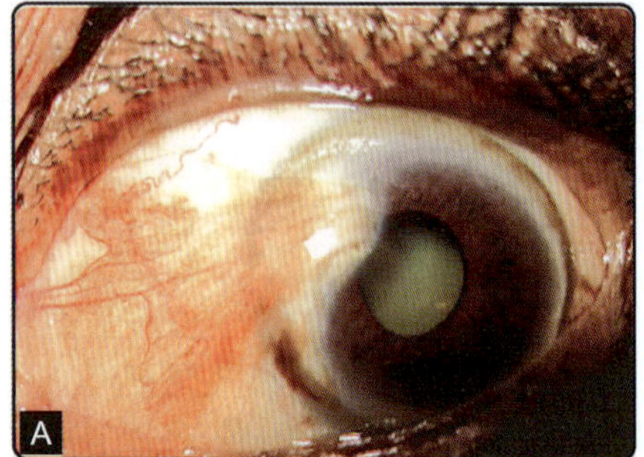

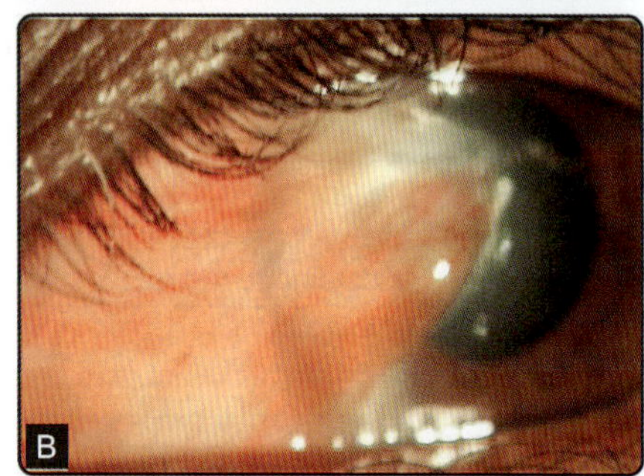

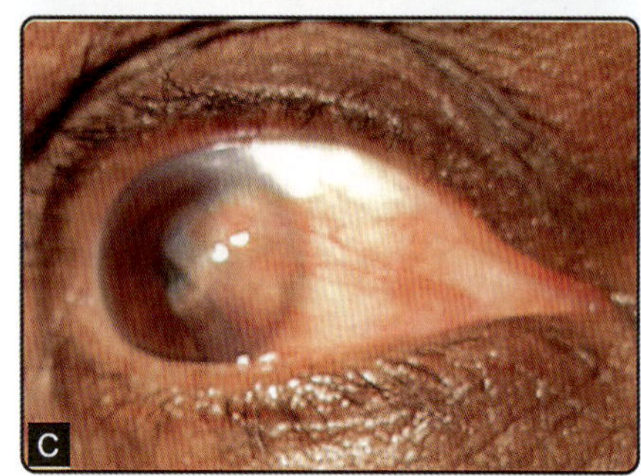

Figs 4.46A to C: Progressive pterygium. **A.** Encroaching up to pupillary margin; **B.** Encroaching up to midpupillary area. **C.** Crossing pupillary area.

9. What are the indications for excision of pterygium?

a. Optical: Pterygium causing diminution of vision either due to corneal astigmatism or due to obstruction of the visual axis.
b. Cosmetic: For cosmetic reasons.
c. Therapeutic: Recurrent inflammation of pterygium.

10. What are the complications of pterygium?

- Recurrent inflammations (inflamed pterygium) causing recurrent episodes of pain, redness, etc.
- Cystic degeneration (Fig. 4.47)
- Neoplastic change to epithelioma and fibrosarcoma (very rare complication).

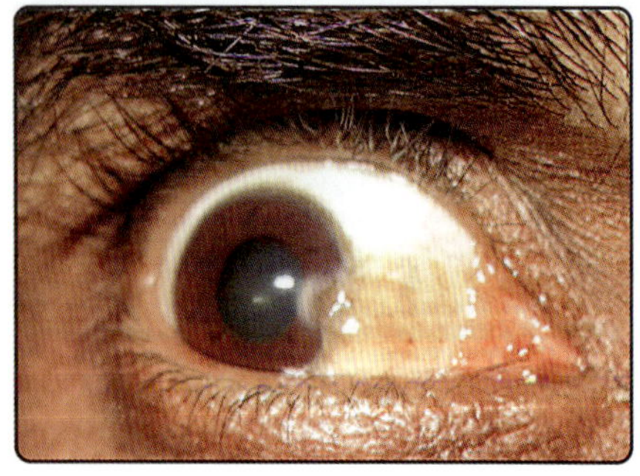

Fig. 4.47: Pterygium with cystic degeneration

11. Describe the treatment for pterygium.

Surgical excision is the treatment of choice for pterygium. The various methods of pterygium excision are as follows.

Simple pterygium excision

- Simple pterygium excision with primary closure of the conjunctiva
- Pterygium excision with bare sclera technique.

Pterygium excision with grafting

- Pterygium excision with free conjunctival graft
- Pterygium excision with amniotic membrane graft
- Pterygium excision with mucous membrane graft
- Pterygium excision with limbal conjunctival graft
- Pterygium excision with rotational conjunctival graft
- Pterygium **PERFECT**—**P**terygium **E**xtensive **R**emoval **F**ollowed by **E**xtended **C**onjunctival **T**ransplant.

Surgeries to prevent recurrence of pterygium

Pterygium recurrence is attributed to the fact that pterygium is due to altered limbal stem cells, which continue to proliferate resulting in recurrence. The recurrence rate is in the range of 30–50%. It is highest with simple pterygium excision by bare sclera technique and least with limbal conjunctival grafting as in the latter method altered stem cells are replaced by normal ones.

McReynolds operation

Transplantation of the head of the pterygium under bulbar conjunctiva. This will change the direction of pterygium in which it grows thereby prevents corneal encroachment, but cosmetically it may not be acceptable.

Other methods

a. Pterygium excision with adjunct antimetabolites:
   - Thiotepa eyedrops four times daily for 6 weeks
   - Mitomycin C (0.02%) applied topically to the bare sclera during surgery.
b. Pterygium excision with beta irradiation.
c. Treatment of pterygium encroaching the pupillary area of cornea: Surgical excision of pterygium is followed by treatment of the residual opacity. Residual corneal opacity is treated by phototherapeutic keratectomy or lamellar keratoplasty.

Pterygium cannot be removed without leaving scar on the cornea, as it involves Bowman's membrane. Any lesion, which involves Bowman's membrane will leave scar. The scar left behind depending on the density requires phototherapeutic keratectomy or lamellar keratoplasty.

12. What is recurrence of pterygium?

Recurrence of pterygium is the most common complication after pterygium excision:

- Recurrence rate is 30–50%
- Bare sclera excision has got maximum recurrence rate
- Pterygium excision by other methods has got relatively less recurrence rates
- Pterygium excision with limbal conjunctival graft has got least recurrence rate.

13. What are the causes for recurrence of pterygium?

Recurrence of pterygium is because of proliferation of granulation tissue, as the conjunctiva is incised during excision of pterygium.

Recent hypothesis for recurrence of pterygium is regarded as due to problem in the stem cells, present in the limbal area and because of proliferation of these stem cells pterygium recurs (i.e. why pterygium excision with limbal conjunctival grafting, which replaces these damaged stem cells has got least amount of recurrence).

Listeria, Actinomyces), gram-negative bacilli (e.g. *Pseudomonas, Proteus, Haemophilus*), gram-negative cocci (e.g. *Neisseria gonorrhoeae*).

b. Fungi including filamentous such as *Fusarium, Aspergillus, Cephalosporium, Penicillium,* yeasts and fungi such as *Candida* and *Cryptococcus.*

c. Viruses including herpes simplex, *Varicella zoster.*

d. Protozoa including *Acanthamoeba.*

Non-infective causes

a. Trauma including chemical injury, mechanical injury.

b. Neurological, i.e. neurotrophic keratitis (fifth nerve lesion), neuroparalytic keratitis (seventh nerve lesion).

c. Immunological diseases such as collagen vascular disorders and Mooren's ulcer.

d. Dermatological lesions, i.e. rosacea, pemphigoid.

e. Nutritional, i.e. keratomalacia.

f. Post infectious, i.e. metaherpetic keratitis.

3. What are the stages of corneal ulcer?

- Stage of infiltration (Fig. 4.49A)
- Stage of ulceration (Fig. 4.49B)
- Stage of regression (Fig. 4.49C)
- Stage of healing (Fig. 4.49D).

4. Name the bacteria that can penetrate intact corneal epithelium.

- *Neisseria gonorrhoeae*
- *Corynebacterium diphtheriae*
- *Listeria monocytogenes*
- *Haemophilus influenzae.*

Fungi cannot penetrate intact corneal epithelium, but they can penetrate intact Descemet's membrane and endothelium, hence hypopyon in case of fungal corneal ulcer is not sterile, i.e. fungi can be seen in anterior chamber.

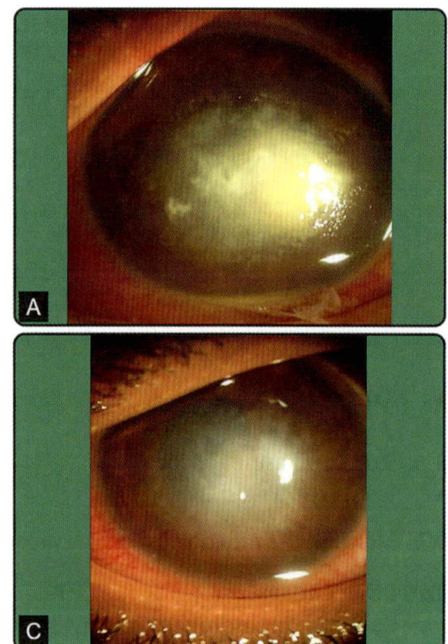

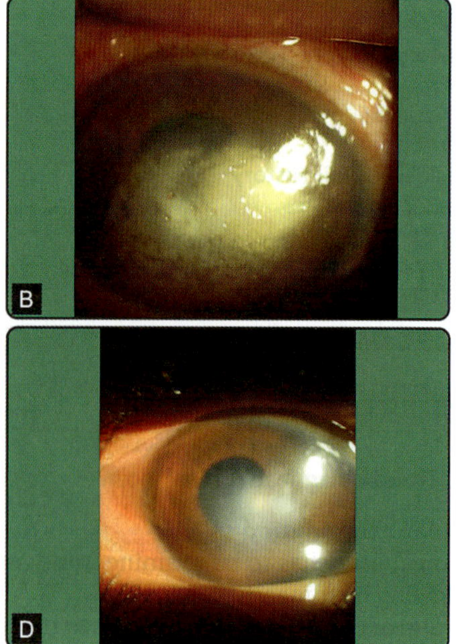

Figs 4.49A to D: Stages of corneal ulcer. **A.** Stage of infiltration; **B.** Stage of ulceration; **C.** Stage of regression; **D.** Stage of healing.

5. What are the predisposing factors for bacterial corneal ulcer?

Cornea has got defense mechanisms to prevent infections. The defense mechanisms in cornea are:

a. Protective action of the eyelids, antimicrobial activity of tear film due to presence of lysozymes, immunoglobulins and presence of intact corneal epithelium.
b. Disruption of these normal defense mechanisms predisposes to infection of cornea as occurring in the following conditions.
c. Damage to corneal epithelium as caused by vitamin A deficiency, corneal edema, exposure keratopathy, loss of corneal sensation, use of topical steroids.
d. Corneal abrasions caused by injury to cornea and contact lens associated trauma.
e. Diseases of eyelids such as entropion leading to repeated corneal erosions, ectropion and lagophthalmos leading to exposure keratopathy.
f. Diseases affecting tear film such as dry eye.

6. What is hypopyon corneal ulcer or ulcus serpens?

The characteristic corneal ulcer produced by pneumococcus is called hypopyon corneal ulcer. The ulcer caused by pneumococcus creeps over cornea in a serpiginous fashion and associated with a hypopyon and it is called hypopyon corneal ulcer or ulcus serpens. It is seen commonly in old debilitated patients and alcoholics. The source of infection is usually chronic dacryocystitis.

Hypopyon corneal ulcer

The ulcer creeps over cornea in a serpiginous fashion and hence called ulcus serpens.

The ulcer is usually greater at the edges and the ulcer spreads on one side and at the other side, cicatrization may be seen.

Severe iridocyclitis with hypopyon is usually seen.

Corneal ulcer with hypopyon

Corneal ulcer associated with hypopyon due to other organisms such as *Pseudomonas,* gonococci, staphylococci, streptococci, fungi are included in this list. These ulcers would not show the characteristic features of hypopyon corneal ulcer caused by *Pneumococcus* as described above.

Hypopyon

Collection of pus (inflammatory exudates consisting of predominantly leukocytes) in anterior chamber is called hypopyon. Hypopyon is because of associated iritis (caused by toxins causing corneal ulcer) causing outpouring of leukocytes from the vessels, which gravitate and collect at the bottom of the anterior chamber as hypopyon.

Bacteria cannot penetrate corneal endothelium, hence hypopyon in case of bacterial corneal ulcer is sterile. Fungi can penetrate intact corneal endothelium, hence hypopyon in case of fungal corneal ulcer is not sterile.

7. What are the sources of infection for corneal ulcer?

a. Exogenous route is the commonest mode of infection. The infection may be acquired from external injuries with infected vegetative matter or foreign bodies.
b. The infection may be acquired by contiguous spread from the neighboring structures such as conjunctiva, sclera, uveal tract.
c. Endogenous route is rarely seen because of avascularity of cornea.

8. What are the complications of corneal ulcer?

a. Ectatic cicatrix: It results because of spreading of the infection resulting in sloughing and thinning of the cornea, which bulges out because of influence of intraocular pressure.
b. Descemetocele: It is the herniation of Descemet's membrane as a transparent vesicle through the floor of the corneal

ulcer. It is because of deeper penetration of the corneal ulcer and the resistance offered from Descemet's membrane. It may rupture leading to perforated corneal ulcer.

c. Perforated corneal ulcer: It is because of penetration of the corneal ulcer involving the full thickness of cornea. It results because of rupture of descemetocele because of minimal trauma or because of sudden exertion leading to increase in intraocular pressure.
d. Anterior staphyloma: It is abnormal protrusion of uveal tissue through weak outer coat of the eyeball. It occurs secondary to localized or diffuse thinning of the outer coat of the eyeball, cornea or sclera. The uveal tissue, which lies below the cornea or sclera bulges out leading to staphyloma.
e. Endophthalmitis: It occurs in case of high virulence of the causative organism because of extension of infection to involve the inner coats and cavities of the eye.
f. Panophthalmitis: It also occurs in case of high virulence of the causative organism because of extension of infection to involve the all the three coats and cavities of the eye.
g. Secondary glaucoma: It is because of inflammatory exudates blocking the trabecular meshwork.
h. Corneal opacity: It is the end result of healing of corneal ulcer. The grade of corneal opacity depends on the depth of penetration of the ulcer.

9. What are the complications of perforated corneal ulcer?

a. Iris prolapse: In case of small perforations, iris can plug the perforated site leading to adherent leukoma after healing of the corneal ulcer. In case of bigger perforations, it can lead to anterior staphyloma.
b. Extrudation or anterior dislocation of the lens because of sudden anterior movement of the iris lens diaphragm.
c. The intraocular extension of infection leading to endophthalmitis or panophthalmitis.

10. Describe the work up of a patient with corneal ulcer.

Detailed history regarding mode of onset of the ulcer:

- General physical examination to know any systemic predisposing factors such as diabetes, immunodeficiency and malnutrition
- Ocular examination to rule out infection of the surrounding structures such as conjunctivitis, chronic dacryocystitis (lacrimal syringing is mandatory in all cases of corneal ulcer)
- Slit-lamp examination of corneal ulcer after staining with 2% fluorescein to look for the morphology of the ulcer.

Laboratory investigations

- Blood sugar/Urine sugar to rule out diabetes
- Corneal scraping and Gram staining, Giemsa staining, KOH mount, culture on blood agar, Sabouraud's dextrose agar.

11. Describe the morphological characters of corneal ulcers (Table 4.6).

Bacterial corneal ulcer

Gram-negative bacilli such as *Pseudomonas* are known to produce corneal ulcers with rapid necrosis, presenting as sloughing corneal ulcer. Presence of greenish yellow mucopurulent discharge is typical of pseudomonas infection.

Gram-positive cocci such as staphylococci are known to produce localized oval or round grayish white ulcer with distinct margins.

Contd...

Contd...

Fungal corneal ulcer (DEFGHI) (Figs 4.50A to C)
- **D**ry looking
- **E**levated margins
- **F**eathery finger-like extensions
- **G**rayish white in color
- Big **H**ypopyon
- **I**mmune ring and independent satellite lesions.

Viral corneal ulcer
- Herpes simplex—dendritic ulcer with markedly reduced corneal sensation
- Herpes zoster—pseudodendritic ulcer with characteristic vesicular skin lesions not crossing the midline.

Acanthamoeba corneal ulcers
These are usually seen as a complication of contact lens wear present as multiple stromal infiltrates with severe pain because of radial keratoneuritis.

12. What is the treatment protocol for corneal ulcer?

Non-specific treatment

a. Cycloplegic agents such as atropine 1% eye ointment, homide eyedrops or cyclopentolate eyedrops.

b. Oral anti-inflammatory drugs such as diclofenac sodium, ibuprofen, etc. for relief from pain and for treatment of associated inflammatory symptoms.

Table 4.6: Differences between bacterial, fungal and viral corneal ulcers

Features	Bacterial	Fungal	Viral
Etiology	Corneal epithelial defect, ocular infections	Injury by vegetative matter, animal tail, etc. Immunocompromised state	Close contact with infected individuals
Symptoms	Marked	Mild	Moderate
Signs	Symptoms = Signs	Signs > Symptoms	Symptoms = Signs
Ulcer	Yellowish white to grayish white with wet look	Grayish white with dry look, feathery extensions and elevated	Dendritic pattern
Hypopyon	Sterile and mobile	Nonsterile and stationary	Rarely seen
Keratic precipitates (KPs)	Not seen	Not seen	Common
Recurrences	Nil	Nil	Common
Steroids	Contraindicated	Contraindicated	Contraindicated in infective epithelial keratitis; indicated in disciform keratitis and zoster ophthalmicus
Immune ring	Uncommon	Common	May be seen
Satellite lesions	Not seen	Seen	Not seen
Skin lesions	Not seen	Not seen	Seen
Diagnosis	Culture and sensitivity	Culture and sensitivity	PCR, ELISA, etc.

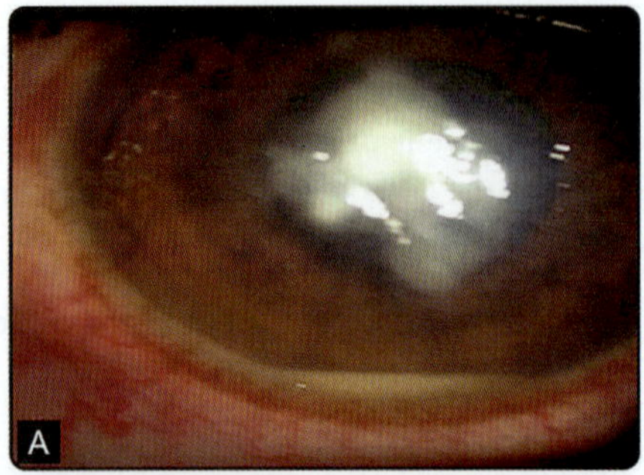
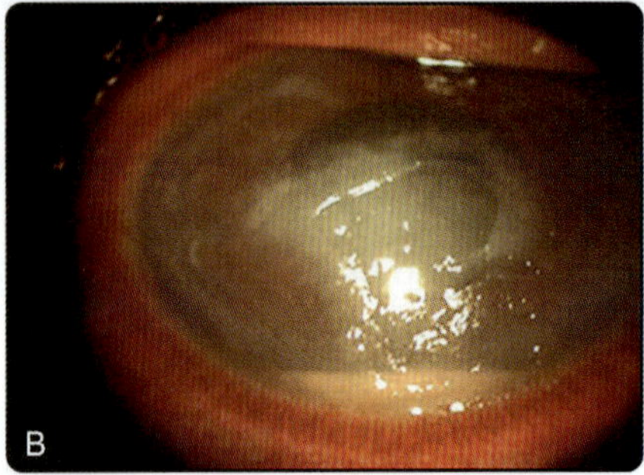
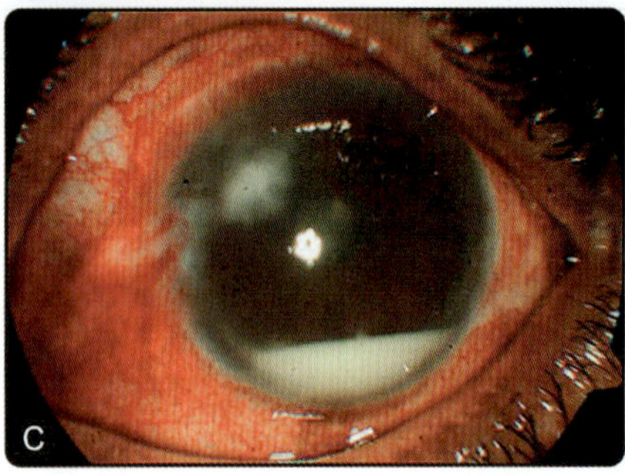

Figs 4.50A to C: Fungal corneal ulcer (*Note:* Corneal ulcer with features suggesting fungal etiology such as dry, elevated, grayish white, feathery extensions, hypopyon).

Specific treatment

Treatment depends on the cause of corneal ulcer, i.e. bacteria, fungi, virus, etc.

Bacterial corneal ulcer

Specific treatment is by use of topical antibiotics in the form of eyedrops and eye ointments. Broad-spectrum antibiotic eyedrops are started initially and later the antibiotic eyedrops are replaced by specific antibiotics according to the culture and sensitivity report. The eyedrops are instilled as frequently as half hourly depending on the severity of the ulcer. Usually, fortified preparations of the eyedrops are preferred over the commercially available preparations. The commonly used fortified preparations are fortified tobramycin 14 mg/mL, fortified cefazolin 75 mg/mL, fortified ceftriaxone 50 mg/mL and commercially available preparations contain less concentration of the antibiotics compared to fortified preparations.

Systemic antibiotics are indicated in patients with total corneal ulcer, marginal corneal ulcer, perforated corneal ulcer and corneal ulcer associated with hypopyon.

Fungal corneal ulcer

For Fusarium keratitis

a. Natamycin 5% eyedrops initially hourly and then gradually tapered.
b. Oral fluconazole 100 mg twice a day in case of deep keratitis.
c. Broad-spectrum topical antibiotic eyedrops, i.e. 0.3% ciprofloxacin to prevent secondary bacterial infection.

For Aspergillus and Candida keratitis

a. Amphotericin B 0.15% eyedrops.
b. Oral fluconazole 100 mg twice a day in case of deep keratitis.
c. Broad-spectrum topical antibiotic eyedrops to prevent the secondary bacterial infection.

Viral corneal ulcer

For herpes simplex keratitis

a. Acyclovir 3% eye ointment five times per day.
b. Broad-spectrum topical antibiotic eyedrops to prevent secondary bacterial infection.

For herpes zoster keratitis

a. Systemic acyclovir 800 mg five times per day.

b. Topical acyclovir 3% eye ointment five times per day.
c. Oral steroids in case of neurological complications such as third nerve palsy, iridocyclitis and scleritis.

Acanthamoeba keratitis

Chlorhexidine digluconate and polyhexamethylene biguanide commonly used antiseptic agents are the first-line drugs and they are active against both trophozoite and cysts of *Acanthamoeba.* Propamidine isethionate and neomycin are also effective against *Acanthamoeba:*

a. Azoles such as fluconazole, itraconazole are used for systemic treatment.
b. Patients not responding to medical line of treatment are treated by surgical treatment in the form of keratoplasty.

13. What is the role of atropine in the treatment of corneal ulcer?

Atropine decreases pain by relieving ciliary spasm, decreases exudation by decreasing hyperemia, prevents formation of synechiae because of associated iridocyclitis, increases blood supply to uvea and brings more antibodies to the aqueous humor.

14. What are the causes for non-healing corneal ulcer?

a. Systemic causes such as uncontrolled diabetes mellitus, treatment with immunosuppressive drugs and steroids, malnutrition, immunosuppressive diseases.
b. Ocular causes such as untreated dacryocystitis, diseases of the corneal, i.e. corneal edema, corneal dystrophies, corneal degenerations, presence of predisposing factors for corneal ulceration such as entropion leading to repeated corneal erosions, ectropion and lagophthalmos leading to exposure keratopathy.
c. Inadequate treatment or wrong treatment.

15. What is the treatment of non-healing corneal ulcer?

a. Evaluation to look for underlying causes for non-healing corneal ulcer and treatment of predisposing causes if any.
b. Treatment based on the culture and sensitivity report if not started before.
c. Mechanical debridement of the ulcer under topical anesthesia.
d. Cauterization of the ulcer by using thermal cautery or chemical cauterization by using carbolic acid.
e. Therapeutic keratoplasty in cases not responding to medical line of management.

16. What is the treatment of perforated corneal ulcer?

a. It depends on the size of the perforation.
b. Small perforation can be treated by tissue adhesive glues or by covering with bandage contact lens.
c. Larger perforation needs tectonic keratoplasty.
d. Perforation can be prevented by taking precautions in the form of:
   - Lowering IOP by antiglaucoma medications
   - Asking the patient to avoid straining such as sneezing, coughing violently
   - Therapeutic keratoplasty.

17. What is atheromatous corneal ulcer?

Degenerative corneal ulcer seen in old leukomatous grade corneal opacities is called atheromatous corneal ulcer.

18. What is dendritic ulcer?

An ulcer, which is irregular with linear branching with knobs at the ends typically seen in herpes simplex epithelial keratitis is called dendritic ulcer. The ulcer stains prominently with fluorescein and margins stain with rose bengal.

19. What is trophic corneal ulcer?

Inflammation of cornea secondary to degenerative changes in the corneal epithelium as a result of decreased cornel sensation or drying of cornea leading to altered metabolic activity of the corneal epithelium is called trophic corneal ulcer or trophic keratitis. Trophic keratitis is of three types:

a. Neurotrophic keratitis: Inflammation/Ulceration of cornea secondary to degenerative changes in the corneal epithelium as a result of decreased cornel sensation is called neurotrophic keratitis.
b. Exposure keratitis: Inflammation/Ulceration of cornea because of exposure of cornea leading to drying and desiccation of corneal epithelium.
c. Neurotrophic keratitis and Neuroparalytic keratitis: These are used interchangingly for similar conditions.

Neuroparalytic keratitis is similar to neurotrophic keratitis, the only difference being it includes only those causes, which lead to paralysis of the sensory nerve supply of cornea such as paralysis of trigeminal nerve as a result of surgery, trauma, neoplasms. Neuroparalytic keratitis can be the first sign of intracranial neoplasms because of paralysis of trigeminal nerve caused by the tumor.

20. What is pseudodendritic ulcer?

An ulcer, which is broader and plaque-like, elevated with absence of knobbed ends seen in zoster keratitis is called pseudodendritic ulcer. It shows little or minimal staining with fluorescein and does not stain with rose bengal.

21. What is disciform keratitis?

Inflammation of stroma of cornea presenting as a disk-shaped edema because of delayed hypersensitivity reaction to Herpes simplex virus antigen is called disciform keratitis.

22. What are the indications for topical steroids in keratitis?

- Herpes zoster keratitis associated with iridocyclitis, scleritis, optic neuritis
- Disciform keratitis
- Mooren's corneal ulcer
- Interstitial keratitis.

23. What is interstitial keratitis?

Non-suppurative inflammation of the corneal stroma without involvement of corneal epithelium and endothelium is called interstitial keratitis. The common causes are:

- Bacterial infections such as syphilis, tuberculosis, leprosy
- Viral infections such as herpes simplex, herpes zoster
- Parasitic infections such as leishmaniasis, trypanosomiasis
- Systemic diseases such as Cogan's syndrome
- Collagen vascular diseases such as sarcoidosis, rheumatoid arthritis.

PTOSIS

The word ptosis is derived from Greek and it means falling downwards or drooping of any organ.

CASE PROFORMA (Box 4.9)

Box 4.9: Proforma for ptosis

Biodata

Here is a male/female patient aged about..........years,..........by occupation, from..........

Presenting Complaints

His/Her presenting complaints are drooping of upper eyelid of right eye (RE)/left eye (LE)/both eye (BE) since months/years.

History of Presenting Illness

....

....

- History will differentiate congenital and acquired ptosis. Congenital ptosis will be present at birth with or without family history
- In cases of acquired ptosis, enquiry has to be made to find out the etiology
- History of trauma or surgery to rule out aponeurotic ptosis
- History of swelling over the upper lid to rule out mechanical ptosis
- Ptosis may cause diminution of vision when the ptotic eyelid covers the visual axis (this may cause stimulus deprivation amblyopia in children).

Ocular History

....

....

Past History

....

....

Family History

Family history is significant in cases of congenital ptosis.

Personal History and Socioeconomic History

....

....

CASE DISCUSSION

1. How ptosis is diagnosed?

Ocular examination

a. Ptosis has to be examined under the following headings:
   - Look for microphthalmos, anophthalmos, phthisis bulbi, enophthalmos to exclude pseudoptosis
   - Palpebral fissure height in straight/ primary gaze
   - Palpebral fissure height in downgaze.

> Palpebral fissure height in primary gaze will be decreased on the ptotic side (Fig. 4.51).

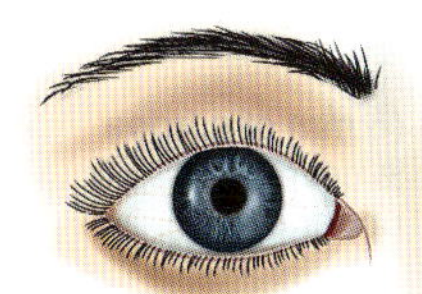
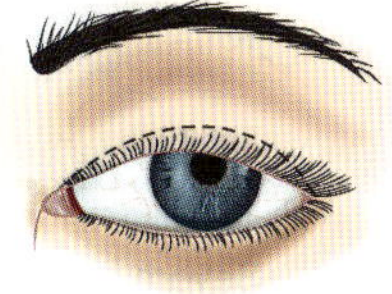

Fig. 4.51: Palpebral fissure height in primary gaze decreased on ptotic side (left side)

If jaw-winking phenomenon is present, levator resection surgery should not be done as it will increase the jaw winking.

Strabismus: Presence of strabismus particularly hypotropia should be specifically looked for by doing cover and uncover tests.

Hypotropia is one of the causes for pseudoptosis (because of depression of the eye). Hence, correction of hypotropia has to be made first before operating for ptosis.

2. Define blepharoptosis.

Blepharoptosis is defined as drooping of the upper eyelid from its normal position. In ophthalmology, blepharoptosis is generally referred as ptosis. Normally upper eyelid covers 2 mm of cornea. In ptosis, the upper eyelid covers more than 2 mm of cornea.

3. Classify ptosis.

Ptosis can be classified into different types based on the etiology or onset and pathology or cause.

Based on etiology
- Congenital ptosis
- Acquired ptosis.

Based on the pathology
- Neurogenic ptosis
- Myogenic ptosis
- Aponeurotic ptosis
- Mechanical ptosis.

4. What is the pathophysiology of ptosis?

Ptosis or drooping of the upper eyelid is because of the weakness of the elevators/retractors of the upper eyelid (levator palpebrae superioris and Müller's muscle). The cause for weakness may be in the muscle, aponeurosis, neuromuscular junction or in the nerves supplying the muscle.

5. What is Marcus Gunn jaw-winking syndrome?

It is also called congenital synkinetic ptosis (Marcus Gunn jaw-winking ptosis). It is because of misdirection of mandibular division of the V cranial nerve or III cranial nerve to the levator muscle. It is characterized by retraction of the ptotic eyelid resulting in elevation of the eyelid seen with stimulation of ipsilateral pterygoid muscle as in chewing, clenching the teeth or opening of mouth.

6. What is Horner's syndrome?

Horner's syndrome is because of oculosympathetic paresis. It is characterized by ptosis, miosis of pupil, inverse ptosis of lower eyelid, anhidrosis of ipsilateral face and enophthalmos. It is diagnosed by phenylephrine test.

7. Describe phenylephrine test.

Phenylephrine test is done by instilling one drop of phenylephrine into the conjunctival sac of both eyes after measuring the amount of ptosis. Improvement in ptosis and dilatation of the miotic pupil more than the normal pupil because of denervation supersensitivity after 5 minutes indicates Horner's syndrome.

8. What is ocular myasthenia gravis?

Myasthenia gravis is an autoimmune disorder characterized by abnormal fatigability of the muscles because of deficiency of acetylcholine receptors as a result of destruction of acetylcholine receptors by the antibodies directed against them. Ocular myasthenia gravis presents with history of variable degree of ptosis, increasing with fatigue.

Contd...

Contd...

Diagnosis

Myasthenia gravis is diagnosed by following tests.

Ice test: Ice pack is applied to the eyelid for 5–10 minutes. Improvement in the amount of ptosis is seen in myasthenia gravis. It is because of the fact that cold temperature enhances neuromuscular transmission by inhibiting the action of acetylcholinesterase.

Neostigmine test: The neostigmine is a reversible acetylcholinesterase inhibitor. The test is done by intramuscular injection of neostigmine 4 mg. Improvement in the amount of ptosis is seen in myasthenia gravis.

Tensilon test (edrophonium test): The edrophonium is also reversible acetylcholine esterase inhibitor. The test is done by intravenous injection of 10 mg of edrophonium. Improvement in the amount of ptosis is seen in myasthenia gravis. Edrophonium is safer than neostigmine.

Serum assay for acetylcholine receptor antibodies and electromyography: These are the laboratory investigations required for confirmation of myasthenia gravis.

9. What is the treatment for ptosis?

Congenital ptosis

Surgery is the treatment of choice.

Timing of surgery

Mild-to-moderate ptosis: Surgery may be delayed till 4 years of age, so that accurate measurements can be taken when the child can cooperate for ptosis measurements.

Severe ptosis: Surgery should be performed as early as possible to prevent amblyopia.

Type of surgery

The type of surgery is determined by:

- Amount of ptosis
- Levator muscle action.

Principle of surgery

The principle of surgery is to strengthen the retractors of the upper eyelid.

Fasanella-Servat operation: It is done in mild ptosis with good levator muscle function. Here a part of tarsal plate and Müller's muscle are excised (resected) to strengthen the Müller's muscle.

Levator resection: It is done in moderate-to-severe ptosis with good-to-moderate levator function. It is the surgery of choice for most of the cases of ptosis with good levator function, since levator palpebrae superioris (LPS) is the primary retractor of the upper eyelid. Here LPS is shortened (resected) to strengthen the LPS muscle.

Frontalis sling operation: It is done in severe ptosis with poor levator muscle function. Here, upper eyelid is anchored to the frontalis muscle by a sling. Synthetic sutures or autogenous fascia lata are used as sling.

Treatment of associated conditions in ptosis

Blepharophimosis syndrome is treated by medial canthal tendon plication for telecanthus, and epicanthus and frontalis sling operation for ptosis.

Marcus Gunn jaw-winking syndrome is treated by levator resection in mild cases and by levator disinsertion and frontalis sling suspension in severe cases.

Mechanical ptosis

The condition is treated by treatment of the mechanical factor causing ptosis.

Acquired ptosis

Treatment is done by identifying the underlying cause of ptosis and treatment of the causative disease. Surgery is done only after the primary disease causing ptosis is treated. Surgery if required is chosen as for the congenital ptosis.

Chapter 5

Diagnostic Tests in Ophthalmology

Chapter Outline

- Tonometry
- Slit-lamp Examination
- Ophthalmoscopy
- Keratometry
- Retinoscopy
- Gonioscopy
- Perimetry
- Ultrasonography
- Ultrasound Biomicroscopy
- Vital Stains
- Specular Microscopy
- Fundus Fluorescein Angiography
- Indocyanine Green Angiography
- Optical Coherence Tomography
- Heidelberg Retinal Tomography
- Corneal Topography
- Electrophysiological Tests
- Retinal Function Tests
- Macular Function Tests
- Tests for Evaluation of a Case of Watering Eye
- Tests for Evaluation of a Case of Squint
- Tests for Evaluation of Tear Film

TONOMETRY

Measurement of intraocular pressure (IOP) is called tonometry.

Intraocular Pressure

1. Intraocular pressure is defined as pressure exerted by fluids inside the eyeball.
2. Intraocular pressure (IOP) between 10 and 21 mm Hg with a mean IOP of 16 mm Hg with standard deviation of 3 mm Hg is considered as normal IOP.
3. Persistent IOP above 21 mm Hg or below 7 mm Hg will produce structural and functional changes in the eye.

Digital Tonometry

Measurement of intraocular pressure (IOP) can be roughly estimated by palpating the eyeball with index fingers of both hands after asking the patient to look down over the upper eyelid above the tarsal plate. Index finger of one hand indents the eyeball, while the index finger of the other hand feels the pressure changes produced by the indenting finger.

It provides a rough estimation of the IOP of the eye. In cases of raised IOP, the eyeball is felt hard, i.e. stony hard and in cases of decreased IOP, the eyeball is felt soft, i.e. water bag.

Indentation Tonometry

Indentation tonometry is done by Schiötz tonometer.

Principle

The tonometry works on the principle of indentation. A fluid filled sphere when indented by a plunger, the plunger will indent the sphere till the pressure of the plunger equals the pressure inside the sphere.

Parts of Schiötz Tonometer

- Footplate
- Plunger
- Indicator needle
- Scale
- Holder
- Weight (Fig. 5.1).

Technique of Schiötz Indentation Tonometry

The technique is done under topical anesthesia with 4% lignocaine eyedrops with patient lying in supine position. The footplate of the Schiötz tonometer is placed gently over the cornea and the deflection of the indicator on the scale is noted. Procedure is started with the fixed 5.5 g weight, if the deflection is less than 3 on the scale, 7.5 g, 10 g, 15 g weights one after the other are used and the average of the three readings is taken as mean IOP. IOP in mm Hg is derived by comparing the scale reading and plunger weight using Friedenwald nomogram, a conversion table (Fig. 5.2).

Disadvantages: Indentation is influenced by scleral rigidity; hence it is not an accurate method.

Advantages: As it is cheaper and easy to use, it continues to be in use in spite of the drawbacks.

Applanation Tonometry

Goldmann Applanation Tonometer

Principle: This is based on Imbert-Fick law. It states that the pressure inside the sphere (P) is equal to the force necessary to flatten the surface (F) divided by the area of flattening (A), i.e. P = F/A.

Structure: It consists of a double prism mounted on a slit lamp.

Technique: It is done under topical anesthesia with 4% lignocaine eyedrops. It requires the tear film to be stained with fluorescein and it is done using slit lamp. Patient is seated in front of the slit lamp and asked to look straight ahead with both eyes kept wide open. Biprism are illuminated from slit lamp with light intensity kept to maximum with cobalt blue filter. Slit lamp is moved forward till the biprism touch the cornea in the center. When the prisms touch the cornea, two semicircles are seen through the eyepiece of slit lamp and the applanation force

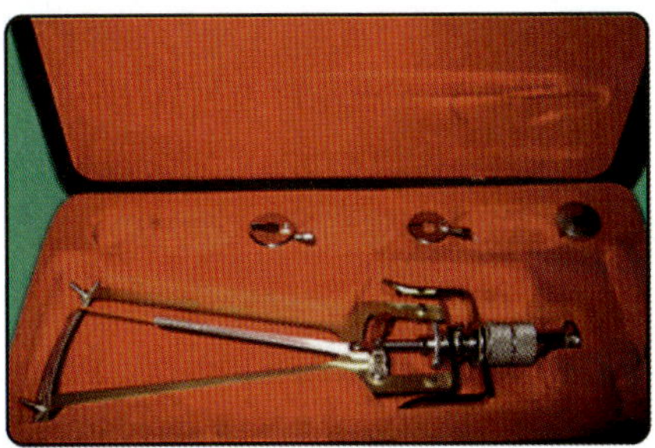

Fig. 5.1: Schiötz tonometer

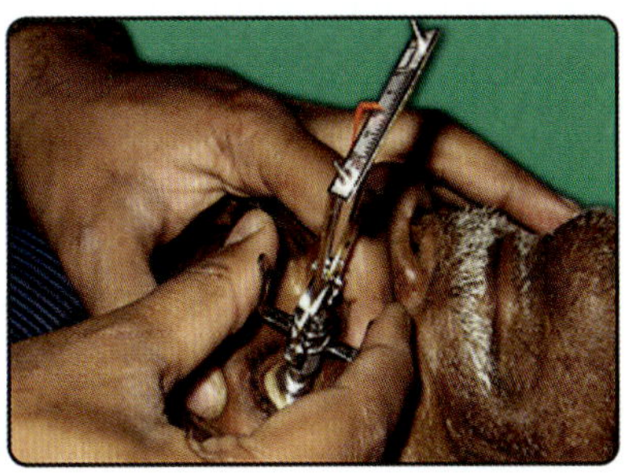

Fig. 5.2: Schiötz tonometry

is adjusted till the inner edges of the semicircles touch (Fig. 5.3). The IOP is derived by multiplying the reading on the dial by 10.

Advantages: It is most accurate method considered as gold standard for measurement of IOP because it is not affected by scleral rigidity.

Other applanation tonometer: Perkins hand-held applanation tonometer (Fig. 5.4), air-puff tonometer, Tono-Pen, non-contact tonometer.

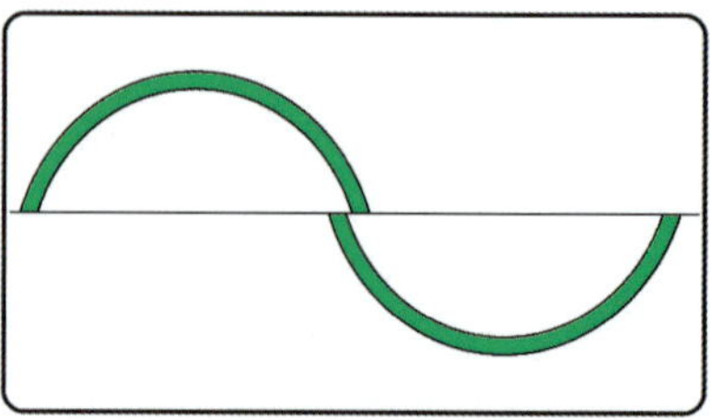

Fig. 5.3: End point of applanation tonometry—inner edges of semicircles touching each other

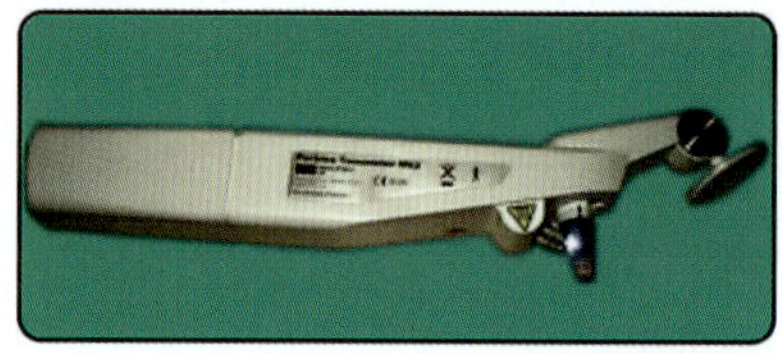

Fig. 5.4: Perkins hand-held applanation tonometer

SLIT-LAMP EXAMINATION

Slit lamp is the most important of all the ophthalmological instruments as the complete ophthalmological examination can be done with this instrument by combining it with other accessories.

Parts: Slit lamp consists of illumination system, engineering support and observation system.

Optics: Slit lamp works on the principle of compound microscope. Slit lamp consists of +22 D objective lens, +10 to +16 D eyepiece. Magnification produced by the equipment is in the range of 10–16 times (newer slit lamps with zoom magnification provide magnification in the range of 7–35 times).

Slit lamp provides both illumination and magnification, which is required for ophthalmological examination.

Filters: Slit lamp consists of:

- Blue filter to look for fluorescence after staining with fluorescein dye
- Green filter to examine the nerve fiber layer of retina (Figs 5.5 to 5.8).

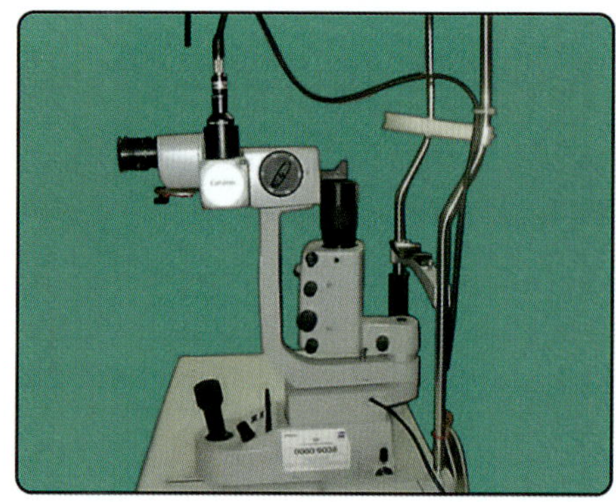

Fig. 5.5: Slit lamp

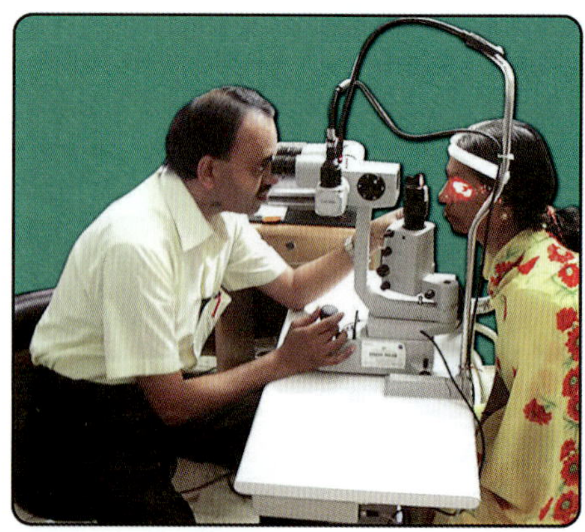

Fig. 5.6: Slit-lamp examination

Uses

- Anterior segment is examined by slit lamp by diffuse illumination, direct illumination, indirect illumination and retroillumination

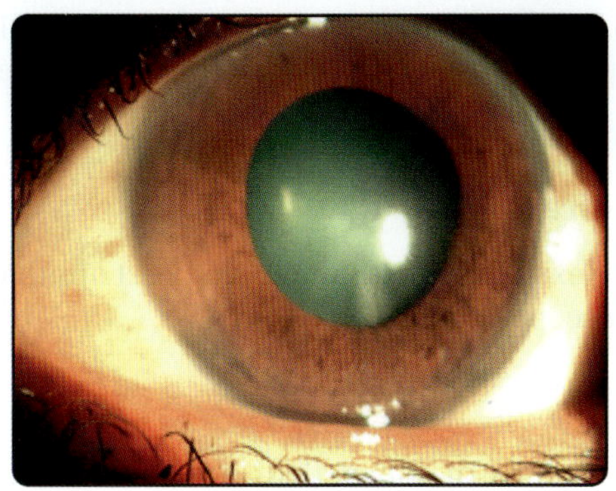

Fig. 5.7: Diffuse illumination

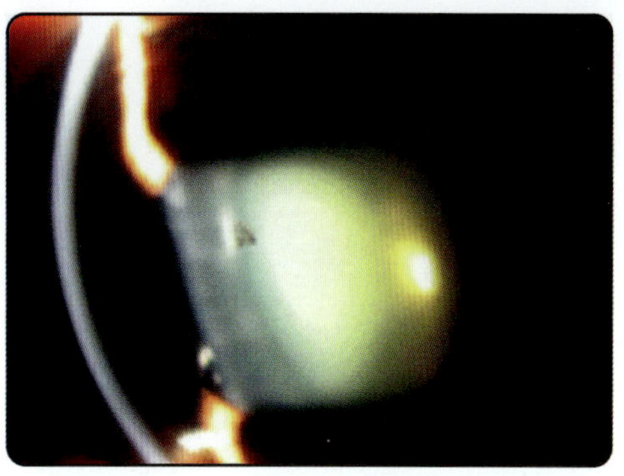

Fig. 5.8: Optical section (slit view)

- Angle of the anterior chamber is examined by using Gonio lens with slit lamp
- Thickness of cornea is measured by using pachymeter with slit lamp
- The IOP is measured by using Goldmann applanation tonometer with slit lamp
- Retina is examined by slit lamp with lenses such as +78 D, +90 D and –58.6 D lens.

OPHTHALMOSCOPY

Examination of the eye by ophthalmoscope is called ophthalmoscopy (Table 5.1). Ophthalmoscopy is done for:

- Examination of vitreous and retina (fundus)
- To detect opacities in ocular media.

Direct Ophthalmoscopy

The examination is done by direct ophthalmoscope (Fig. 5.9).

Technique

1. For ophthalmoscopy (all types) darkroom/semi-darkroom is preferred as pupil dilates in dim light and the examination is easier.
2. Patient is seated and asked to see straight ahead.
3. Examiner stands on the side of the eye to be examined and uses the same side eye as that of patient, i.e. to examine right eye

Table 5.1: Differences between direct and indirect ophthalmoscopy

Features	Direct ophthalmoscopy	Indirect ophthalmoscopy
Procedure	Uniocular	Binocular
Dilatation of pupils	Not required/Optional	Required
Patient posture	Patient sitting	Patient supine
Examiner	Standing in front	Standing at the head end
Examination distance	As close to patient as possible	At arm's length
Magnification	15 time	3–5 time
Image	Virtual and erect	Real and inverted
Condensing lens	Not required	Required
Area of field seen	Central fundus (up to equator)	Complete fundus (up to ora serrata)
Uses	Only diagnostic purpose	Diagnostic and therapeutic (for doing lasers)

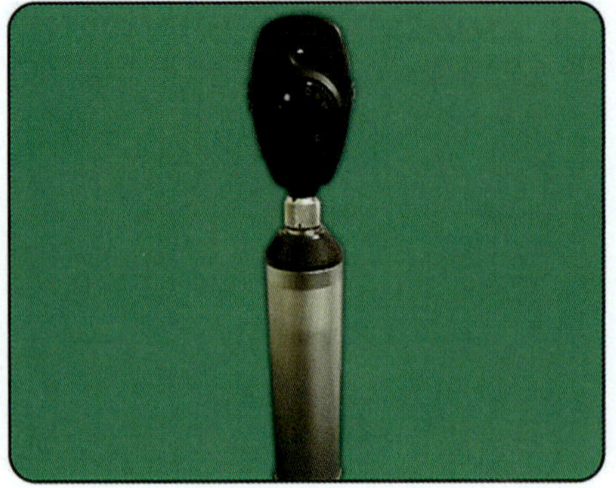

Fig. 5.9: Direct ophthalmoscope

examiner stands on right side and uses his/her right eye.

4. Light from ophthalmoscope is directed into patient's pupil, after seeing red reflex, examiner moves as close as possible to patient's eye (anterior focal length of eye 15 mm) and examines optic disk and macula.
5. Direct ophthalmoscope provides about 15 times magnification and the image formed is virtual and erect (Figs 5.10A to C).

Indirect Ophthalmoscopy

The examination is done by indirect ophthalmoscope (Fig. 5.11).

Technique

1. Pupils of the patient are dilated with tropicamide.
2. Patient is asked to lie in supine position.
3. Indirect ophthalmoscope is worn on the head, light is directed into patient's eye from a distance of an arm length and a +20 D lens is interposed in the path of the light, so that when light is focused on the retina of patient, an image is formed between the patient and the examiner.

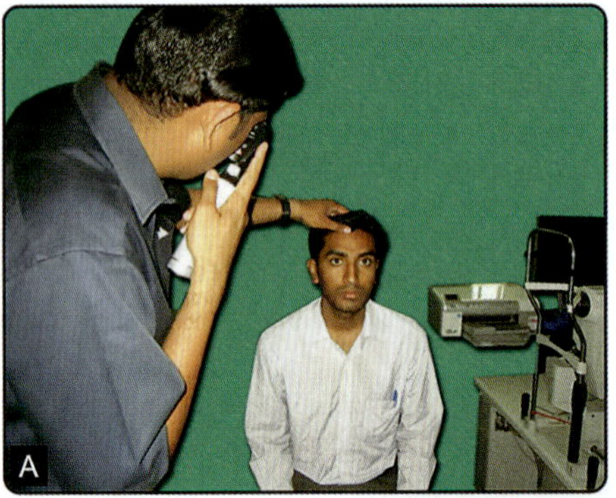

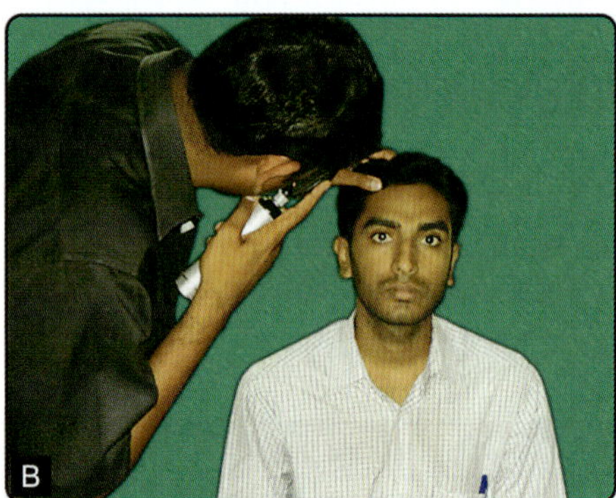

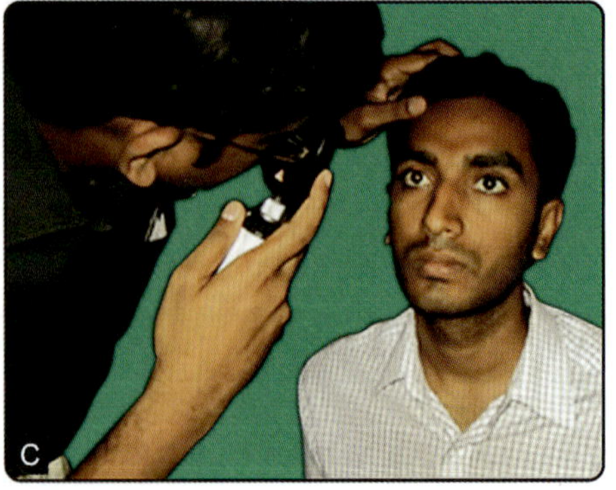

Figs 5.10A to C: Procedure of direct ophthalmoscopy

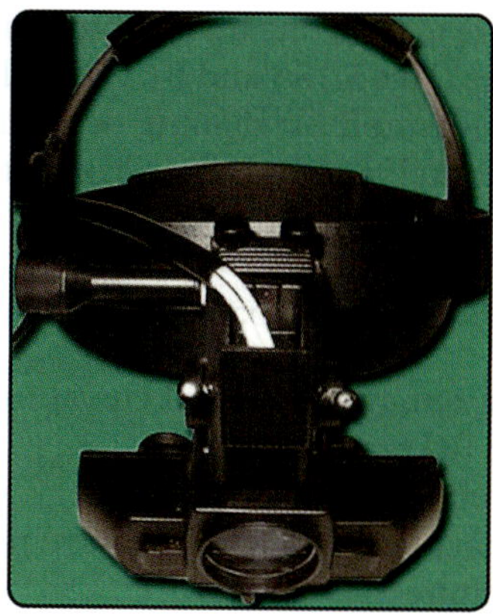

Fig. 5.11: Indirect ophthalmoscope

4. It provides three times magnification and the image formed is real and inverted.
5. Image magnification is the ratio of power of the eye to power of the condensing lens (60/20 = 3) (Figs 5.12A and B).

Distant Direct Ophthalmoscopy

Distant direct ophthalmoscopy is performed to detect opacities in the media. It is performed by direct ophthalmoscope or by a plain mirror.

Technique

1. Light is directed into patient's eye from a distance of 25 cm and the features of red glow are studied.
2. Any opacity in the media appears as black shadow.
3. Any opacity in the pupillary plane will not move with movement of light, the opacity in front of pupillary plane moves in the same direction and the opacity behind the pupillary plane moves in opposite direction.

KERATOMETRY

Keratometry (Figs 5.13A and B) is the measurement of curvature of cornea by an instrument called keratometer.

Keratometry is based on the principle that the anterior surface of cornea acts as convex mirror. So the size of the image produced varies with its curvature, hence from the size of the image corneal curvature can be estimated. Javal-Schiötz keratometer and Bausch and Lomb keratometer are used in clinical practice.

In Bausch and Lomb (B and L) keratometer mires (Fig. 5.14) consists of a circle with two plus signs in horizontal meridian and two minus signs in vertical meridian. This is projected on to the patient's cornea on which the reflected image is formed (first Purkinje image). Because of presence of doubling prisms in the objective, the examiner sees three images,

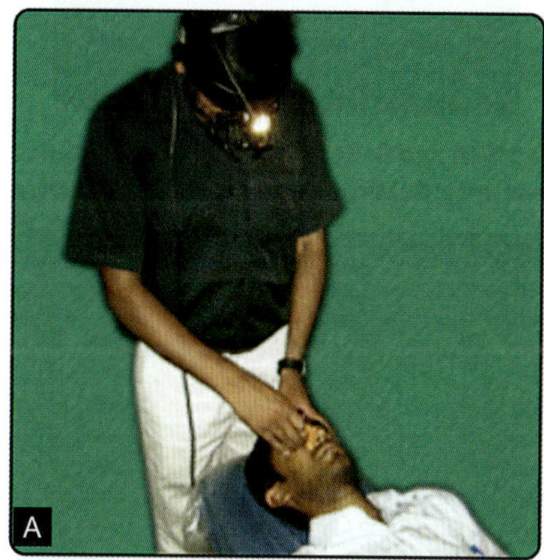

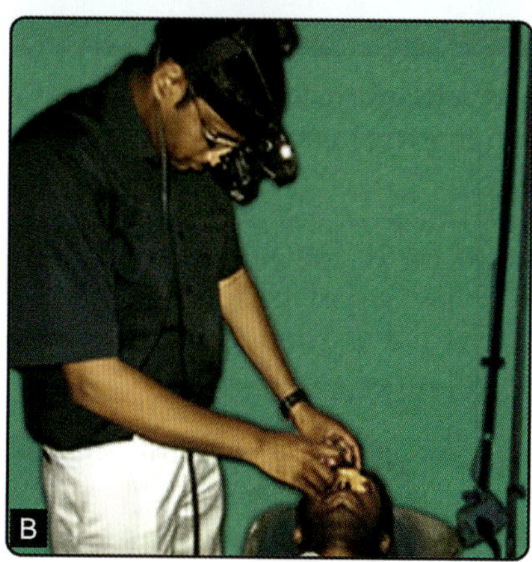

Figs 5.12A and B: Procedure of indirect ophthalmoscopy

Uses

Assessment of posterior segment in the presence of opaque media and for evaluating vitreoretinal and orbital mass lesions.

C-scan (Coronal Scan)

C-scan is similar to B-scan differing from B-scan by the fact that here echoes are recorded from coronal plane, thus C-scan displays soft tissues in the coronal plane of the orbit.

ULTRASOUND BIOMICROSCOPY

In ultrasound biomicroscopy (UBM) higher frequencies 50–100 MHz providing higher resolution (roughly it equals to that provided by microscope, i.e. about 50 microns, hence called ultrasound biomicroscopy). But the penetration of UBM is only up to 5 mm, hence only structures of the anterior segment can be examined.

Uses

Evaluation of mass lesions of anterior segment. Examination of anterior chamber depth, angle of anterior chamber.

VITAL STAINS

- Fluorescein
- Rose Bengal
- Lissamine Green.

Fluorescein stains epithelial defects. It is appreciated better under blue filter of the slit lamp as it appears brilliant green due to fluorescence.

Rose Bengal and Lissamine Green stain devitalized cells.

Fluorescein is a large molecule, which will not cross tight junctions of intact epithelium and hence it stains epithelial defects.

Rose Bengal and Lissamine Green being smaller than fluorescein, can penetrate intact epithelium and stain devitalized epithelial cells.

Rose Bengal causes more ocular irritation than Lissamine Green, hence, Lissamine Green can be used in its place when patient is not able to tolerate Rose Bengal.

Uses of Vital Stains

- Vital staining is used for evaluation of a patient with dry eye
- Tear film break up time (T-BUT) using fluorescein
- Rose Bengal staining.

Tear Film Break Up Time

Tears are stained with fluorescein dye and the time interval between a complete blink to the appearance of first dry spot in the tear film is T-BUT:

- Normal: 15–30 seconds
- Abnormal: Less than 5 seconds.

Rose Bengal Staining

Eye is stained with Rose Bengal. Ocular surface is divided into three zones:

1. Cornea.
2. Nasal bulbar conjunctiva.
3. Temporal bulbar conjunctiva.

Each zone is evaluated for the density of stain and given score of:

- 0: None
- 1: Mild staining
- 2: Moderate staining
- 3: Severe staining.

A total score of more than 3.5 is taken as positive for dry eye.

Fluorescein

Fluorescein is an orange water soluble dye (Figs 5.25A and B). It exhibits the property of fluorescence.

Fluorescence is the property of molecules to emit light energy of a longer wavelength when stimulated by a light of shorter wavelength.

Fluorescein responds to light energy between 465 and 490 nm (blue light) and fluorescence at a wave length of 520–530 nm (green light). Hence, if blue light is directed at fluorescein it emits green light. Because of this property of fluorescence, fluorescein is better appreciated under blue filter of slit lamp (Figs 5.26 to 5.28).

Uses of Fluorescein

- For identification of corneal epithelial defects by fluorescein staining
- For examination of corneal ulcer to study morphology of the ulcer
- In dry eye evaluation for performing T-BUT
- In evaluation of patient with watering eye for fluorescein dye disappearance test and Jones tests
- Seidel's test to identify leak from anterior chamber (in traumatic corneal tear or postoperative shallow anterior chamber after cataract surgery)
- Fundus fluorescein angiography to study retinal and choroidal circulation.

Other Dyes Used in Ophthalmology

1. Indocyanine green used for indocyanine green angiography.
2. Trypan blue used to stain anterior capsule in cataract surgery for performing capsulorhexis.

Seidel's Test

Seidel's test is done under slit lamp. The suspected site of wound leak is stained with fluorescein and the fluorescein pattern is observed for dilution, which indicates leak of aqueous (aqueous if leaking mixes with fluorescein thereby diluting fluorescein) from anterior chamber.

SPECULAR MICROSCOPY

Specular microscope is a reflected microscope, which employs the technique of specular reflection, i.e. where angle of incidence is equal to angle of reflection to study corneal endothelium (Fig. 5.29).

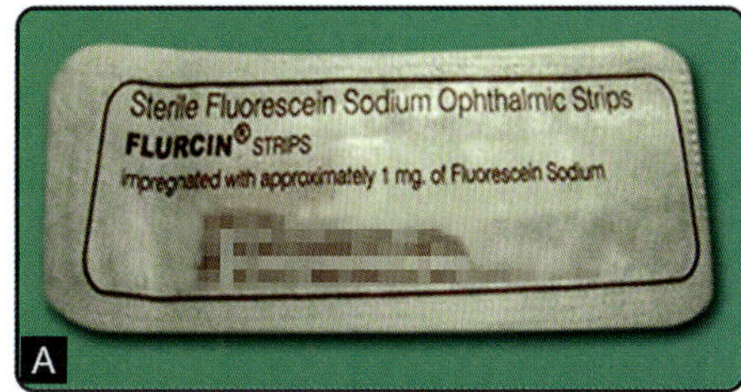

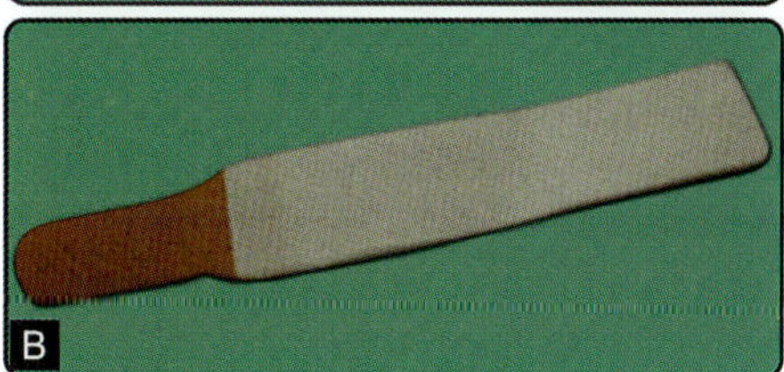

Figs 5.25A and B: Fluorescein strip

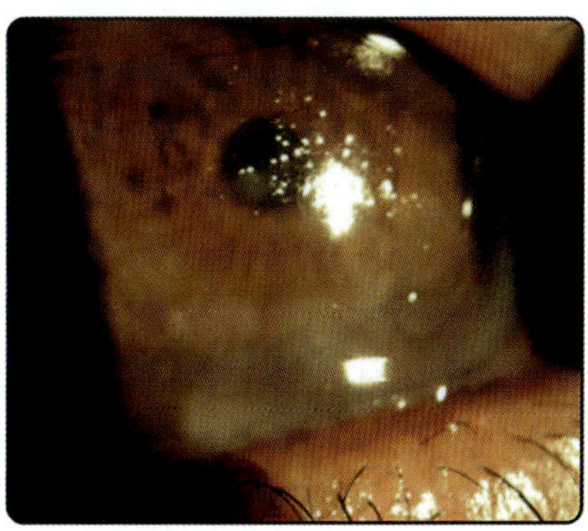

Fig. 5.26: Under diffuse light

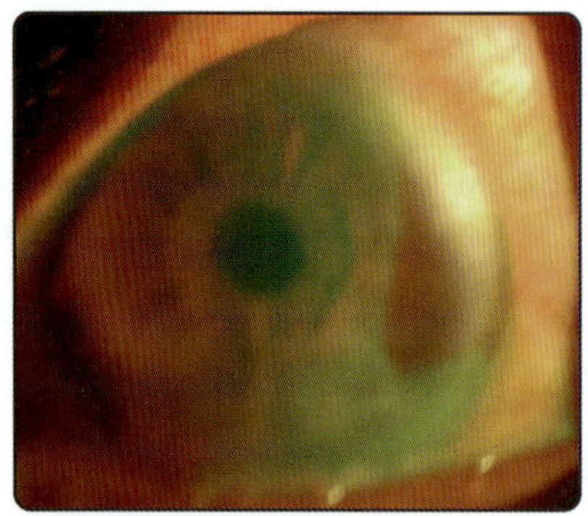

Fig. 5.27: Under diffuse light after staining with fluorescein

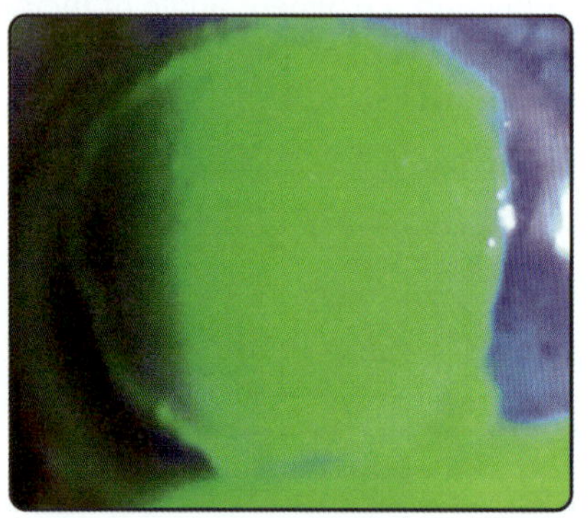

Fig. 5.28: Under blue light after staining with fluorescein

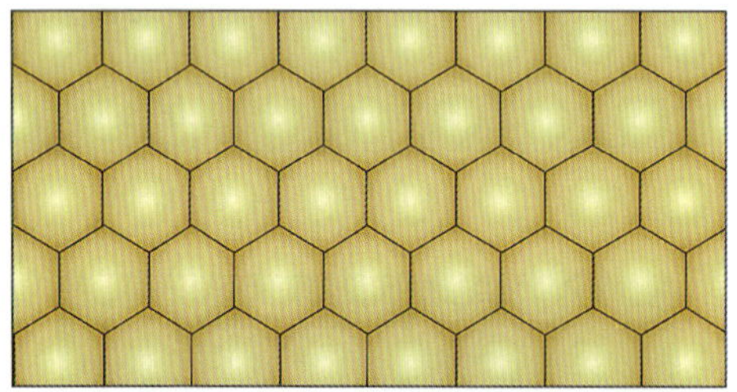

Fig. 5.29: Normal hexagonal corneal endothelium as seen on specular microscopy

Uses

- Evaluation of donor corneal endothelium in eye bank
- Early diagnosis of endothelial dystrophies such as Fuchs endothelial dystrophy.

FUNDUS FLUORESCEIN ANGIOGRAPHY

Fundus fluorescein angiography is photographic surveillance (Figs 5.30 and 5.31) of the passage of fluorescein through the retinal and choroidal circulations after fluorescein is injected into antecubital vein.

Fluorescein (5 mL of 10% or 10 mL of 5%) is injected into antecubital vein and photos are taken with a fundus camera after 5 seconds every second for next 20 seconds and every 5 seconds for next 1 minute.

Normally, fluorescein does not cross the blood-retinal barrier and it rapidly diffuses through the choriocapillaris. The photographs are studied for hyperfluorescence and hypofluorescence.

Hypofluorescence is seen in blockage of arteries, veins, capillaries like artery occlusion and filling defects of the veins.

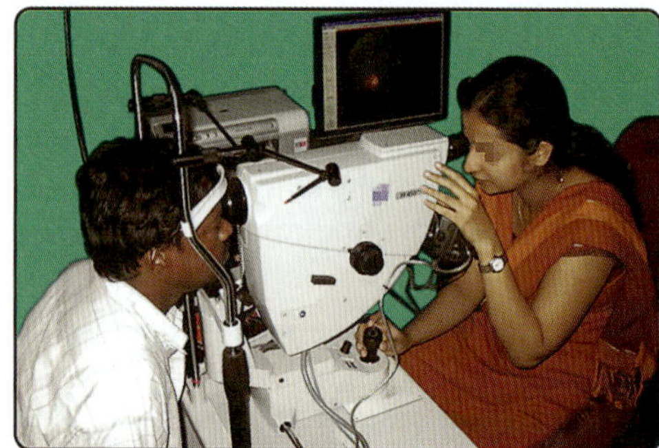

Fig. 5.30: Fundus camera and fundus photography

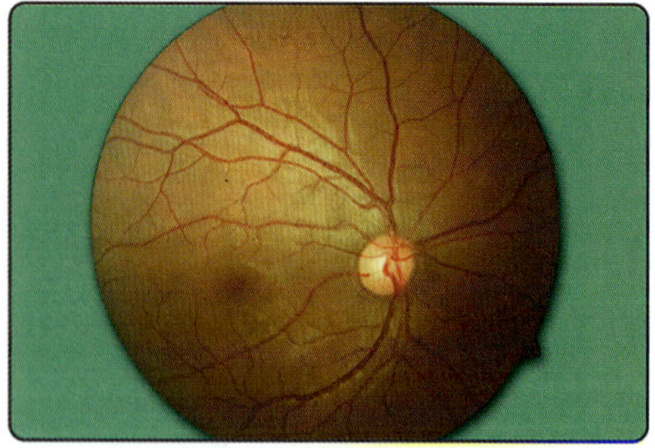

Fig. 5.31: Fundus photograph

Hyperfluorescence is seen because of leakage of dye as in diabetic retinopathy, central serous retinopathy.

Uses

In retinal disorders such as:
- Diabetic retinopathy
- Central serous retinopathy (inkblot pattern and smokestack pattern)
- Cystoid macular edema (flower petal appearance)
- Vein/Artery occlusions of retina
- Eales disease, i.e. age-related macular degeneration (ARMD).

INDOCYANINE GREEN ANGIOGRAPHY

Indocyanine dye remains in the choriocapillaris in contrast to fluorescein, which extravasates from choriocapillaris, hence it allows imaging of choroid.

Uses

For diagnosis of choroidal disorders such as choroidal neovascularization, polypoidal choroidal vasculopathy.

OPTICAL COHERENCE TOMOGRAPHY

Optical coherence tomography (OCT) permits high resolution cross-sectional imaging of retina using coherence light.

Uses

1. For examination of macular diseases such as macular hole, macular edema, epiretinal membrane, central serous retinopathy, age-related macular degeneration, vitreomacular traction syndrome.
2. For measurement of nerve fiber layer thickness in patients with glaucoma for assessment of glaucoma.

HEIDELBERG RETINAL TOMOGRAPHY

Heidelberg retinal tomography is a confocal scanning laser ophthalmoscopy for imaging of optic nerve head and nerve fiber layer.

Uses

In patients with glaucoma/glaucoma suspects for early detection of glaucomatous damage and progression.

CORNEAL TOPOGRAPHY

Analysis of corneal shape (curvature) is done by corneal topography.

Uses

For diagnosis and monitoring the progression of keratoconus. It is a mandatory test before refractive surgeries

ELECTROPHYSIOLOGICAL TESTS

Electrophysiological tests are done for objective evaluation of the retinal functions.

Electroretinography

Electroretinography (ERG) is the record of electric potential changes in the retina induced by a flash of light. It depicts the response of the outer layer of the retina.

Uses

In detecting functional abnormalities of the outer retina before ophthalmoscopic signs appear. ERG is useful in diagnosis of 'diseases, which involve outer retina such as retinitis pigmentosa and other chorioretinal degenerations.

It is done as retinal function test when fundus examination is not possible because of opacities in the media.

Electrooculography

Electrooculography measures the resting potential between cornea and back of the eye. It has similar uses as to that of ERG.

Visually Evoked Potential

Visually evoked potential measures the changes in the resting potential induced by a flash of light at the occipital lobe.

Uses

It is used to objectively assess the functional state of the visual system beyond the retinal ganglion cells.

RETINAL FUNCTION TESTS

Described in Chapter 4 under 'Cataract Case Presentation'.

MACULAR FUNCTION TESTS

Described in Chapter 4 under 'Cataract Case Presentation' (Fig. 5.32).

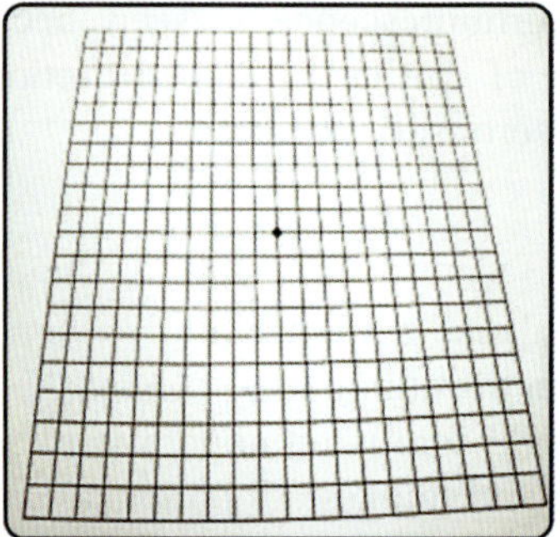

Fig. 5.32: Amsler's grid consists of 400 small squares with a central fixation point. Patient is asked to close one eye and to see at Amsler's chart with the other eye, holding the chart at normal reading distance. Patient is asked to look for any distortion in the grid while looking at the central fixing dot. Distortion indicates macular pathology. The test is repeated in the other eye.

TESTS FOR EVALUATION OF A CASE OF WATERING EYE

Described in Chapter 4 under 'Adult Dacryocystitis'.

TESTS FOR EVALUATION OF A CASE OF SQUINT

Hirschberg Corneal Reflex Test (Fig. 5.33)

- Hirschberg conrneal reflex test is a rough method for estimation of amount of squint
- Patient is asked to fixate at a point light held at a distance of 33 cm, normally corneal light reflex (Purkinje first image) is at the center of the pupil

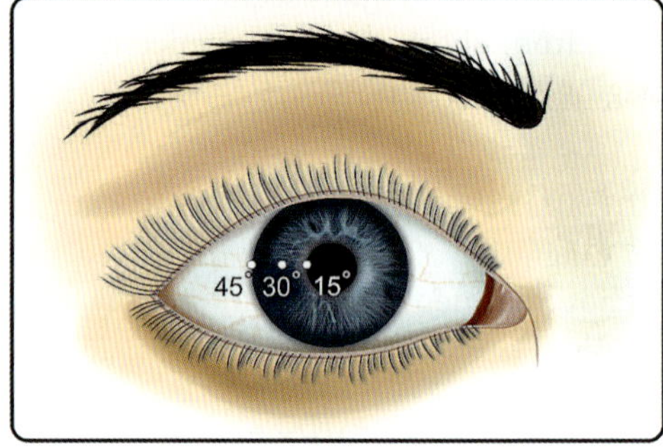

Fig. 5.33: Hirschberg corneal reflex test

- Each millimeter of shift of corneal light reflex from center of pupil is equal to 7.5° or 15 prism diopters of squint
- In esotropia the light reflex falls on the temporal side as the eyeball is deviated nasally and reverse in case of exotropia
- Light reflex at pupillary margin = 2 mm shift of corneal reflex = 15°
- Light reflex in between pupillary margin and limbus = 4 mm shift = 30°
- Light reflex at limbus = 6 mm shift of corneal reflex = 45°.

Cover Test

Cover test is done to detect the presence of manifest squint and to differentiate it from pseudosquint (Fig. 5.34):

1. It is performed both for near and distance (patient fixing at a target of 33 cm for near and 6 meters for distance).
2. Normal eye (undeviated eye) is covered and the movement of deviated eye is noted.
3. No movement of the uncovered eye pseudosquint, i.e. no squint—orthophoria.
4. Inward movement of the uncovered eye (outward deviated eye)—exotropia (Figs 5.35A to C).
5. Outward movement of the uncovered eye (inward deviated eye)—esotropia (Figs 5.36A to C).
6. Downward movement of the uncovered eye (upward deviated eye)—hypertropia.
7. Upward movement of the uncovered eye (downward deviated eye)—hypotropia.

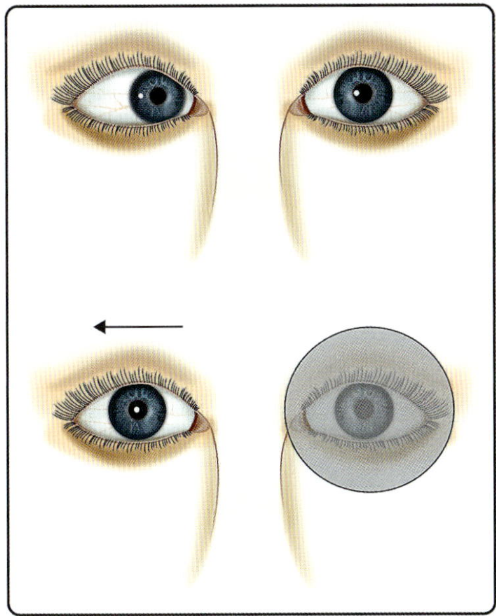

Fig. 5.34: Cover test (*Note:* Outward movement of uncovered eye, on covering normal eye).

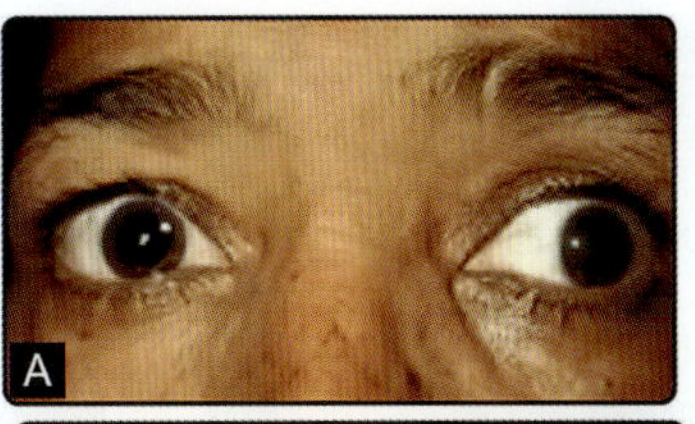

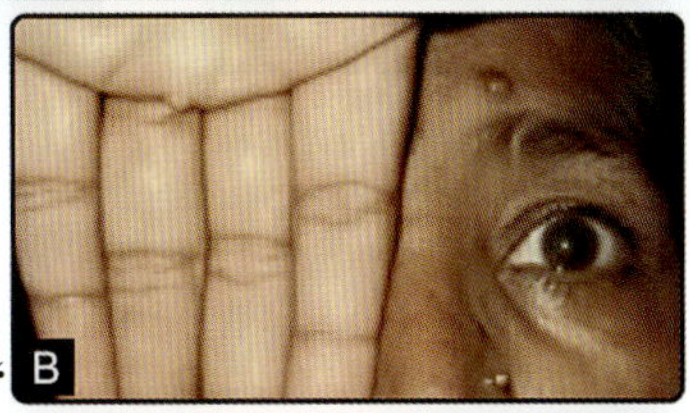

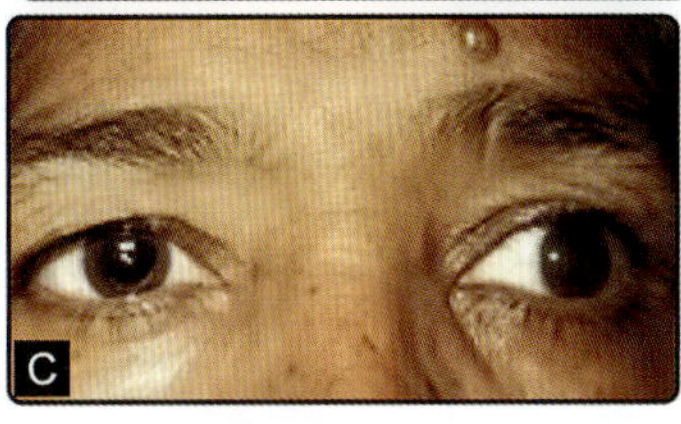

Figs 5.35A to C: Cover test for exotropia. **A.** Left eye—exotropia (deviated outwards); **B.** On covering right eye, left eye takes fixation; **C.** On uncovering right eye, left eye deviates again.

Cover-uncover Test (Fig. 5.37)

- Cover-uncover test is done to detect latent squint
- It is performed both for near and distance
- Here the eye is covered for less than 2 seconds and the cover is removed and the refixation movement of eye under cover is observed
- No movement of the eye under cover—orthophoria
- Inward refixation movement of the eye under cover—exophorpia
- Outward refixation movement of the eye under cover—esophoria.

Alternate Cover Test

1. Alternate cover test is done to detect total squint, i.e. manifest squint and latent squint.

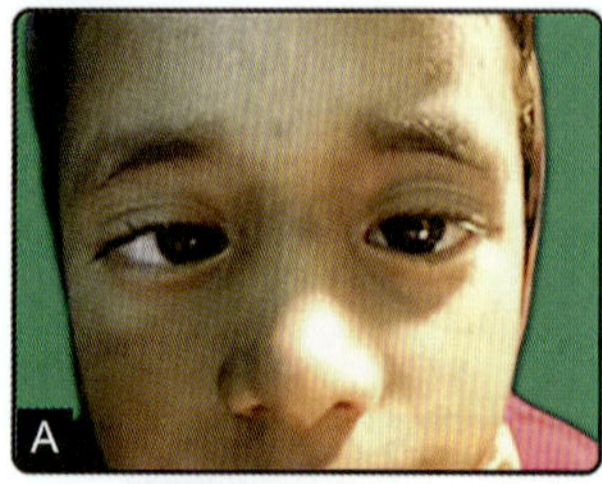

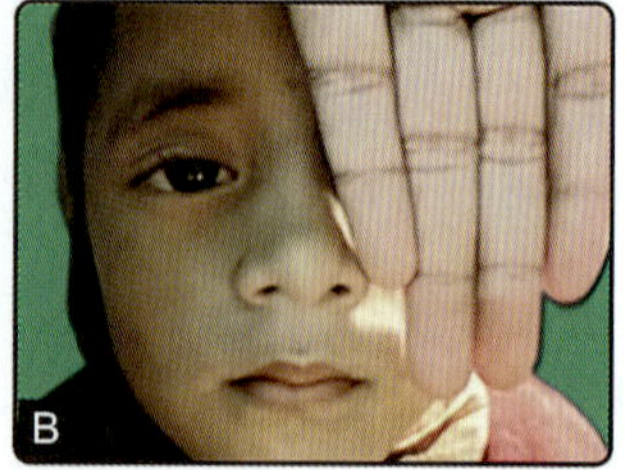

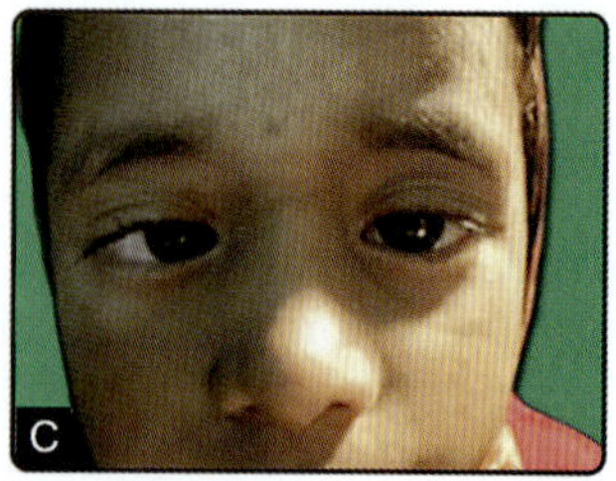

Figs 5.36A to C: Cover test for esotropia. **A.** Right eye—esotropia (deviated inwards); **B.** On covering left eye, right eye takes fixation; **C.** On uncovering left eye, right eye deviates again.

2. It is performed both for near and distance.
3. Here eye is covered for more than 2 seconds and the cover is immediately shifted to other eye while observing the movement of the covered eye, this is repeated several times. The principle is to break fusion and to make the latent squint to manifest, hence it measures the total amount of squint or deviation.

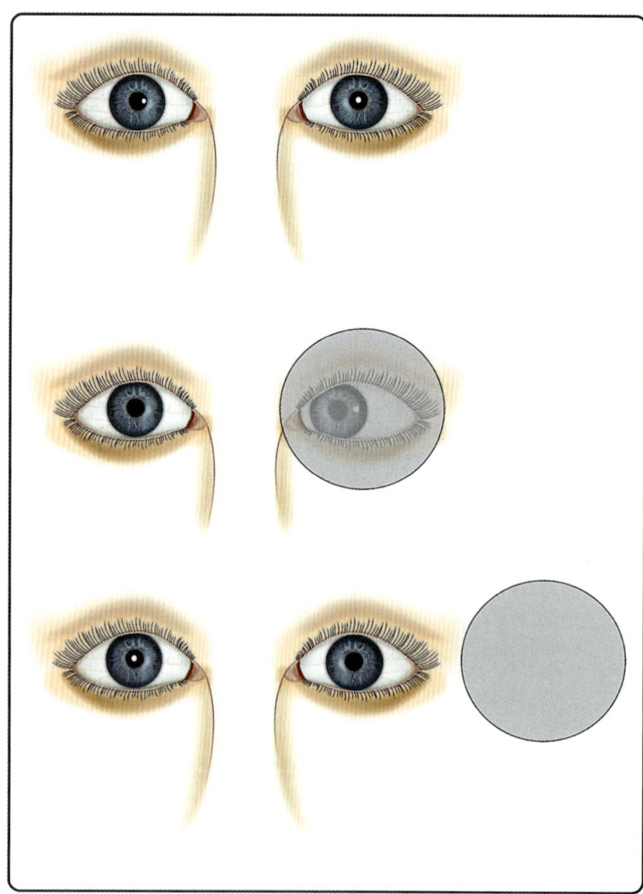

Fig. 5.37: Cover-uncover test (*Note:* Outward refixation movement of eye under cover—esophoria).

In cover test the movement of uncovered eye is observed. It is done to detect tropia or manifest squint. In cover-uncover test refixation movement of covered eye is observed. It is done to detect phoria or latent squint.

In alternate cover test refixation movement of the covered eye is observed. It is done to detect total squint (phoria+tropia).

Prism Bar Cover Test

Prisms of increasing strengths are placed in front of one eye with apex of the prism directed towards the deviation. Cover test and cover-uncover test are done till there is no refixation movement of the eye under cover. The strength of the prism at this point gives the amount of deviation (Fig. 5.38).

Krimsky Corneal Reflex Test

Prisms of increasing strengths are placed infront of one eye with apex of the prism directed towards the deviation, till the Hirschberg corneal reflex test is centered. The strength of the prism at this point gives the amount of deviation.

Maddox Wing Test

Maddox wing works by presenting dissimilar images to two eyes thereby breaking fusion and thus measures phoria (latent squint).

It is done from a distance of 33 cm hence it measures phoria for near.

The instrument is constructed in such a way that the right eye sees only white vertical arrow and a red horizontal arrow, the left eye sees only horizontal and vertical rows of numbers. The patient is asked to tell the number on the horizontal line, which the vertical white arrow is pointing to measure the horizontal deviation.

Vertical deviation is measured by asking the patient to say the number on the vertical line pointed by red arrow. The amount of cyclophoria is calculated by asking the patient to align the arrow with horizontal line of numbers.

Maddox Rod Test

Maddox rod consists of a series of parallel high power plus cylinders that convert point light as a red straight line at right angle to the axis of the rod.

It also works by presenting dissimilar images to two eyes there by breaking fusion and thus measures phoria (latent squint).

It is done from a distance of 6 m, hence it measures phoria for distance.

Maddox rod is placed in front of the right eye and asked to see point source of light. This dissociates the two eyes as he/she will be seeing red line in right eye and a point source of light in left eye. The number on Maddox tangent scale where the red line falls gives the amount of heterophoria in degrees (Fig. 5.39).

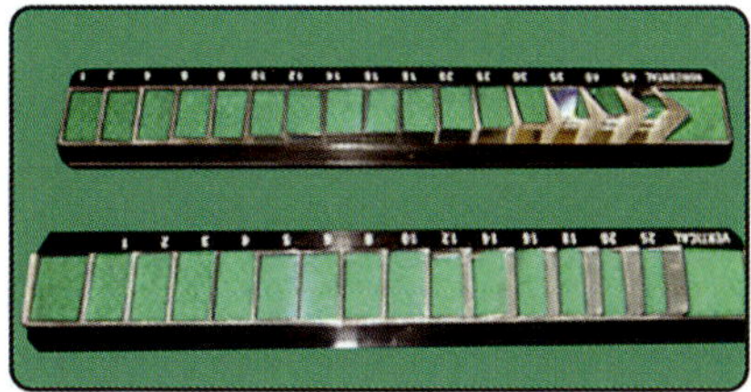

Fig. 5.38: Prism bars

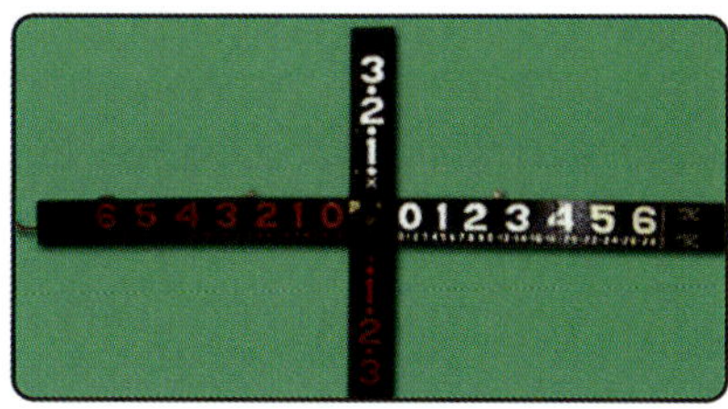

Fig. 5.39: Maddox tangent scale

TESTS FOR EVALUATION OF TEAR FILM

Schirmer's Test (Fig. 5.40)

Schirmer's Test I

1. Schirmer's test I measures the total tear secretions.
2. It is performed with Schirmer's test strip, (a Whatman filter paper 5 by 35 mm strip), which is folded at 5 mm and kept in lower conjunctival fornix. The test strip is kept in the lower fornix for 5 minutes and the amount of wetting on the filter paper is noted.
3. Wetting up to or more than 15 mm—normal.
4. Wetting between 10 and 15 mm—borderline or mild dry eye.
5. Wetting between 5 and 10 mm—moderate dry eye.
6. Wetting less than 5 mm—severe dry eye.

Schirmer's Test II

1. Schirmer's test II is done to measure reflex secretions.

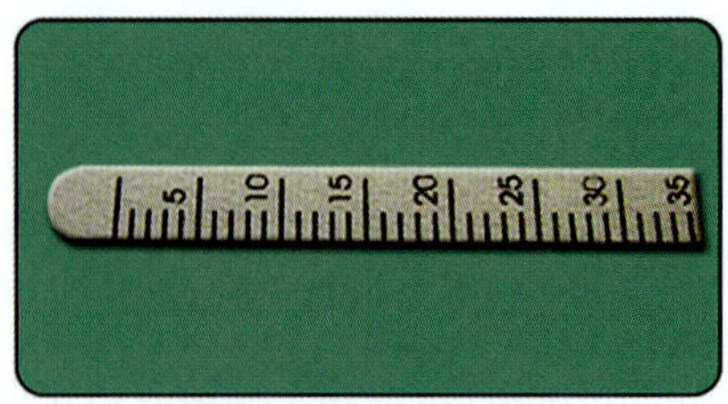

Fig. 5.40: Schirmer's test strip

2. It is performed in similar way as first test except that nasal mucosa is rubbed by a cotton bud to irritate it to measure reflex secretions.

Schirmer's Basal Secretion Test

Schirmer's basal secretion test is performed similar to test I except that conjunctival fornix is anesthetized before performing the test.

Tear film break up time: Described under 'Vital Staining'.

Vital staining: Described under 'Vital Staining'.

Chapter 6

Ophthalmic Instruments

Chapter Outline

- Lid Speculum
- Needle Holder
- Forceps
- Scissors
- Knives (Blades)
- Instruments for Incision and Curettage of Chalazion
- Instruments for Lens Removal
- Instruments for Irrigation and Aspiration of Cortical Matter During Cataract Surgery
- Instruments for Enucleation
- Instruments for Evisceration
- Instruments for Lacrimal Sac Surgery
- Hooks and Retractors
- Castroviejo Calipers
- Iris Repositor
- Thermal Ball Point Cautery
- Cystitome or Capsulotome

LID SPECULUM

Lid speculum is used to keep the lids apart during surgeries on eyeball such as pterygium excision, corneal surgeries, glaucoma surgeries and cataract surgery. Minor outpatient procedures such as corneal foreign body removal and scraping of corneal ulcer. It is called universal speculum because it can be used for both right and left eyes. It has to be inserted with open end facing medial canthus and the closed end towards the lateral canthus (Figs 6.1 to 6.3).

NEEDLE HOLDER

Needle holders are meant to grasp/hold needles during suturing.

Castroviejo-Kalt Needle Holder and Stevens Needle Holder

Castroviejo-Kalt needle holder and Stevens needle holder are larger in size and have a locking mechanism (Fig. 6.4).

These are used for holding the needle for suturing during extraocular surgeries such as lid surgeries and for passing superior rectus bridle suture.

Barraquer and Castroviejo Needle Holder

Barraquer and Castroviejo needle holder are used for holding the needle during suturing in surgeries on conjunctiva, cornea, sclera and extraocular muscles. These have a spring action for holding the needles (Fig. 6.5).

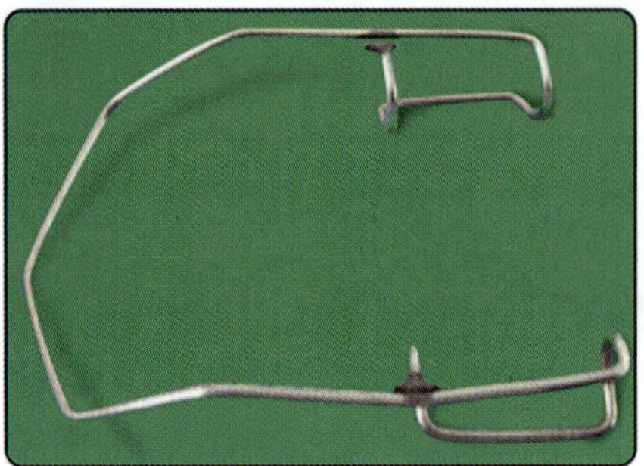

Fig. 6.1: Barraquer wire speculum

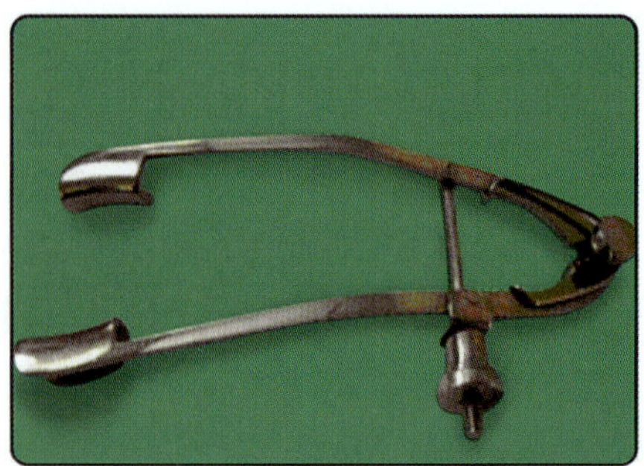

Fig. 6.2: Wire speculum with spring mechanism and solid blades

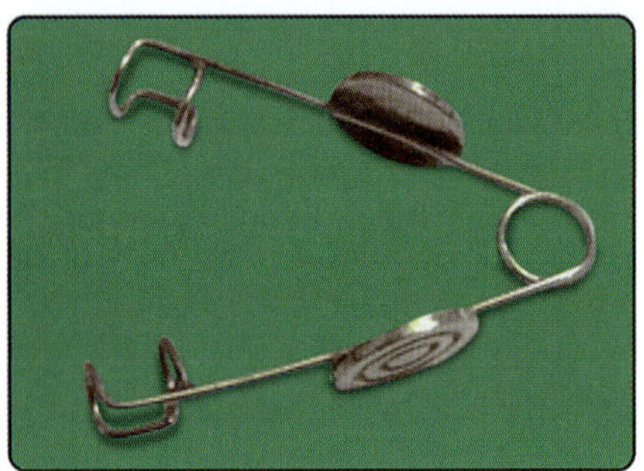

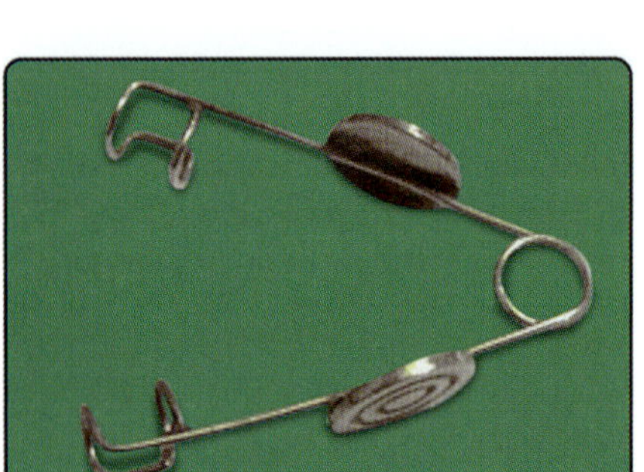

Fig. 6.3: Pediatric speculum

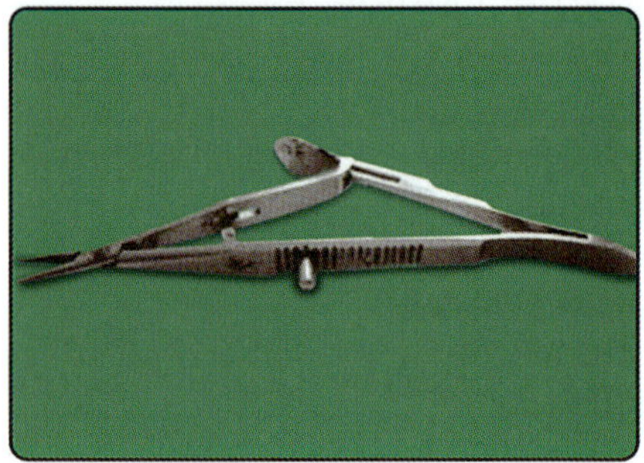

Fig. 6.4: Castroviejo-Kalt needle holder

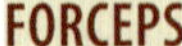

FORCEPS

Forceps are instruments designed for holding tissues and sutures.

Superior Rectus Holding Forceps

Superior rectus holding forceps is toothed forceps with a double curve near the tip resembling the alphabet 'S' (Figs 6.6A and B).

It is used to hold superior rectus muscle for passing bridle suture for fixation of globe to stabilize eyeball during intraocular surgeries such as cataract surgery, corneal surgery and glaucoma surgery.

Superior rectus along with other recti muscles originate from common tendinous ring at the apex of the orbit and get inserted into sclera at 7.7 mm from the limbus.

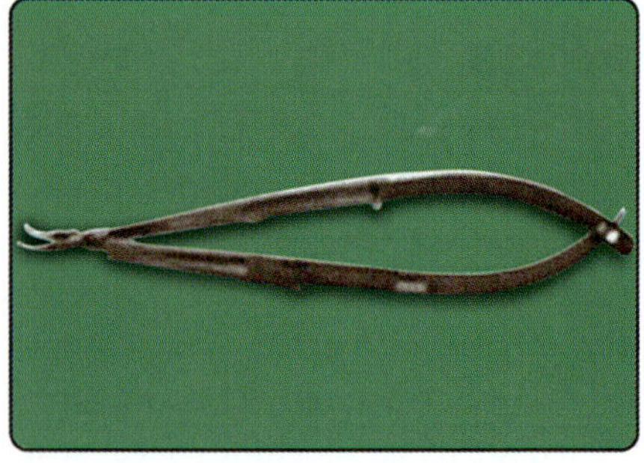

Fig. 6.5: Barraquer needle holder

The distance of insertion of rectus muscles from limbus are:

- Medial rectus: 5.5 mm
- Inferior rectus: 6.5 mm
- Lateral rectus: 6.9 mm
- Superior rectus: 7.7 mm.

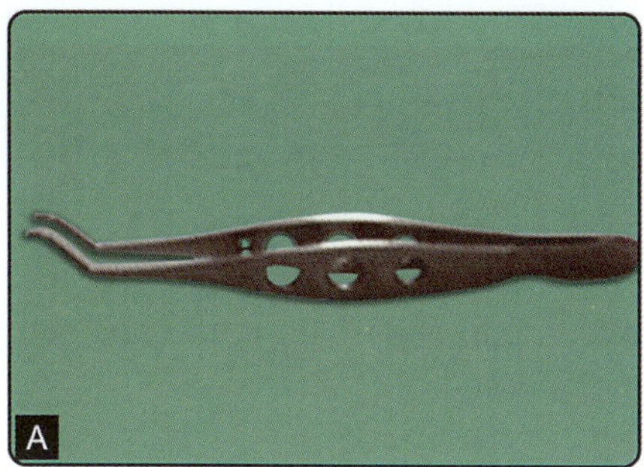

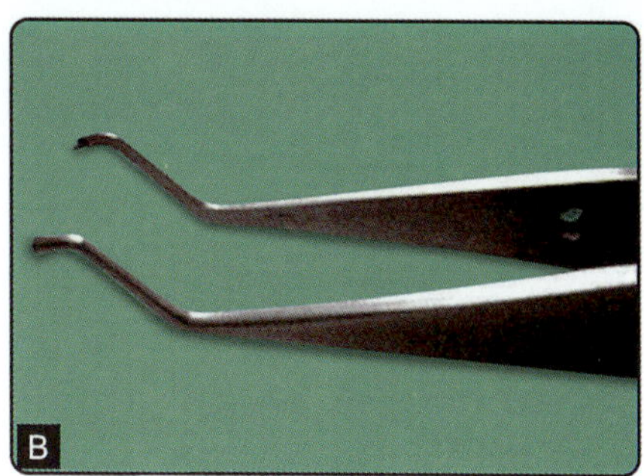

Figs 6.6A and B: Superior rectus holding forceps

Spiral of Tillaux

Spiral of Tillaux is an imaginary line joining the insertions of the four rectus muscles, which resembles a spiral pattern with insertion of medial rectus being nearest and the insertion of superior rectus being farthest away from the limbus.

Fixation Forceps

Fixation forceps (Figs 6.7A and B) have tooth at the tip and used to hold conjunctiva and episcleral tissues for fixing the globe during ocular surgeries.

Corneoscleral Forceps

Corneoscleral forceps are having fine teeth at the tip and are used to hold cornea and sclera for suturing during surgeries such as extracapsular cataract extraction (ECCE), keratoplasty and trabeculectomy.

Pierse Type Microforceps

Pierse type microforceps is a straight forceps with fine teeth at the tip (Fig. 6.8).

Lim's Forceps

Lim's forceps has a tying platform at the tip (Figs 6.9A and B).

Tying Forceps

Tying forceps are used for tying sutures (8-0 to 11-0) during surgeries such as ECCE, keratoplasty, trabeculectomy, sclerocorneal tear repair and conjunctival suturing during pterygium surgery.

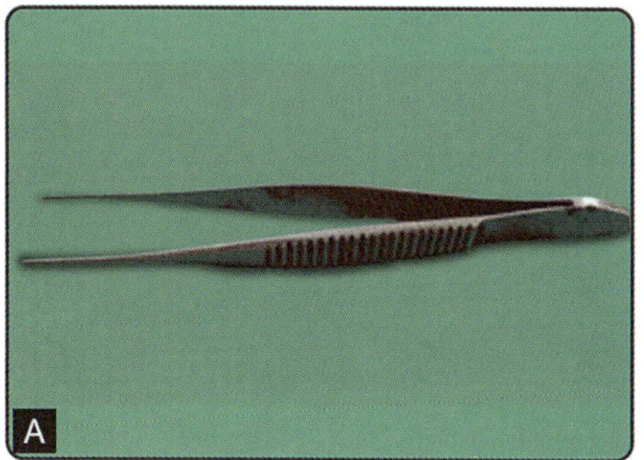

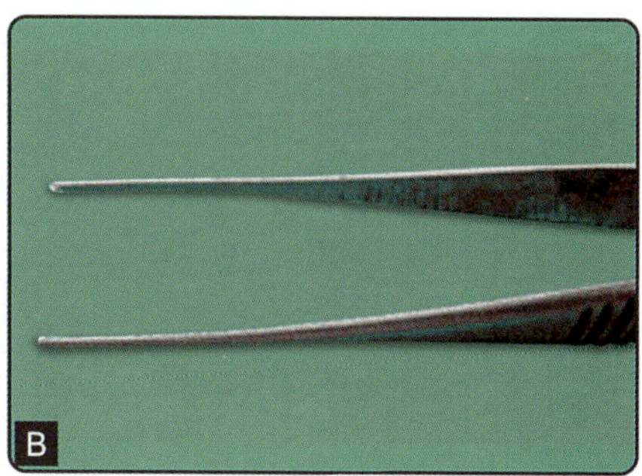

Figs 6.7A and B: Fixation forceps

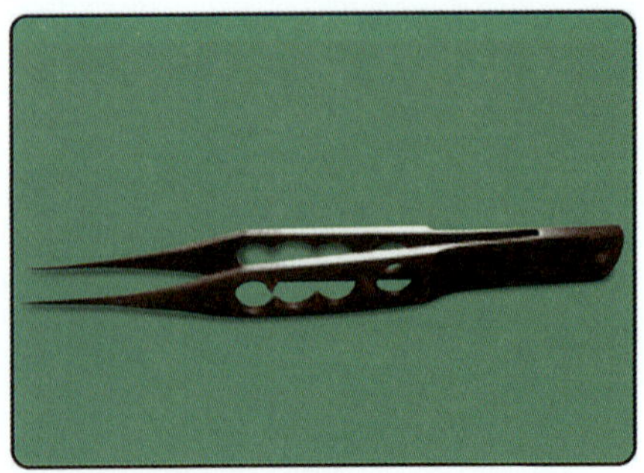

Fig. 6.8: Pierse microforceps

Kelman-McPherson Forceps (Figs 6.10A and B)

Other than for tying sutures it is also used to:
- Insert intraocular lens (IOL) (Fig. 6.11)
- To tear off the anterior capsular flap in ECCE.

McPherson Tying Forceps

McPherson typing forceps is used only for tying sutures (Figs 6.12A and B).

Jaffe Tying Forceps

Jaffe typing forceps is used for tying sutures (Figs 6.13A and B).

Iris Forceps

Iris forceps is used to hold iris for doing iridectomy during surgeries, e.g. trabeculectomy (Figs 6.14A and B).

Artery Forceps

Artery forceps is used for hemostatic purpose to catch the bleeding vessels to prevent

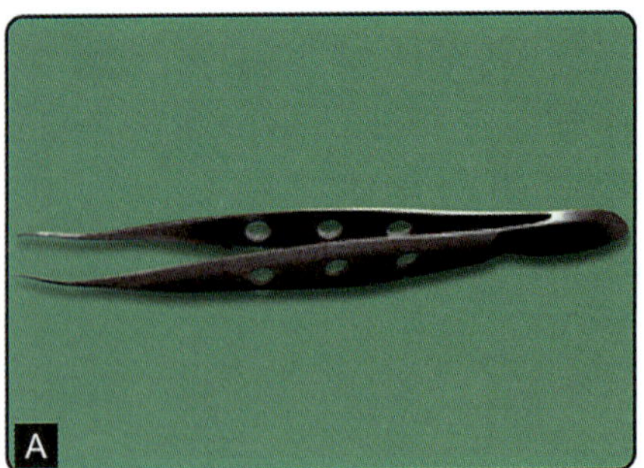

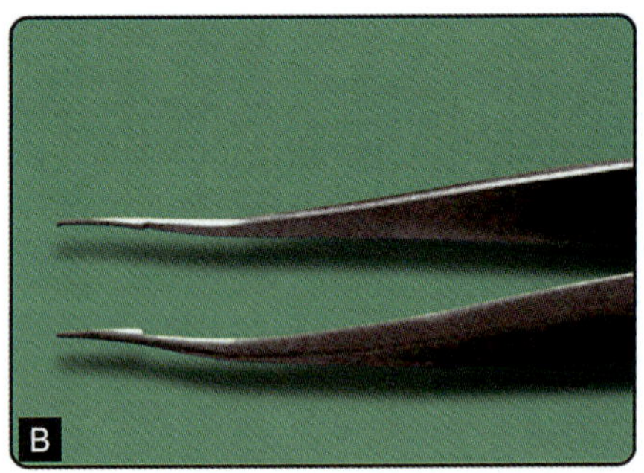

Figs 6.9A and B: Lim's forceps

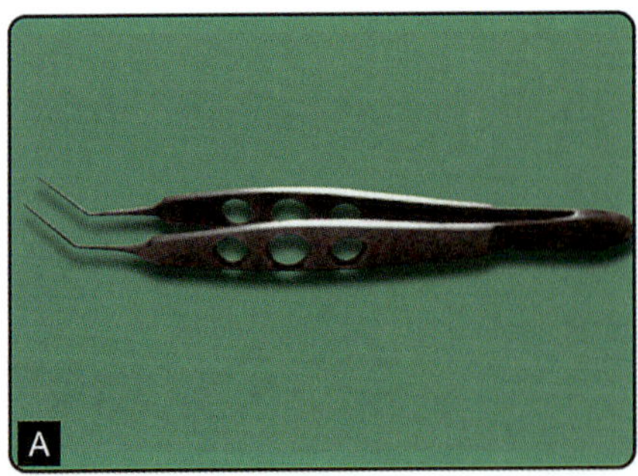

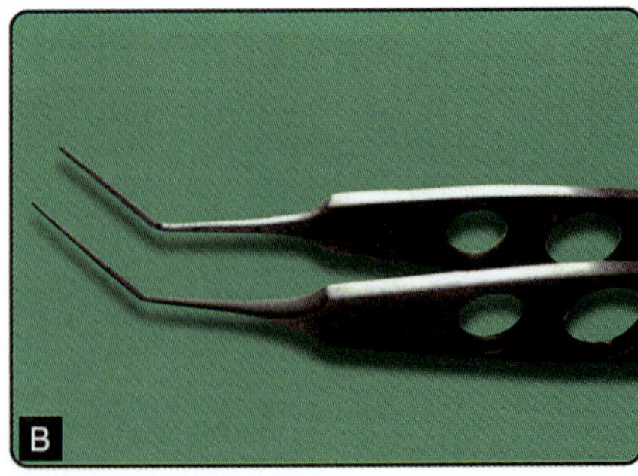

Figs 6.10A and B: Kelman-McPherson forceps

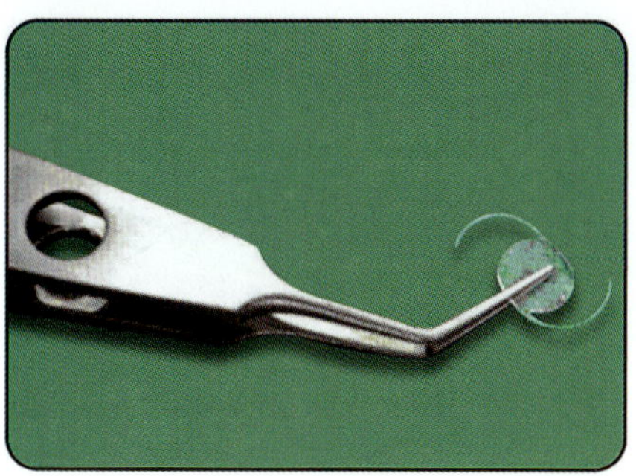

Fig. 6.11: Kelman-McPherson forceps with intraocular lens

bleeding during lid surgeries and lacrimal sac surgeries. It is used to hold bridle suture for fixation of globe (Figs 6.15 and 6.16).

SCISSORS

Scissors are instruments designed to cut tissues and sutures.

Conjunctival Scissors

Conjunctival scissors is a fine curved scissor with blunt tip, the blades of the scissors are kept apart by spring action (Figs 6.17A and B).

It is used to cut conjunctiva in various surgeries such as pterygium excision, ECCE, small incision cataract surgery (SICS), trabeculectomy and squint surgeries.

The tip of the conjunctival scissors is blunt to prevent formation of button hole of the conjunctiva. This is used to lift the conjunctiva during cutting and thereby to prevent injury to the underlying sclera.

Corneal Scissors

Corneal scissors is a fine curved scissor with sharp tip, the blades of the scissors are kept apart by spring action (Figs 6.18A and B).

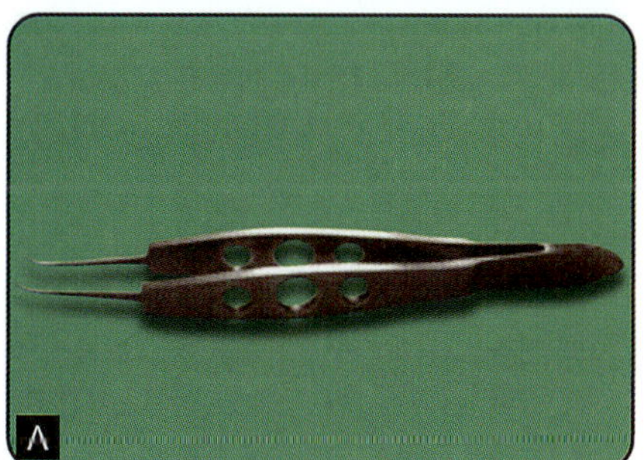

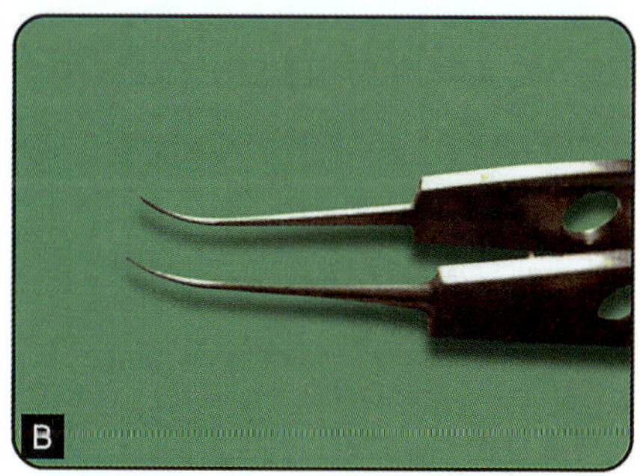

Figs 6.12A and B: McPherson tying forceps

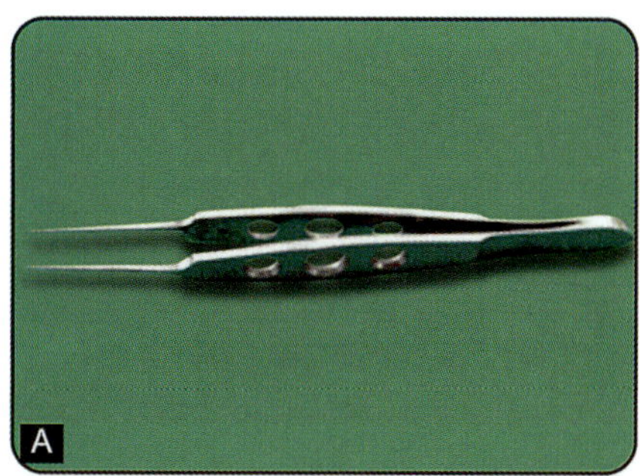

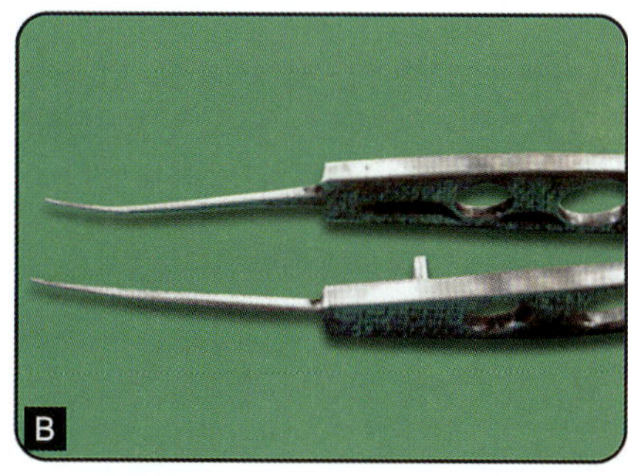

Figs 6.13A and B: Jaffe tying forceps

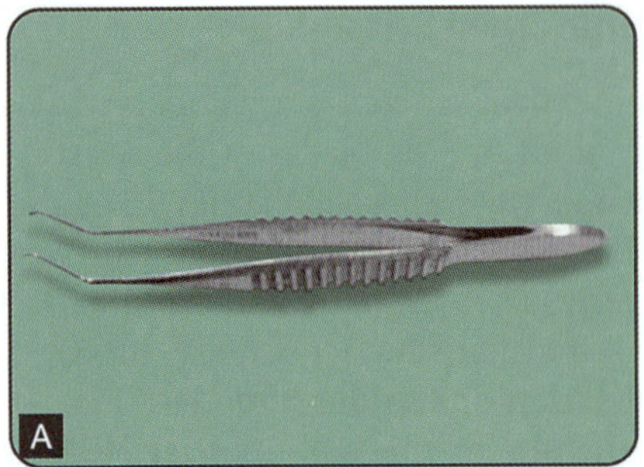

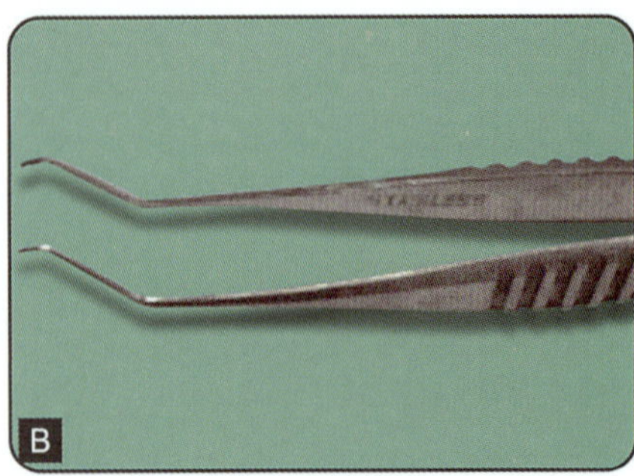

Figs 6.14A and B: Iris forceps

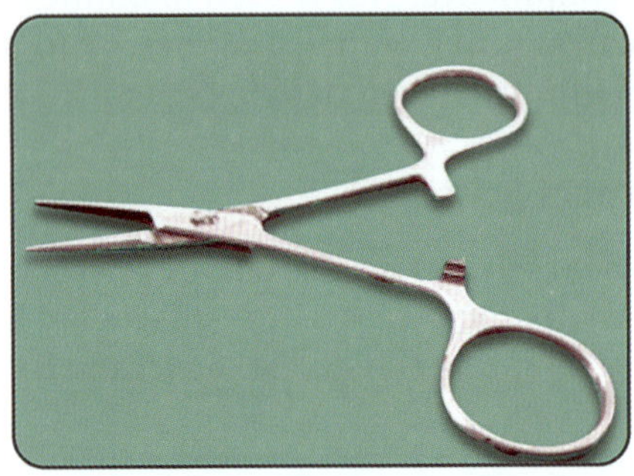

Fig. 6.15: Straight artery forceps

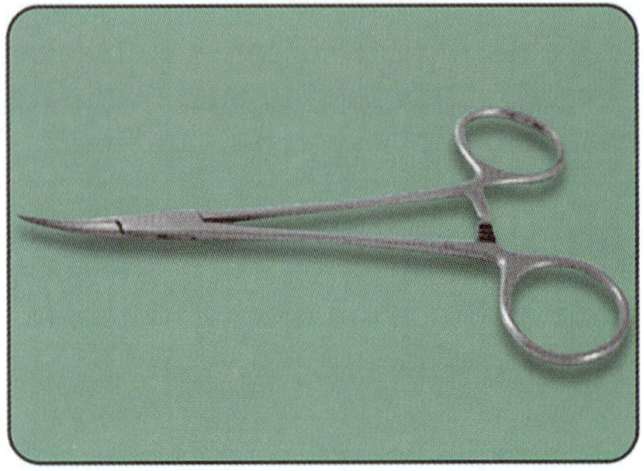

Fig. 6.16: Curved artery forceps

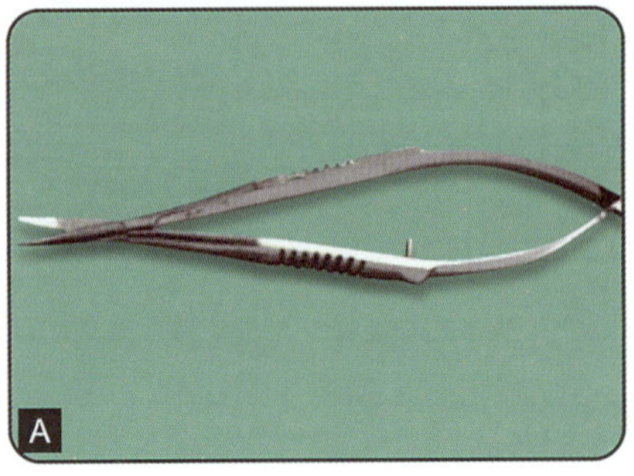

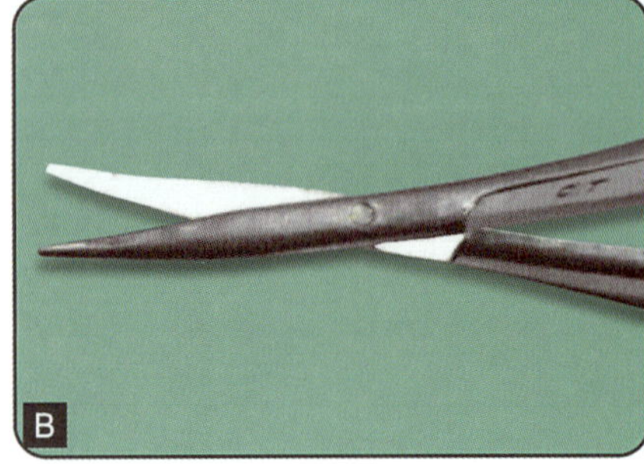

Figs 6.17A and B: Conjunctival scissors

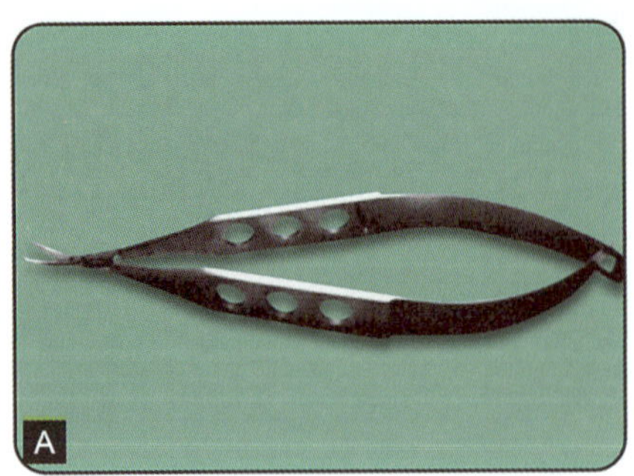

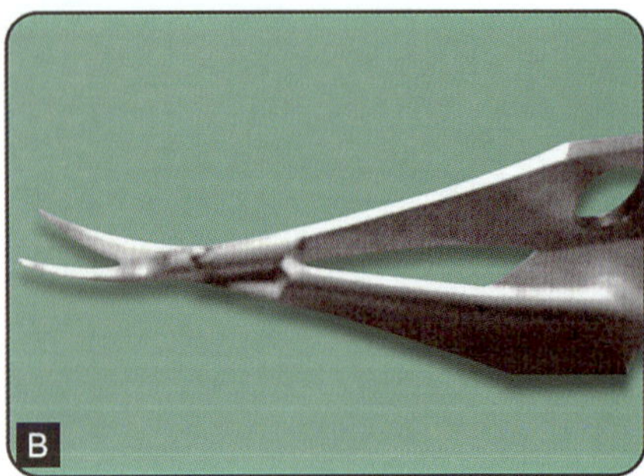

Figs 6.18A and B: Corneal scissors

It is used to cut cornea in surgeries such as conventional ECCE, keratoplasty. The tip of the corneal scissors is sharp to have precise cut to prevent irregular, ragged edges of the cornea, which can lead to astigmatism.

Vannas Scissors

Vannas scissors is a fine scissor with small cutting blades. The spring action separates the blades (Figs 6.19A to C).

In Vannas scissors, blades can be straight or curved called Vannas straight and curved scissors respectively. It is used to cut:

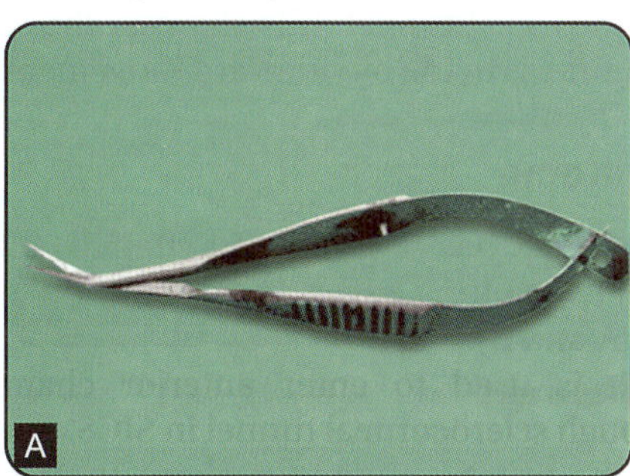

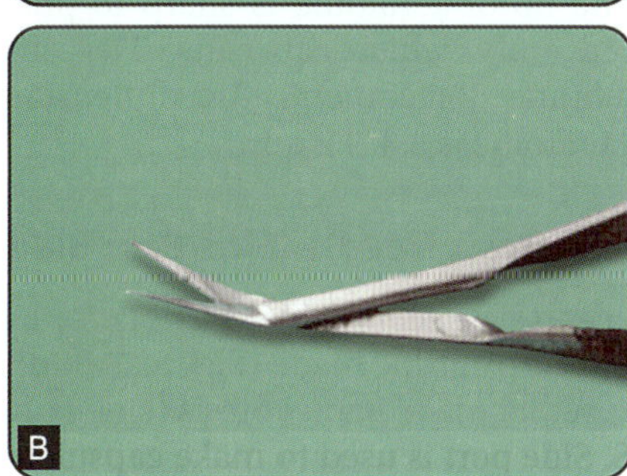

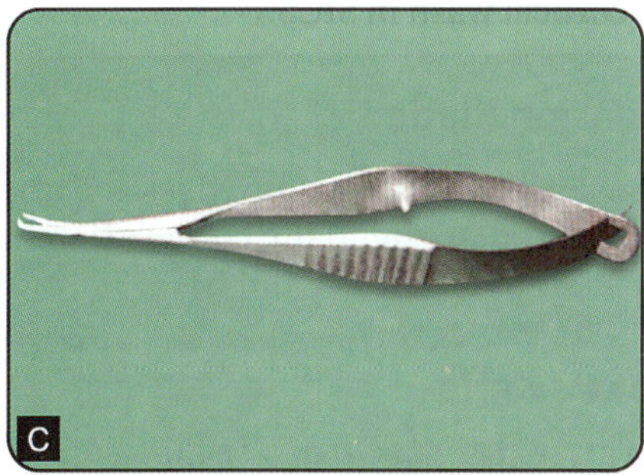

Figs 6.19A to C: Vannas scissors

- Anterior capsule during ECCE
- To cut 10-0 and 9-0 nylon sutures
- To cut sphincter pupillae for sphincterotomy
- To cut iris for performing iridectomy.

de Wecker Scissors

de Wecker scissors is a fine scissor with small blades perpendicular to the arms (Fig. 6.20). It is used to cut iris for performing iridectomy, to cut prolapsed vitreous during vitreous loss in surgeries such as intracapsular cataract extraction (ICCE), ECCE with vitreous loss, SICS with vitreous loss.

Enucleation Scissors

Enucleation scissors is a long, curved scissors. It is used to cut optic nerve during enucleation (Figs 6.21A and B).

Plain Straight Scissors

Plain straight scissors is used to cut skin sutures after lid surgeries, dacryocystectomy (DCT), dacryocystorhinostomy (DCR) (Fig. 6.22).

KNIVES (BLADES)

Crescent Blade

Crescent blade is sharp at the sides with blunt tip (Figs 6.23A and B). It is used to do self-sealing sclerocorneal tunnel in SICS. It is blunt

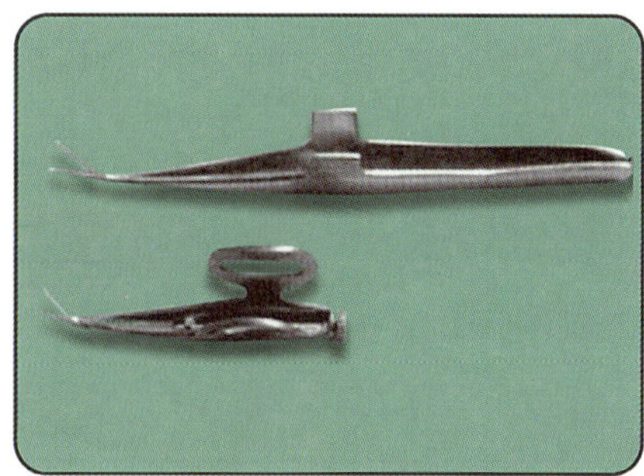

Fig. 6.20: de Wecker scissors

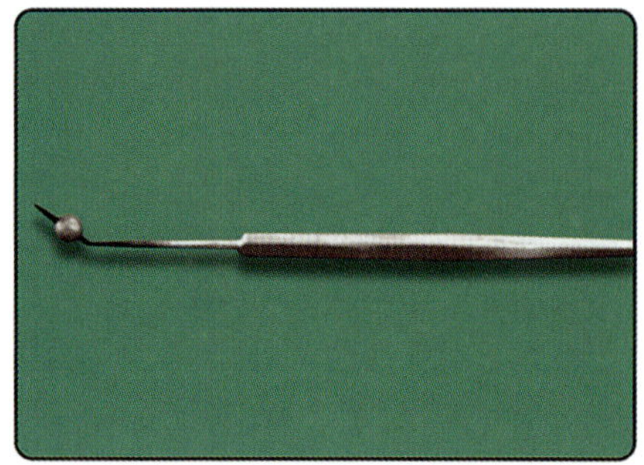

Fig. 6.48: Thermal ball point cautery

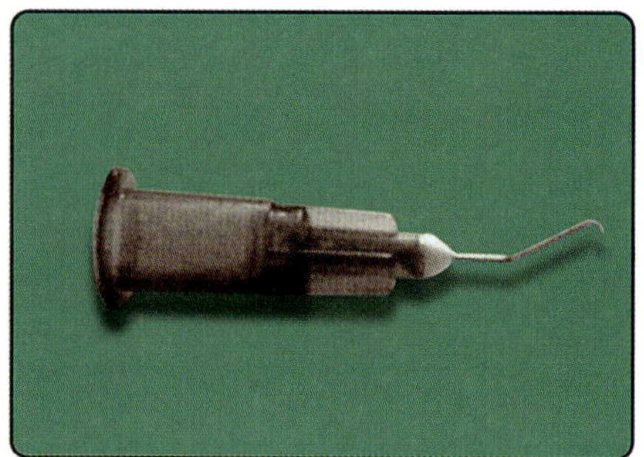

Fig. 6.49: Cystitome

The posterior smooth part of the ciliary body is called pars plana. It is 5 mm wide temporally and 3 mm wide nasally.

IRIS REPOSITOR

Iris repositor is a blunt-tipped instrument (Fig. 6.47) used in eye surgeries.

Uses

To reposit the iris into anterior chamber if it prolapses out during surgeries such as cataract surgery, keratoplasty and corneal tear repair.

THERMAL BALL POINT CAUTERY

The instrument consists of a copper ball and a tip with a long handle. The instrument is heated with the copper ball held in the flame of spirit lamp and the heat, which is retained by the copper ball is transmitted to the tip that is used to achieve hemostasis by thermal coagulation (to cauterize conjunctival and episcleral vessels) (Fig. 6.48).

Uses

To cauterize bleeding vessels in surgeries involving conjunctival periotomy such as cataract surgery, pterygium excision and trabeculectomy.

CYSTITOME OR CAPSULOTOME

About 26 gauge needle is bent twice, once at the tip and one more bent perpendicular to first one (Fig. 6.49).

Uses

For doing capsulotomy/capsulorhexis during ECCE.

Chapter 7

Ophthalmic Lenses

Chapter Outline

- Lens
- Pinhole
- Stenopaic Slit
- Priestley Smith's Retinoscope Mirror
- Jackson Cross Cylinder
- Maddox Rod
- 20 D Lens
- +78 D Lens

LENS

A transparent refractive medium with two surfaces, which form a part of a sphere or a cylinder is called lens.

Types

Spherical Lenses

Spherical lenses (Fig. 7.1) are bounded by two surfaces, which form a part of a sphere. Spherical lens can be:

- Convex spherical lens (plus lens)
- Concave spherical lens (minus lens).

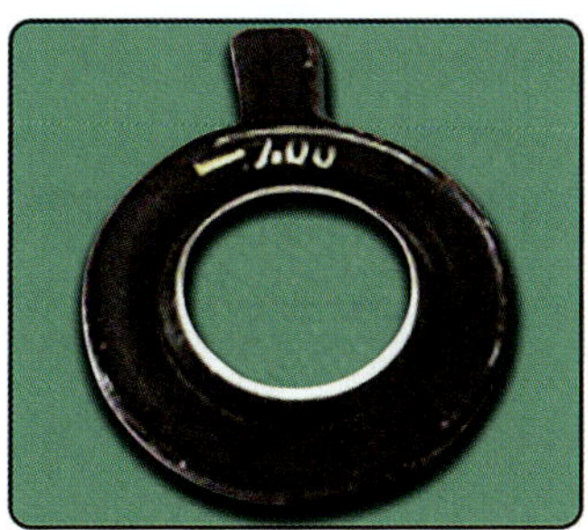

Fig. 7.1: Spherical lens

Cylindrical Lenses

Cylindrical lenses (Fig. 7.2) are bounded by two surfaces, which form a part of cylinder. Cylindrical lenses can be:

- Convex cylindrical lens
- Concave cylindrical lens.

Lens

The following questions have to be answered:

- How to identify the type of lens?
- What are the uses of the lens?

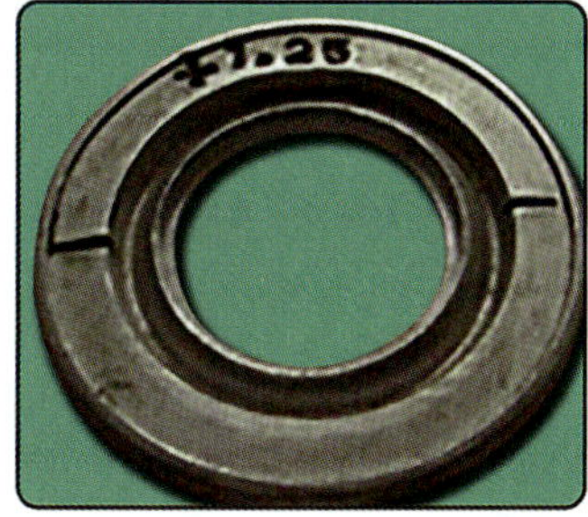

Fig. 7.2: Cylindrical lens

How to Identify the Type of Lens?

Those with handle are spherical lenses and those without handle, and with a line marked on the frame holding the lens are cylindrical lenses (in cylindrical lenses handle is absent to facilitate smooth rotatory movement to check the axis of the cylinder and line marked on it to identify the axis of the cylinder).

But do not identify lens by this method, what is expected to see is, what is happening to the object when seen through the lens?

Magnification: Convex lens.

Minification: Concave lens.

Movement of the object when lens is moved:

- Object moves in both the axis—sphere
- Object moves in only one axis—cylinder
- Object moves in opposite direction as the lens—convex lens
- Object moves in same direction as the lens—concave lens
- Distortion of the image when the lens is rotated—cylinder.

Spherical lens: Object seen through it moves in both axis and there is no distortion of object on rotating the lens.

Cylindrical lens: Object seen through it moves in one axis (direction right angle to the axis). Line marked on a cylindrical lens indicates the principal axis, i.e. along which the lens does not have any power, i.e. no action along this axis. There is distortion of object on rotating the lens.

Convex Spherical Lens (Lens 1)

- Object when seen through the lens appears magnified (Figs 7.3A and B)
- Object moves in both the axis and in opposite direction as the lens when moved
- No distortion of the image when the lens is rotated
- Lens is thicker in the center and thin at the periphery. Hence, the lens is convex spherical.

Uses

- For correction of hypermetropia, presbyopia, aphakia
- 20 D lens in indirect ophthalmoscopy
- +78 D, +90 D lens for slit lamp biomicroscopy examination of the fundus
- In loupe and lens examination—focal illumination for examination of structures of anterior segment of eye.

Concave Spherical Lens (Lens 2)

- Object when seen through the lens appears minified (Fig. 7.4)
- Object moves in both the axis and in same direction as the lens when moved
- No distortion of the image when the lens is rotated
- Lens is thin in the center and thick at the periphery. Hence, the lens is concave spherical.

Uses

- For correction of myopia
- Hruby lens—58.6 D lens for slit lamp biomicroscopic examination of the fundus.

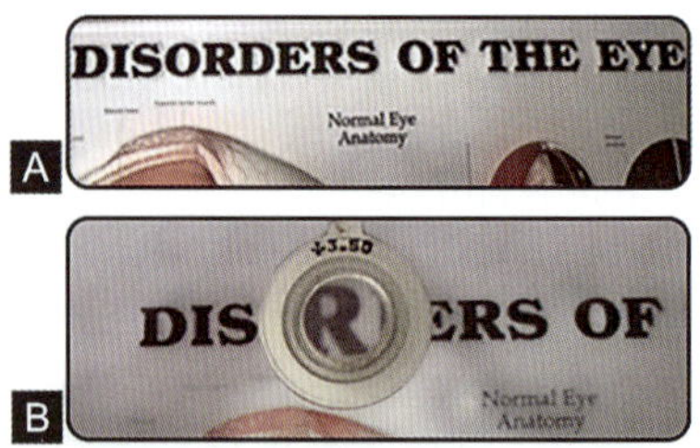

Figs 7.3A and B: Spherical convex lens. **A.** Without lens; **B.** Magnification of image through spherical lens.

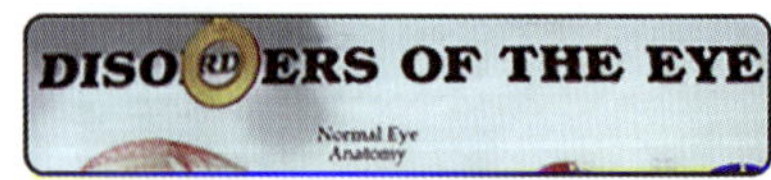

Fig. 7.4: Minification of image through spherical concave lens

Convex Cylindrical Lens (Lens 3)

- Object when seen through the lens appears magnified (Fig. 7.5A)
- Object moves in one axis and in opposite direction as the lens when moved
- Distortion of the image when the lens is rotated (Fig. 7.5B)
- Lens is thicker in the center and thin at the periphery. Hence, the lens is convex cylinder.

Uses

- For correction of hypermetropic astigmatism
- In Jackson cross cylinder for verification of subjective refraction.

Concave Cylindrical Lens (Lens 4)

- Object when seen through the lens appears minified (Fig. 7.6A)
- Object moves in one axis and in same direction as the lens when moved
- Distortion of the image when the lens is rotated (Fig. 7.6B)
- Lens is thin in the center and thick at the periphery. Hence, the lens is concave cylinder.

Uses

- For correction of myopic astigmatism
- In Jackson cross cylinder for verification of subjective refraction.

PINHOLE

Pinhole (Fig. 7.7) is used for pinhole test.

Pinhole Test

If the distance vision is less than 6/6, all patients should be asked to look through a pinhole and improvement, if any visual acuity, should be recorded. A pinhole cuts off all the peripheral rays and allows only central parallel beam of rays to enter eye and visual improvement is seen in cases of refractive errors. If the cause for diminution of vision is not refractive error as in case of cataract or retinal diseases then improvement is not seen. The size of the pinhole is 1 mm.

STENOPAIC SLIT

Stenopaic slit (Fig. 7.8) is used for stenopaic slit test.

Stenopaic Slit Test

Stenopaic slit allows clearest vision when it is rotated into the axis of astigmatism. It is done for checking the correction of astigmatism. If the vision improves with stenopaic slit when it is rotated into the axis of astigmatism, it indicates under correction. The size of the slit is 1 mm.

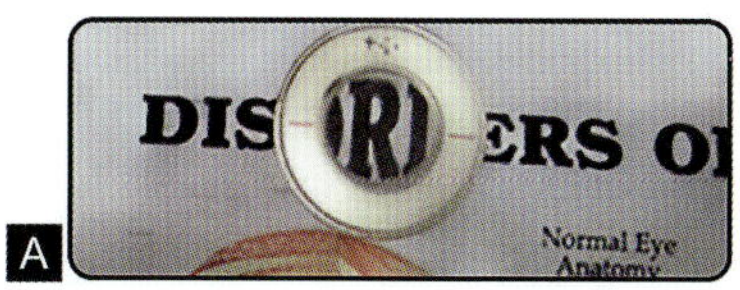

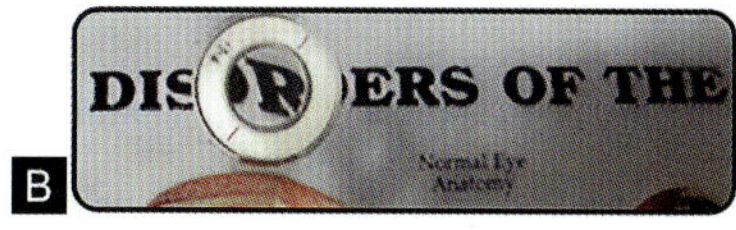

Figs 7.5A and B: Convex cylindrical lens. **A.** Magnification of image; **B.** Distortion on rotating.

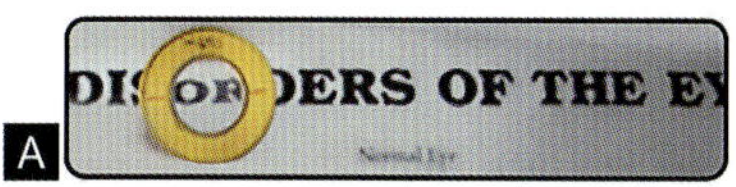

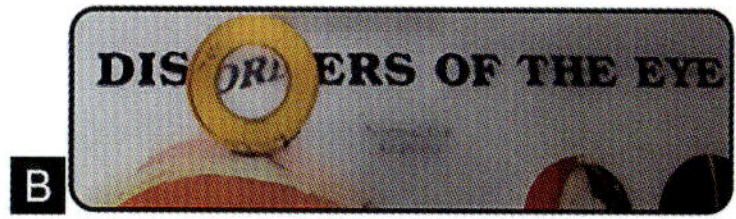

Figs 7.6A and B: Concave cylindrical lens. **A.** Magnification of image; **B.** Distortion on rotating.

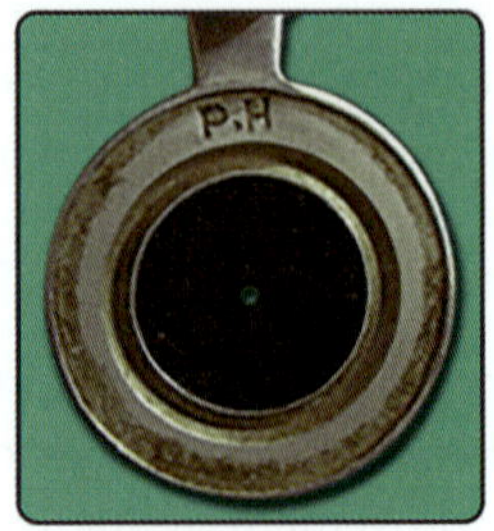

Fig. 7.7: Pinhole

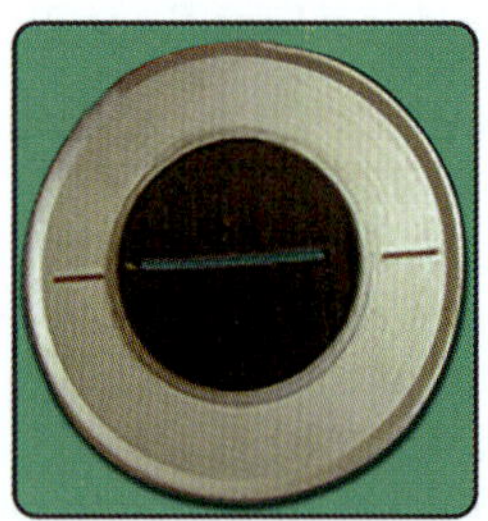

Fig. 7.8: Stenopaic slit

PRIESTLEY SMITH'S RETINOSCOPE MIRROR

Smith's mirror (Figs 7.9 to 7.11) is a combination of plane mirror and concave mirror. It is used for doing retinoscopy. Plane mirror is used in all patients for retinoscopy and in patients with hazy media concave mirror is preferred (as concave mirror converges the light rays).

JACKSON CROSS CYLINDER

Jackson cross cylinder (Fig. 7.12) is combination of two cylinders of equal strength with opposite signs with their axis at right angles to each other. Commonly used powers are +/–0.25 D and +/–0.5 D. It is used for verification of cylinder power and axis.

MADDOX ROD

Maddox rod (Fig. 7.13) consists of plus cylinders arranged parallel, which convert point light into a straight line of light at right angle to the axis of the rod.

Maddox Rod Test for Assessing

Macular Function

Patient is asked to look through a Maddox rod at a bright light; if the patient sees continuous unbroken and undistorted redline then the macula is normal; if the line is broken it shows some pathology of macula.

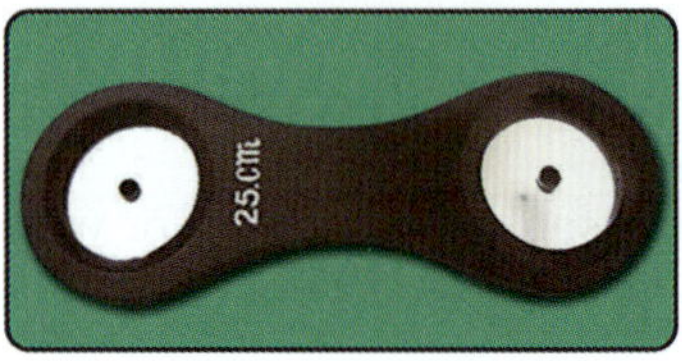

Fig. 7.9: Mirror retinoscope

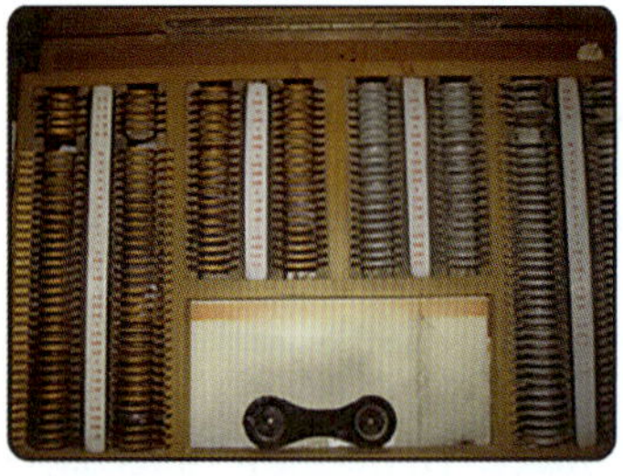

Fig. 7.10: Trial lens set

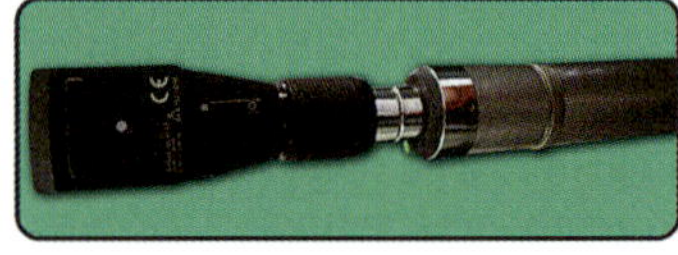

Fig. 7.11: Streak retinoscope

Fig. 7.12: Jackson cross cylinder

Maddox Rod Test for Measurement of Latent Squint

Maddox rod test works by presenting dissimilar images to two eyes there by breaking fusion and measures phoria (latent squint).

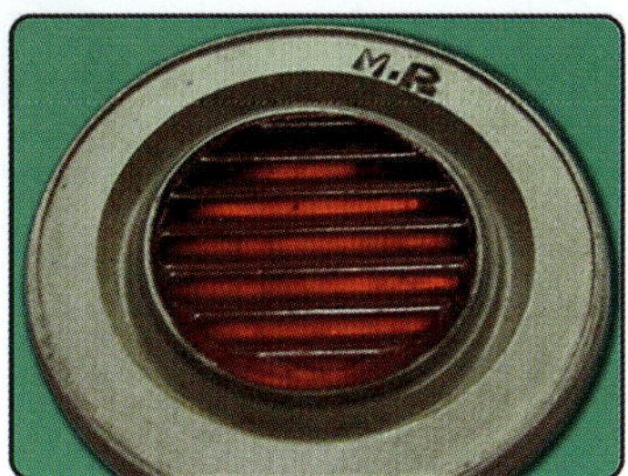

Fig. 7.13: Maddox rod

It is done from a distance of 6 m hence, it measures phoria for distance. Maddox rod is placed in front of the right eye and asked to see point source of light. This dissociates the two eyes as he/she will be seeing redline in right eye and a point source of light in left eye. The number on Maddox tangent scale where the redline falls gives the amount of heterophoria in degrees.

Double Maddox Rod Test

Double Maddox rod test is done to diagnose torsional squint (cyclotropia). Two Maddox rods are placed as one each in front of each eye with the axis horizontally so that the patient sees vertical lines. Patient without cyclotropia see the lines parallel to each other. In incyclotropia, the 12 O'clock position of the line is seen turned nasally and in excyclotropia is seen turned temporally.

20 D LENS

The 20 D lens (Fig. 7.14) is used for indirect ophthalmoscopy for examination of fundus. It provides magnification of three times.

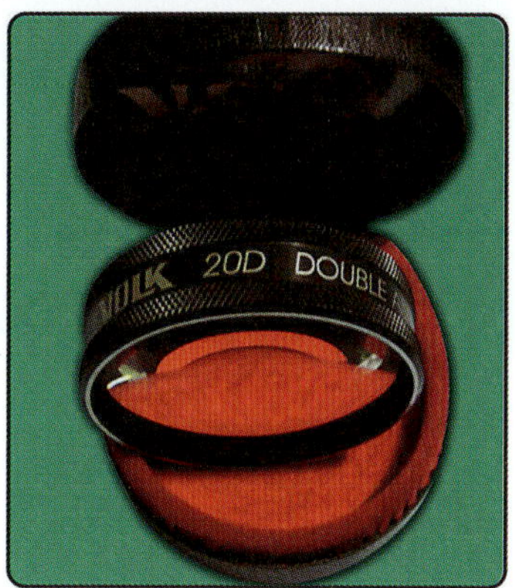

Fig. 7.14: 20 D lens

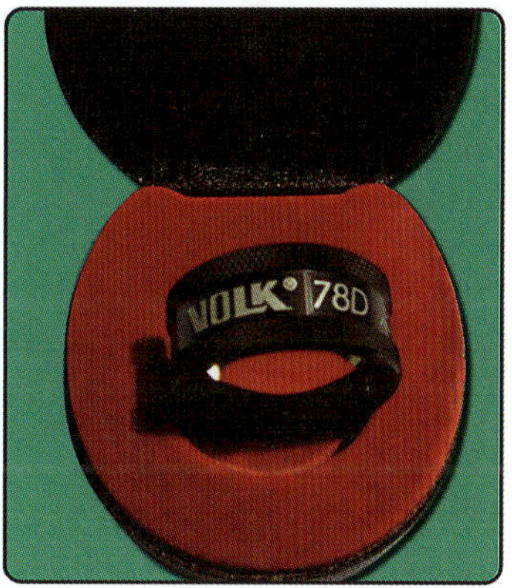

Fig. 7.15: +78 D lens

+78 D LENS

The +78 D lens (Fig. 7.15) is used for slit lamp biomicroscopic examination of retina. Other lenses used for slit lamp biomicroscopic examination of retina are +90 D lens and –58.6 D lens.

Chapter 8

Drugs Used in Ophthalmology

Chapter Outline

- Antiglaucoma Drugs
- Mydriatics and Cycloplegics
- Corticosteroids
- Antibacterial Drugs
- Antiviral Drugs
- Antifungal Drugs
- Non-steroidal Anti-inflammatory Drugs
- Local Anesthetic Drugs
- Hyaluronidase Injection
- Viscoelastics
- Artificial Tears
- Sutures
- Dyes
- Antiallergic Drugs

ANTIGLAUCOMA DRUGS

The main objective of drug treatment in glaucoma is to reduce intraocular pressure (IOP), so that optic nerve damage and visual field defects are prevented. Antiglaucoma drugs are classified as:

1. Adrenergic agonists (sympathomimetics):
   - Non-selective α-adrenergic agonists:
     - Epinephrine.
   - Selective α-adrenergic agonists:
     - Apraclonidine
     - Brimonidine.
2. Adrenergic antagonists:
   - Non-selective beta blocker:
     - Timolol
     - Levobunolol.
   - Selective beta-1 blocker:
     - Betaxolol.
3. Parasympathomimetic drugs:
   - Pilocarpine
   - Carbachol.
4. Hyperosmotic agents:
   - Oral glycerine
   - Intravenous (IV) Mannitol and urea.
5. Prostaglandins:
   - Latanoprost
   - Bimatoprost
   - Travoprost
   - Unoprostone.
6. Carbonic anhydrase inhibitors:
   - Oral acetazolamide
   - Topical dorzolamide.
7. Neuroprotective agents:
   - Calcium channel blockers
   - Antioxidants
   - Vasodilators.
8. Pilocarpine: Nearly 1%, 2%, 4% four times per day. Pilocarpine is a natural alkaloid obtained from pilocarpus microphyllus.

Mechanism of Action

Increased outflow through trabecular meshwork by contraction of longitudinal fibers of the ciliary muscles leading to opening of trabecular pores in open-angle glaucoma. Peripheral iris is pulled away from trabecular meshwork by constriction of pupil thereby preventing the crowding of iris at the angle of anterior chamber in narrow-angle glaucoma.

Indications

- Primary open-angle glaucoma
- Angle-closure glaucoma
- Non-inflammatory secondary glaucoma
- Intraoperatively to achieve meiosis of pupil.

Pilocarpine was the first-line drug till 1980s, now it is replaced by beta blockers and prostaglandin analogs.

Contraindications

Inflammatory glaucoma.

Adverse Side Effects

Ocular

- Myopia due to ciliary muscle contraction
- Retinal hole
- Retinal detachment
- Iris cysts
- Ocular pemphigoid.

Pilocarpine has to be avoided in patients with risk factors for retinal detachment such as high myopics and patients with retinal holes.

Systemic

Increased systemic muscarinic activity due to systemic absorption across the nasolacrimal duct causing lacrimation, salivation, diarrhea, vomiting and bronchospasm.

Timolol

Approximately 0.25%, 0.5% two times per day.

Mechanism of Action

Timolol is a nonspecific beta-1 and beta-2 blocker, it acts by decreasing the production of aqueous humor.

Indications

All varieties of glaucoma—open-angle, narrow-angle glaucoma and secondary glaucoma.

Timolol is the most common drug used to lower IOP in all kinds of glaucoma.

Contraindications

Asthma, chronic obstructive pulmonary disease (COPD), bradycardia, congestive heart failure.

Adverse Effects

1. Ocular: Allergic conjunctivitis, keratoconjunctivitis sicca, corneal anesthesia, superficial punctate keratitis.
2. Systemic: Bronchospasm, bradycardia, central nervous system (CNS) side effects, e.g. depression, anxiety, disorientation.

Timolol has to be used with caution in diabetics as it masks the signs of hypoglycemia.

Betaxolol

Approximately 0.25 %, 0.5 % two times per day. It is similar to timolol in its mechanism of action and its uses except that it selectively blocks beta-1 receptors. It is less effective in reducing IOP as the ciliary body adrenoreceptors are predominantly beta-2.

Since, it selectively blocks beta-1 receptors, it can be safely used in patients with asthma, COPD, where timolol is contraindicated; however cardiac side effects are more with betaxolol.

Brimonidine is selective α-2 adrenergic agonist acts by decreasing aqueous production. Its efficacy is similar to timolol.

Hyperosmotic Agents

Mechanism of Action

Hyperosmotic agents act by increasing the osmolarity of plasma leading to absorption of water from ocular tissues thus decreasing the IOP.

Indications

- Acute glaucomas where IOP is very high and need to be reduced immediately
- Oral glycerol 1.5–3 mL/kg body weight and IV Mannitol 1–2 g/kg body weight are the commonly used hyperosmotic agents.

Prostaglandins

Mechanism of Action

Increased uveoscleral outflow by altering the extracellular matrix of ciliary muscle (increase in spaces and decrease in the resistance to outflow).

Latanoprost

- Latanoprost 0.005%, one drop once daily is the most commonly used prostaglandin
- Latanoprost has got more efficacy than timolol and is among the first-line drugs for glaucoma
- Latanoprost should be stored below room temperature and in darkness as it has thermal and solar instability.

Adverse Effects

- Brownish discoloration of iris, e.g. iris sun tan syndrome
- Conjunctival hyperemia
- Iritis
- Cystoid macular edema
- Trichomegaly, i.e. increase in the length of eye lashes.

Carbonic Anhydrase Inhibitors

Mechanism of Action

1. Inhibition of carbonic anhydrase present in the epithelium of ciliary body, thus preventing bicarbonate anions and sodium influx thereby decreasing aqueous production.
2. Oral acetazolamide 250 mg four times per day is the recommended dosage.

Adverse Effects

Metallic taste to food, depression, kidney stones, metabolic acidosis, hypokalemia and bone marrow depression are the adverse effects of carbonic anhydrase inhibitors.

MYDRIATICS AND CYCLOPLEGICS

Mydriatics and cycloplegics are anticholinergic drugs, which cause dilatation of pupil and paralyze the action of ciliary muscle.

Tropicamide: It is the shortest acting mydriatic, which does not have cycloplegic action. Its action lasts for 4–6 hours. It is available as 0.5% eyedrops and used for dilatation of pupil before indirect ophthalmoscopy, before cataract surgery, and for retinoscopy in patients with hazy media aged more than 18 years.

Cyclopentolate: It is both mydriatic and cycloplegic, and its action lasts for 24 hours. It is used for retinoscopy in children aged between 12 and 18 years in treatment of iridocyclitis and corneal ulcer.

Homatropine: It is both mydriatic and cycloplegic and its action lasts for 72 hours. It is used for retinoscopy in children aged between 7 and 12 years in treatment of iridocyclitis and corneal ulcer.

Atropine: It is the strongest and longest acting mydriatic and cycloplegic agent. It is available as 1% eye ointment and eyedrops. Its action lasts for 21 days. It is used in retinoscopy in children less than 7 years, treatment of iridocyclitis and corneal ulcer.

Role of Atropine and Other Cycloplegics in Treatment of Iridocyclitis and Corneal Ulcer

- Atropine relieves ciliary spasm by causing paralysis of ciliary muscle action
- It increases blood supply by relieving pressure on ciliary arteries, decreases exudation by decreasing vascular permeability and prevents the formation of synechiae
- Atropine eyedrops have to be avoided because of risk of systemic toxicity by absorption via nasolacrimal duct.

Side Effects and Toxicity of Atropine

Dry mouth, difficulty in talking, dry flushed hot skin, difficulty in micturation, dilated pupil, delirium, rapid cardiovascular collapse and convulsions.

Atropine and other cycloplegics are contraindicated in narrow angle of the anterior chamber as they may precipitate angle-closure glaucoma.

CORTICOSTEROIDS

Corticosteroids have potent anti-inflammatory and antiallergic action. Commonly used corticosteroids are:

- Hydrocortisone (short acting < 12 hour)
- Prednisolone and methyl prednisolone (intermediate acting 12–36 hour)
- Dexamethasone and betamethasone (long acting > 36 hour).

Indications

1. Topical steroids are used in allergic conjunctivitis, scleritis, episcleritis, Mooren's ulcer, iridocyclitis and postoperative period after cataract surgery, pterygium surgery and keratoplasty.
2. Systemic steroids are used in optic neuritis, traumatic optic neuropathy, posterior uveitis, pseudotumor of orbit, thyroid ophthalmopathy and sympathetic ophthalmitis.

Adverse Effects

1. Ocular: Glaucoma, cataract.
2. Systemic: Gastric ulcer, osteoporosis, cushingoid status, aggravation of diabetes mellitus, psychiatric disturbances (mild euphoria is the most common) and susceptibility to infection.

Steroids are contraindicated in all infective conditions caused by bacteria, viruses and fungi.

- Topical steroids when used for longer duration are known to cause glaucoma because of deposition of mucopolysaccharides in the trabecular meshwork leading to rise in IOP
- Oral/Systemic steroids when used for longer duration are known to cause posterior subcapsular cataract.

ANTIBACTERIAL DRUGS

The commonly used antibiotic drugs are as follows.

Sulfonamides

Mechanism of Action

Being structural analogue of para-aminobenzoic acid (PABA), it acts by inhibiting bacterial folate synthetase. It is bacteriostatic in nature.

Indications

- Treatment of chlamydial infections such as trachoma and inclusion conjunctivitis
- Treatment of ocular toxoplasmosis.

Aminoglycosides (Gentamicin, Tobramycin)

Mechanism of Action

Aminoglycosides are bactericidal, which primarily act against gram-negative bacteria. They act by inhibiting protein synthesis by binding to ribosomes.

Indications

In infective conditions of eye such as bacterial corneal ulcer, bacterial conjunctivitis, postoperatively after surgeries such as cataract surgery, keratoplasty as prophylactic to prevent secondary bacterial infections.

Fluoroquinolones (Ciprofloxacin, Ofloxacin, Moxifloxacin)

Mechanism of Action

Fluoroquinolones act by inhibiting bacterial deoxyribonucleic acid (DNA) gyrase enzyme.

Indications

In infective conditions of eye such as bacterial corneal ulcer, bacterial conjunctivitis, postoperatively after surgeries such as cataract surgery, keratoplasty as prophylactic to prevent secondary bacterial infections.

ANTIVIRAL DRUGS

Commonly used antiviral drugs are acyclovir, a purine analogue and idoxuridine, a pyrimidine analogue.

Acyclovir

Dosage 3% eye ointment five times per day for topical application and 400–800 mg up to five times per day for oral administration.

Mechanism of Action

Acts by inhibiting DNA polymerase.

Indications

1. Topical eye ointment in:
   - Herpes simplex virus (HSV) blepharitis
   - The HSV conjunctivitis
   - The HSV corneal epithelial keratitis along with steroids in treatment of immune stromal keratitis.
2. Oral acyclovir is indicated in:
   - Herpes zoster ophthalmicus (HZO)
   - Prophylaxis against recurrent corneal epithelial keratitis.

Adverse Effects

- Lacrimal punctual occlusion
- Superficial punctuate keratitis
- Follicular conjunctivitis.

ANTIFUNGAL DRUGS

Antifungal drugs used in ophthalmology are described below.

Polyenes

Natamycin 5%, amphotericin B 0.15%.

Mechanism of Action

Polyenes act by interacting with ergosterol present in cell membrane of fungi making cell membrane to become leaky resulting in loss of vital contents of cell.

Indications

Natamycin 5% is the first choice in Fusarium keratitis, amphotericin B 0.15% is the first choice in Aspergillus keratitis, Candida keratitis, dematiaceous keratitis.

Amphotericin eyedrops are not available commercially, it has to be prepared by IV preparation by adding 5% dextrose.

Triazoles

Fluconazole 0.3%, fluconazole 200 mg, itraconazole 200 mg.

Mechanism of Action

Triazoles act by preventing demethylation of lanosterol by inhibiting the action of demethylase in fungi thereby preventing the formation of ergosterol from lanosterol.

Indications

Triazoles are effective against *Candida*, hence used in Candida keratitis. Oral triazoles are used in all cases of fungal keratitis as second-line drugs along with topical natamycin.

Imidazoles

Ketaconazole 200 mg, ketoconazole 2% eyedrops. Ketaconazole is moderately effective in fungal keratitis, hence used as second-line drug in fungal keratitis. Its mechanism of action is similar to triazoles.

NON-STEROIDAL ANTI-INFLAMMATORY DRUGS

Commonly used non-steroidal anti-inflammatory drugs (NSAIDs) are flurbiprofen 0.3% and ketorolac 0.5%.

Mechanism of Action

The NSAIDs act by inhibiting the enzyme cyclooxygenase, which inhibits prostaglandin synthesis.

Indications

To prevent cystoid macular edema postoperatively after cataract surgery. NSAIDs are started before surgery and continued in the postoperative period up to 6 weeks. NSAIDs also help to maintain the pupillary dilatation during cataract surgery. Other indications are in allergic conjunctivitis, episcleritis and inflamed pterygium.

LOCAL ANESTHETIC DRUGS

Commonly used local anesthetic drugs are lignocaine, bupivacaine and proparacaine.

Mechanism of Action

Local anesthetic drugs act by decreasing the entry of sodium ions during upstroke of action potential. 4% lignocaine and 0.5% proparacaine are used for topical anesthesia. 2% lignocaine (duration of action if 1–2 hour) and 0.5% bupivacaine (duration of action is 3–6 hour) are used for infiltration anesthesia.

Indications

1. Surface anesthesia:
   - For removal of corneal and conjunctival foreign bodies
   - For office procedures such as lacrimal syringing, tonometry, corneal scraping.
2. Infiltration anesthesia: For performing intraocular surgeries such as cataract surgery, trabeculectomy, squint surgery, keratoplasty and pterygium excision.

HYALURONIDASE INJECTION

Hyaluronidase 50 U/mL in peribulbar anesthesia is used to increase diffusion of anesthetic agent by breaking hyaluronic acid present in cell membranes.

VISCOELASTICS

Viscoelastics are substances with dual properties, which act as viscous liquids as well as elastic solids. They are used to prevent damage to corneal endothelium and other vital intraocular structures during intraocular surgery. Methyl cellulose and

Drugs Used Along with Local Anesthetic Agents

1. Adrenaline 1 in 1 lakh units to reduce systemic absorption of local anesthetic agent and to prolong the duration of action.
2. Hyaluronidase 50 U/mL in peribulbar anesthesia to increase diffusion of anesthetic agent by breaking hyaluronic acid present in cell membranes.
3. Peribulbar block is best achieved by using both 2% lignocaine (for rapid onset of action) with 0.5% adrenaline.
4. Bupivacaine (for longer duration of action) with hyaluronidase.

The action of lignocaine lasts for 1-2 hours and the duration of action of bupivacaine is 3-6 hours.

Retrobulbar Anesthesia

The principle is to block the sensory nerves and motor nerves, which supply the extraocular muscles before they innervate the extraocular muscles in the posterior conal space [superior oblique muscle is not anesthetized because cranial nerve (CN) IV has extraconal course and it escapes from the block] (Fig. 9.1).

The anesthesia provides excellent anesthesia and akinesia with quick onset of action.

Disadvantages

Complication rate is higher; the complications associated with it are:

- Retrobulbar hemorrhage
- Ocular perforation
- Injury to optic nerve
- Brainstem anesthesia.

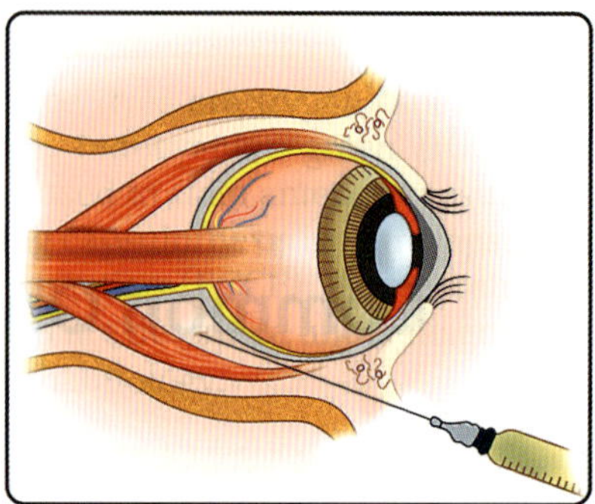

Fig. 9.1: Retrobulbar anesthesia

Peribulbar Anesthesia

The principle is to place local anesthetic agent outside the muscle cone and allow the anesthetic agent to diffuse into muscle cone to cause anesthesia. Injection hyaluronidase is used to assist the anesthetic agent to diffuse across the muscle cone.

The complications rate is low, hence it is the preferred technique over retrobulbar anesthesia (Figs 9.2A and B, 9.3).

Disadvantages

Delayed onset, as the anesthetic agent has to diffuse from peribulbar space to retrobulbar space. All complications of retrobulbar anesthesia can occur with this also, but with very less frequency.

Sub-Tenon's Anesthesia

The principle is to inject anesthetic agent into sub-Tenon's space to block sensory nerve endings to cause anesthesia, but it will not cause akinesia, as it will not block motor nerves.

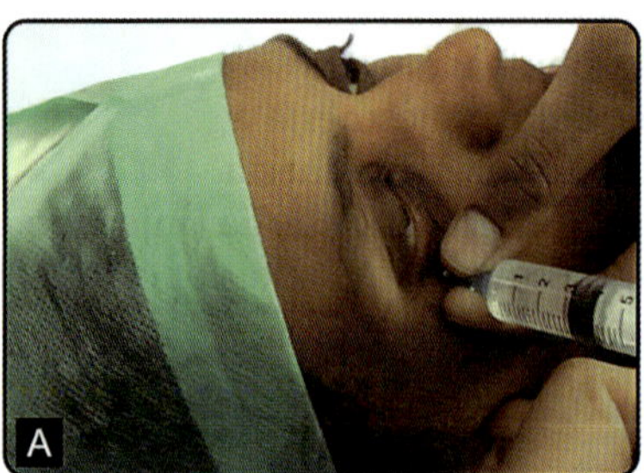

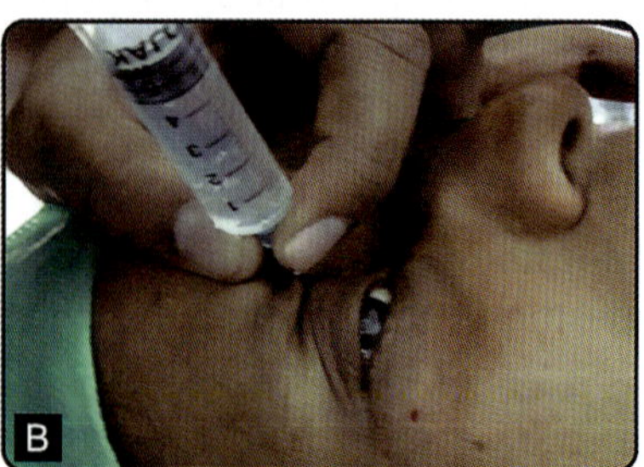

Figs 9.2A and B: Technique of peribulbar block

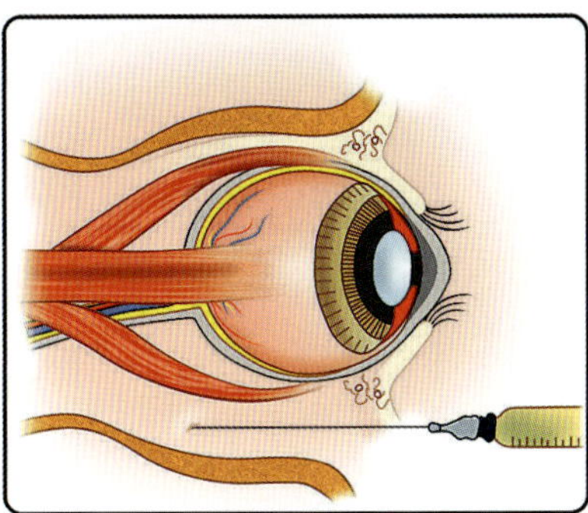

Fig. 9.3: Peribulbar anesthesia

Intracameral Anesthesia

The principle is to inject anesthetic agent into anterior chamber to anesthetize iris and ciliary body to carry out procedures in anterior chamber. It is used in association with topical anesthesia for phacoemulsification.

Facial Block

The principle is to block facial nerve—either its main branch or its peripheral branches to anesthetize orbicularis oculi to prevent squeezing of eyelids during intraocular surgeries.

Van Lint's method: Infiltration of anesthesia along superolateral and inferolateral margin of orbit to block peripheral branches of facial nerve.

Atkinson's method: Facial nerve block over zygomatic arch.

O'Brien's method: Facial nerve block over mandibular condyle.

Nadbath-Rehman method: Facial nerve block (of the main trunk) just below the external auditory meatus (Fig. 9.4).

Other Types of Infiltration Anesthesia

Other types of infiltration anesthesia used in ophthalmology are:

- Frontal nerve block
- Supraorbital nerve block
- Supratrochlear nerve block
- Infratrochlear nerve block
- Lacrimal nerve block
- Infraorbital nerve block.

Anesthesia for Dacryocystorhinostomy (DCR)

- Local skin incision injection
- Infratrochlear nerve block by inserting needle below trochlea
- Infraorbital nerve block by inserting the needle at the junction of inferior orbital margin with anterior lacrimal crest
- Anesthesia of nasal mucosa by packing nose with a gauze piece moistened with lignocaine.

CATARACT SURGERY

The techniques for cataract surgery have undergone evolution starting from couching (applying pressure on the eyeball to dislocate the intact lens into vitreous chamber so that patient becomes aphakic and will have aphakic vision, which is better than vision with mature and hypermature cataracts), which was practiced by Sushruta, father of surgery. The various techniques of cataract surgery are described in Table 9.1.

Indications for Cataract Surgery

Optical: To improve vision when cataract is causing visual impairment.

Therapeutic: As treatment for lens-induced glaucomas and in treatment of posterior

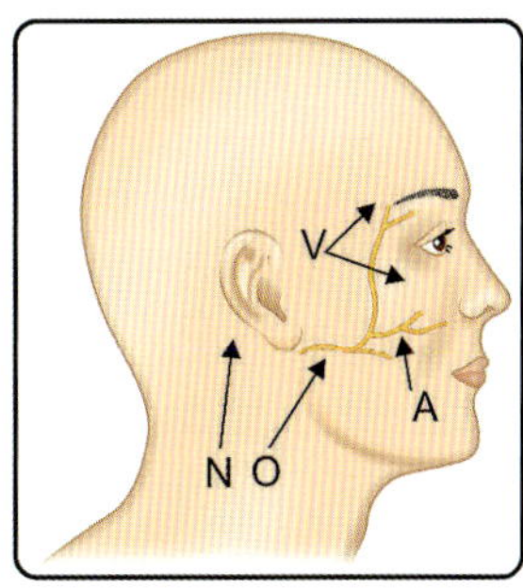

Fig. 9.4: Techniques of facial block (A, site of Atkinson facial block; N, site of Nadbath-Rehman facial block; O, site of O'Brien facial block; V, site of Van Lint facial block).

Table 9.1: Comparison between various techniques of cataract surgery

Type of surgery	Intracapsular cataract extraction (ICCE)	Extracapsular cataract extraction (ECCE) conventional	Small incision cataract surgery (SICS)	Phacoemulsification
Indication	Not done nowadays, indicated only in cases of dislocated lens into anterior or posterior chamber	All other cases	All other cases	All other cases
Principle	Lens is removed completely with both anterior and posterior capsules	Anterior capsule is removed by anterior capsulotomy and lens is removed leaving behind posterior capsule	Anterior capsule is removed by anterior capsulotomy and lens is removed leaving behind posterior capsule	Anterior capsule is removed by anterior capsulorhexis and lens is removed leaving behind posterior capsule; nucleus is emulsified by ultrasonic energy using phacoemulsifier machine
Anesthesia	Peribulbar block	Peribulbar block	Peribulbar block	Peribulbar sub-Tenon's topical anesthesia with intracameral anesthesia
Approach	Superior limbus	Superior limbus	Superior, superotemporal and temporal limbus	Superior, superotemporal, temporal limbus and clear corneal
Size of the incision	10–12 mm	8–10 mm	5.5–6.5 mm	3.5 mm
Methods of lens delivery	Lens is delivered intact (both cortex and nucleus with both anterior and posterior capsules) by cryoextraction or tumbling (pressure and counter pressure)	Nucleus is removed after anterior capsulotomy by pressure and counter pressure method Cortical matter is removed by irrigation and aspiration	Nucleus is expressed through tunnel, after dialing the nucleus into anterior chamber, after anterior capsulotomy or anterior capsulorhexis by phacosandwich or phacofracture, or irrigating vectis or fishhook technique or Blumenthal technique Cortical matter is removed by irrigation and aspiration	Nucleus is emulsified by a vibrating needle using ultrasonic energy

Contd...

Contd...

Type of surgery	Intracapsular cataract extraction (ICCE)	Extracapsular cataract extraction (ECCE) conventional	Small incision cataract surgery (SICS)	Phacoemulsification
Intraocular lens (IOL)	Only anterior chamber IOL can be implanted	Rigid posterior chamber (PC) IOL	Rigid PC IOL	Foldable PC IOL
Sutures	Incision needs to be sutured	Incision needs to be sutured	Sutures not required	Sutures not required
Complications	More because of vitreous disturbances	Less	Less	Less
Astigmatism induced by surgery	Average astigmatism > 2 D	Average astigmatism 1 D–2 D	Average astigmatism 0.5 D–1 D	Average astigmatism is 0.5 D
Visual rehabilitation	8 week	8 week	6 week	4 week
Advantages	It was widely practiced before the advent of microsurgery; now it is completely replaced by microsurgery (surgery using microscope), i.e. ECCE; it was an easy procedure without need for microscope, which was the scenario in underdeveloped and developing countries, especially in eye camps	It has less postoperative complications when compared to ICCE	Because of its self-sealing incision, it is preferred over conventional ECCE and it has got less complications particularly in relation to postoperative astigmatism	Because of its sutureless small incision, it is now the surgery of choice
Disadvantages	More incidence of vitreous-related complications, e.g. vitreous touch syndrome Only anterior chamber IOL can be inserted, which is not the ideal condition	The incision needs suturing, hence carries the risk of surgically induced astigmatism	It stays in between conventional ECCE and phacoemulsification	It is most expensive among all cataract surgeries, hence affordability can be a problem Most skilful and requires mastering over phacoemulsification machine to avoid machine-related complications such as corneal burns, etc.

segment problems such as diabetic retinopathy, retinal detachment, when lens opacity is preventing the treatment of posterior segment problems.

Cosmetic: Cataract surgery to obtain black pupil with no visual prognosis in conditions where cataract is associated with posterior segment diseases such as optic atrophy, etc.

Intracapsular Cataract Extraction

- Entire cataractous lens is removed along with intact capsule
- Not done nowadays
- The indication for intracapsular cataract extraction (ICCE) is dislocated lens into anterior chamber.

> Enzyme alpha-chymotrypsin is used in young patients for performing ICCE to dissolve the zonules, in patients after 50 years of age, this enzyme is not required as the zonules will not be strong.

Steps of Intracapsular Cataract Extraction

1. Local anesthesia—peribulbar block is the preferred one.
2. Preparation of the eyeball by painting the eye with povidone-iodine and draping the eye with eye towel.
3. Insertion of the wire speculum to keep the eyelids apart.
4. Superior rectus stitch or bridle suture for fixation of the globe.
5. Conjunctival peritomy and cauterization of the bleeding vessels.
6. Partial thickness limbal groove 10–12 mm.
7. Corneoscleral section and entry into anterior chamber.
8. Injection of viscoelastic into the anterior chamber.
9. Lens delivery by cryoextraction or tumbling. In cryoextraction, the lens is removed by applying cryoprobe onto the surface of lens. In tumbling, lens is removed by applying pressure and counter pressure at 6 O'clock and 12 O'clock position respectively.
10. Peripheral iridectomy.
11. Anterior chamber IOL insertion.
12. Formation of anterior chamber by balanced salt solution.
13. Closure of the corneoscleral incision by 9-0 or 10-0 nylon suture.
14. Closure of conjunctiva.
15. Subconjunctival injection of antibiotic with steroid.
16. Pad and bandage.

Extracapsular Cataract Extraction

The cataractous lens is removed leaving behind intact posterior capsule. Types of extracapsular cataract extraction (ECCE) are:

- Conventional ECCE
- Small incision cataract surgery (SICS)
- Phacoemulsification.

Steps of ECCE (Conventional ECCE)

1. Anesthesia: Local anesthesia in the form of peribulbar anesthesia.
2. Preparation of the eyeball by painting the eye with povidone-iodine, draping the eye with eye towel.
3. Insertion of the wire speculum.
4. Superior rectus stitch or bridle suture for fixation of the globe.
5. Conjunctival peritomy and cauterization of the bleeding vessels.
6. Partial thickness limbal groove 8–10 mm.
7. Corneoscleral section.
8. Injection of viscoelastic into the anterior chamber.
9. Capsulotomy or capsulorhexis: It is the most important step in ECCE, which differentiates it from ICCE. This step removes the anterior capsule and leaves behind the posterior capsule:
   a. Capsulotomy: It is done by using a bent 26 gauge needle called cystotome.

Multiple radial punctures are made in the anterior capsule in a circular fashion of approximately 6–7 mm in diameter. Capsulotomy is completed by joining these cuts and removing the part of anterior capsule. This is also called canopener capsulotomy or multipuncture capsulotomy.

b. Capsulorhexis: It is done either by a cystotome or a capsulorhexis forceps. This is done by tearing the capsule in a circular fashion of 6–7 mm diameter. Capsulorhexis is better than capsulotomy and preferred, as this can be stretched for in the bag IOL insertion.

10. Enlarging the corneoscleral section.
11. Hydrodissection: This is done by injecting the fluid under the anterior capsule to separate the cortex and nucleus from capsule.
12. Removal of nucleus by pressure and counter pressure method or by using vectis.
13. Removal of cortical matter by irrigation and aspiration.
14. Insertion of posterior chamber IOL.
15. Formation of anterior chamber by balanced salt solution.
16. Closure of the corneoscleral incision.
17. Closure of conjunctiva.
18. Subconjunctival injection of antibiotic with steroid.
19. Pad and bandage.

Phacoemulsification

1. Phacoemulsification is the most popular surgery and is considered as the gold standard surgical procedure for cataract.
2. It was first introduced by Charles D Kelman in 1967.
3. It is the most preferred mode of treatment, as the incision size is less than 3.5 mm, which allows for quick visual rehabilitation. It uses foldable intraocular lenses (Fig. 9.5).

Definition

Phacoemulsification is a surgical procedure for cataract removal, where the cataractous lens is emulsified by ultrasonic energy by using phacoemulsifier machine (Fig. 9.6).

Mechanism

Phacoemulsification handpiece consists of piezoelectric crystals, which convert electrical energy into mechanical vibration (Fig. 9.7). The phacoemulsification needle vibrates at about 40,000 times/second thus emulsifying the nucleus.

Steps of Phacoemulsification

1. Anesthesia: Local anesthesia in the form of peribulbar block or topical anesthesia by 4% lignocaine with intracameral anesthesia by injection of lignocaine into anterior chamber.

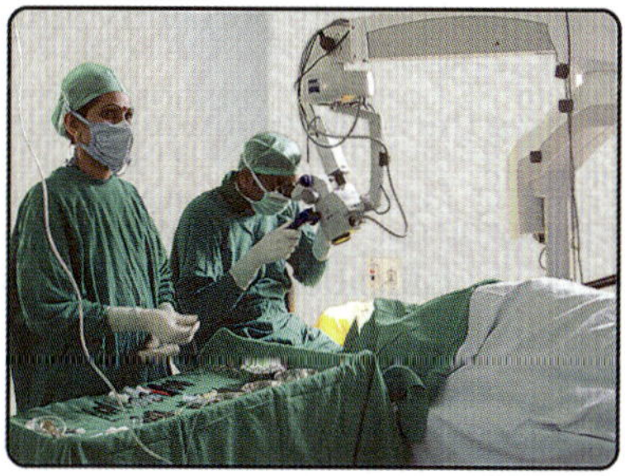

Fig. 9.5: Ophthalmology operation theater surgeon operating under microscope

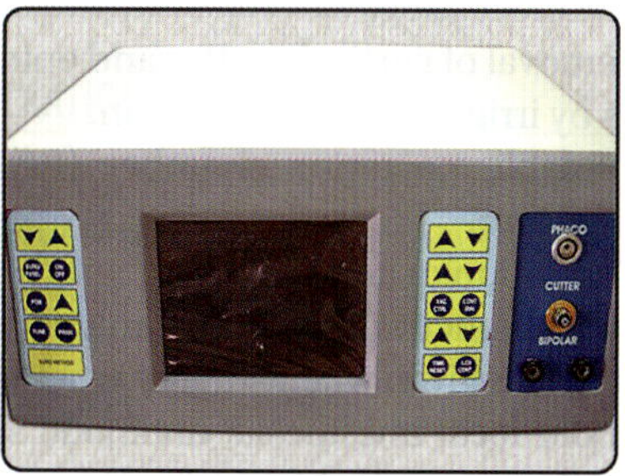

Fig. 9.6: Phacoemulsification machine

Anesthesia Preferred

General anesthesia is preferred, but can also be done under local anesthesia.

Procedure

- After anesthesia and preparing of the eye speculum is inserted
- Dissection of conjunctiva all around the limbus
- Complete excision of cornea with limbus
- Introduction of evisceration scoop to separate uveal tissue from sclera, and uveal tissue and intraocular contents are scooped out
- Hemostasis is achieved with warm saline-soaked gauze
- Silicone ball implant is placed in the scleral cup
- Sclera, Tenon's capsule and conjunctiva are sutured separately
- Pad and bandage.

ENUCLEATION

Enucleation is a surgical procedure, which involves removal of eyeball along with a portion of optic nerve.

Indications

- To collect eyeball from eye donors after their death, is the most common indication
- Malignancies of eye such as retinoblastoma, malignant melanoma
- Sympathetic ophthalmitis
- Endophthalmitis not responding to medical treatment.

Contraindications

Panophthalmitis, as the infection may spread via the cut ends of optic nerve sheath.

Anesthesia Preferred

General anesthesia is preferred, but can also be done under local anesthesia. No anesthesia is required to collect eyeball from donors, which is collected only after death of donors.

Procedure

- After anesthesia and preparing of the eye, the speculum is inserted
- Dissection of conjunctiva all around the limbus
- Four recti muscles are hooked and cut
- Optic nerve is cut with a enucleation scissors
- Oblique muscles are cut
- Eyeball is removed
- Hemostasis is achieved with warm saline-soaked gauze
- Tenon's capsule and conjunctiva are sutured separately
- Pad and bandage.

OTHER SURGERIES

The below mentioned surgeries are described under respective case discussions in Chapter 4 'Case Presentation':

- Pterygium excision
- Keratoplasty
- Dacryocystectomy
- Dacryocystorhinostomy
- Incision and curettage of chalazion (for more details refer Chapter 6 'Ophthalmic Instruments').

Chapter 10

An Approach to a Patient with Red Eye

Chapter Outline

- Acute Red Eye
- Subconjunctival Hemorrhage
- Blepharitis
- Conjunctivitis
- Inflamed Pterygium
- Episcleritis
- Scleritis
- Corneal Abrasion
- Infective and Non-infective Keratitis
- Endophthalmitis
- Panophthalmitis
- Orbital Cellulitis
- Acute Iridocyclitis
- Acute Congestive Glaucoma

ACUTE RED EYE

Differential Diagnosis of Acute Red Eye

Three classical differential diagnosis of this condition are:
1. Acute conjunctivitis.
2. Acute iridocyclitis.
3. Acute congestive glaucoma.

Causes of Red Eye (Table 10.1)

The causes include:
- Blepharitis
- Conjunctivitis
- Subconjunctival hemorrhage
- Episcleritis
- Scleritis
- Corneal abrasion
- Infective and non-infective keratitis
- Endophthalmitis
- Panophthalmitis
- Orbital cellulitis.

SUBCONJUNCTIVAL HEMORRHAGE

The collection of blood under the bulbar conjunctiva is termed as subconjunctival hemorrhage.

Causes

Trauma is the most common cause. The mode of trauma may vary from very trivial one to very serious one such as head injury, orbital wall fractures, etc.

Other causes include hemorrhagic conjunctivitis caused by picornaviruses, pneumococci, bleeding disorders, spontaneous rupture

Table 10.1: Red eye

Painless and with no visual involvement	Mild pain/irritation with no visual involvement	Moderate-to-severe pain with various grades of visual impairment
Subconjunctival hemorrhage	Blepharitis Conjunctivitis Inflamed pterygium Episcleritis	Scleritis Corneal abrasion Infective and non-infective keratitis Endophthalmitis Panophthalmitis Orbital cellulitis Acute iridocyclitis Acute congestive glaucoma

of blood vessels in patients with microvascular diseases such as diabetes and hypertension.

Examination

Posterior limit of the subconjunctival hemorrhage has to be made out clearly, if posterior limit cannot be made out, retrobulbar hemorrhage has to be ruled out particularly in patients with history of moderate-to-severe eye trauma or head injury.

Look out for other causes of subconjunctival hemorrhage in patients with no history of trauma. Evaluate for diabetes and hypertension in patients with spontaneous subconjunctival hemorrhage.

Treatment

Subconjunctival hemorrhage alone will not require treatment other than reassurance and advice that it will resolve over a period of 4 weeks.

BLEPHARITIS

Inflammation of lid margin is called blepharitis.

Causes

- Infective, e.g. staphylococcal ulcerative blepharitis
- Non-infective, e.g. seborrheic or squamous blepharitis
- Meibomianitis.

Examination

Blepharitis usually presents with scales at lid margins in squamous blepharitis, crusts (ulcers on removing crusts) in staphylococcal ulcerative blepharitis and yellowish spots in meibomianitis.

Treatment

Treatment is by lid hygiene, antibiotic/steroid eyedrops/ointment (only antibiotic eyedrops/ointment in ulcerative blepharitis).

CONJUNCTIVITIS

The inflammation of conjunctiva is called conjunctivitis.

Causes

- Infective causes including bacterial conjunctivitis and viral conjunctivitis
- Allergic conjunctivitis
- Traumatic conjunctivitis.

Examination

1. All varieties of conjunctivitis present with conjunctival congestion associated with discharge.
2. Bacterial conjunctivitis presents with mucopurulent or purulent discharge.

3. Viral conjunctivitis presents with watery discharge with follicles in conjunctiva.
4. Allergic conjunctivitis presents with ropy discharge with papillae in conjunctiva mainly in upper palpebral conjunctiva.

Treatment

1. Treatment depends on the causative agent.
2. Bacterial conjunctivitis is treated by appropriate antibiotic eyedrops.
3. Viral conjunctivitis treatment is mainly symptomatic and by antibiotic eyedrops to prevent secondary bacterial infection.
4. Allergic conjunctivitis is treated by antihistamine drugs, mast cell stabilizers, vasoconstrictors and steroid eyedrops.

INFLAMED PTERYGIUM

Pterygium presenting with complaints of inflammation is common in patients with preexisting pterygium usually on exposure to dust, wind, etc.

Treatment

Treatment is by non-steroidal anti-inflammatory agents such as ketorolac eyedrops, flurbiprofen eyedrops or steroidal agents such as fluorometholone eyedrops, dexamethasone eyedrops.

EPISCLERITIS

1. Inflammation of episclera with Tenon's capsule is called episcleritis.
2. It presents with mild pain with sectoral congestion.

Treatment

1. Treatment is by topical steroid eyedrops with or without systemic non-steroidal drugs.
2. Recurrent episcleritis should be evaluated for autoimmune disorders as in case of scleritis.

SCLERITIS

Inflammation of sclera is called scleritis. It presents with moderate-to-severe pain with sectoral congestion. It is important because of its frequent association with autoimmune disorders. Hence, all cases of scleritis have to be evaluated for autoimmune diseases (e.g. rheumatoid arthritis, systemic lupus erythematosus, ankylosing spondylitis), metabolic diseases (e.g. gout, thyroid disease) and granulomatous diseases (e.g. tuberculosis, syphilis, etc.).

Treatment

Treatment is by topical steroids and systemic steroids with non-responsive cases requiring immunosuppressive agents.

CORNEAL ABRASION

Corneal epithelial defect is called corneal abrasion. It presents with severe pain, photophobia, watering and circumcorneal congestion with various grades of visual impairment.

Examination

Search for the cause of corneal abrasion should be made in all cases, particularly look for a retained foreign body in sulcus subtarsalis by everting the upper eyelid. In all cases of corneal abrasion, cornea has to be stained with fluorescein and the size of the abrasion should be noted. Look for corneal dystrophies or degenerations such as epithelial basement dystrophy in patients with recurrent corneal abrasion with no history of trauma.

Treatment

Treatment is mainly by antibiotic eyedrops/ointment to prevent secondary bacterial infection, lubricating eyedrops (e.g. methylcellulose eyedrops) or cycloplegic eyedrops (e.g. homatropine eyedrops) to relieve pain, which is due to ciliary spasm.

Patients with lagophthalmos with corneal abrasion, which is not responding to treatment, may require temporal or permanent tarsorrhaphy.

INFECTIVE AND NON-INFECTIVE KERATITIS

Described under Corneal Ulcer in Chapter 4 'Case Presentation'.

ENDOPHTHALMITIS

Endophthalmitis is defined as severe inflammation of inner coats (uvea and retina) and the intraocular cavities (anterior chamber and vitreous chamber).

Endophthalmitis can be infective following endogenous or exogenous infection by bacteria, fungi or parasite. It can be sterile or toxic as following retained intraocular foreign body, or toxic lens syndrome or phacoanaphylactic uveitis.

Endophthalmitis presents with moderate-to-severe pain with grossly reduced visual acuity, lid edema, ciliary congestion, anterior chamber reaction and vitreous haze because of vitritis with normal extraocular movements.

Treatment

Treatment of sterile endophthalmitis is by controlling the inflammation by topical and systemic steroids. Treatment of bacterial endophthalmitis is guided by endophthalmitis vitrectomy study (EVS), which suggests immediate vitrectomy, if the presenting visual acuity is hand movements or less and in eyes with presenting visual acuity more than hand movements, the initial management is by intravitreal antibiotics (ceftazidime and vancomycin are preferred). The use of systemic antibiotics showed no advantage according to this study and hence not preferred.

Intravitreal antifungal agents (e.g. amphotericin B) are indicated in fungal endophthalmitis initially, if not controlled vitrectomy is indicated.

PANOPHTHALMITIS

Panophthalmitis is defined as severe inflammation of all the three coats of the eye (cornea and sclera, uvea, retina) and the intraocular cavities (anterior chamber and vitreous chamber).

Panophthalmitis is usually an infective condition and follows bacterial infections. All the clinical features of endophthalmitis are present along with added features such as hazy cornea because of involvement of outer fibrous coat and limitation of extraocular movements.

Treatment

1. Medical management involves systemic antibiotics and analgesics to relieve pain, and to prevent intracranial spread of infection.
2. Evisceration is the surgery of choice to prevent intracranial spread of infection, which may be endangering life of the patient.
3. Enucleation is contraindicated in panophthalmitis, as the infection may spread intracranially via cut ends of optic nerve following enucleation; whereas following evisceration, the intact scleral frill provides protection against this.

ORBITAL CELLULITIS

Orbital cellulitis is defined as infection of soft tissues of the orbit, posterior to the orbital septum. It can present as milder form, preseptal orbital cellulitis or severe form postseptal orbital cellulitis.

Preseptal orbital cellulitis presents with periorbital swelling, pain, redness with normal visual acuity and full extraocular movements. Postseptal cellulitis presents with severe proptosis, severe pain, chemosis, markedly reduced visual acuity and restricted ocular movements.

Treatment

Treatment is mainly by systemic antibiotics and analgesic agents.

ACUTE IRIDOCYCLITIS

Acute inflammation of iris and ciliary body is called acute iridocyclitis.

Causes

The causes for acute iridocyclitis are very wide. Causes include infections (e.g. bacterial, viral, fungal, parasitic trauma), hypersensitivity, autoimmune disorders, systemic diseases (e.g. diabetes mellitus, gout) and skin diseases (e.g. psoriasis), etc. Patient presents with moderate-to-severe pain, redness, photophobia, watering and diminution of vision. On examination, the affected eye shows circumcorneal congestion, keratic precipitates, aqueous flare, aqueous cells, hypopyon, iris nodules and posterior synechiae.

Treatment

Treatment is by specific treatment of the cause and by non-specific treatment, which includes cycloplegic drugs such as atropine 1% eye ointment, topical and systemic corticosteroids.

ACUTE CONGESTIVE GLAUCOMA

Glaucoma resulting due to sudden and total closure of the angle of the anterior chamber is called acute congestive glaucoma. Patient presents with severe pain associated with nausea, vomiting, diminution of vision, redness, photophobia and watering.

On examination, the affected eye shows circumcorneal congestion, corneal edema, shallow anterior chamber, mid dilated vertically oval pupil. Patient may give history of previous intermittent attacks and the other eye may show shallow anterior chamber.

Treatment

Acute angle closure glaucoma is an ophthalmological emergency; hence, treatment should be started immediately. The principles of treatment of acute angle closure glaucoma are to:

1. Reduction of intraocular pressure (IOP) and control of inflammation is done by:
   a. Intravenous (IV) Mannitol 20%, 1.5–2 g/kg of the body weight given over period of 45 minutes to 1 hour or oral glycerol, but in cases IV Mannitol is contraindicated.
   b. Oral acetazolamide 250 mg, one or two tablets stat.
   c. Topical timolol 0.5% eyedrops.
   d. Topical steroid eyedrops to control inflammation.
   e. Oral and systemic analgesic drugs to relieve pain.
2. Treatments are aimed at opening of angle of the anterior chamber to increase aqueous outflow.
3. Patient is asked to lie in supine position so that the iris lens diaphragm falls back, thereby increasing the anterior chamber depth.
4. After the IOP is controlled by the above measures, pilocarpine 2–4% eyedrops four times per day are started. Once the IOP is controlled, the corneal edema is subsided and anterior chamber inflammation is controlled, laser iridotomy or surgical iridectomy is done to eliminate pupillary block. If the IOP increases on treatment with pilocarpine as in case of lens-related angle closure, pilocarpine eyedrops are stopped and argon laser iridoplasty is done.
5. Treatment to prevent angle closure in future. After laser iridotomy, or surgical iridectomy or iridoplasty is performed, the patient is examined repeatedly at frequent intervals. At each visit, IOP recording and

gonioscopy are done and depending on the examination findings, following treatment is followed. If the IOP is under control with open angle patient is examined frequently and followed up with optic disk changes, visual field defects as done for open angle glaucoma:

a. If the IOP is elevated with open angle medical treatment similar to open angle glaucoma is continued.
b. If the IOP is elevated with synechial angle closure, less than 180° argon laser trabeculoplasty is carried out.
c. If the IOP is elevated with synechial angle closure, more than 180° trabeculectomy is indicated.
d. If the IOP is still elevated, more complex surgeries, e.g. glaucoma artificial drainage devices are indicated.

6. Treatment of other eye is very important in every patient with acute congestive glaucoma. Other eye should be examined and if the anterior chamber is shallow and angle of the anterior chamber is narrow, prophylactic laser iridotomy has to be done.

Chapter 11

Examination of Retina

Chapter Outline

- Fundus Examination
- Hypertensive Retinopathy
- Diabetic Retinopathy
- Central Retinal Artery Occlusion
- Branch Retinal Vein Occlusion
- Central Retinal Vein Occlusion
- Retinitis Pigmentosa
- Central Serous Retinopathy
- Cystoid Macular Edema
- Myopia
- Papilledema
- Optic Neuritis
- Optic Disk Changes in Glaucoma
- Primary Optic Atrophy
- Secondary Optic Atrophy
- Consecutive Optic Atrophy

FUNDUS EXAMINATION

Retina is examined by following methods:

1. Ophthalmoscopy: Direct ophthalmoscopy and indirect ophthalmoscopy.
2. Slit-lamp biomicroscopy: With accessory lenses such as +78 D, +90 D, –58.6 D lenses, Goldmann three-mirror lens.

The visible portion of retina is referred as fundus (Fig. 11.1). Fundus has to be examined under the headings.

Media

Normally media of the eye is clear or transparent. The media becomes hazy or opaque in case of opacities in the media such as corneal opacity, cataract and vitreous hemorrhage.

Optic Disk

1. Size: Normal size of the optic disk is 1.5 mm in diameter.

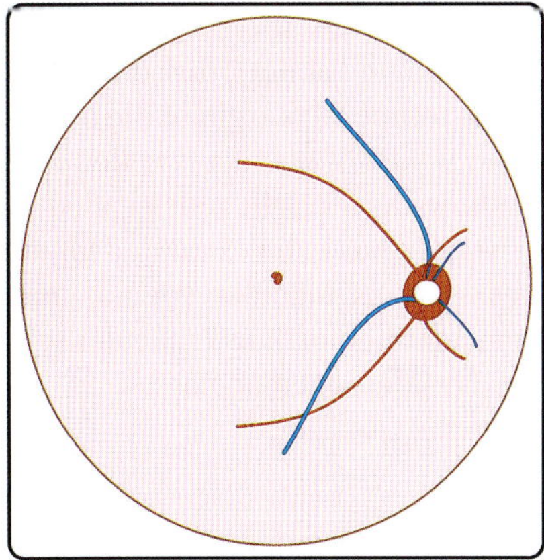

Fig. 11.1: Normal fundus (diagrammatic representation)

2. Shape: Normal disk is circular in shape.
3. Color: Normal color of the optic disk is pink, which is due to capillaries on the optic disk. It is chalky white in primary optic atrophy, dirty white in postneuritic optic atrophy and waxy white in consecutive optic atrophy.
4. Margin: Normal margin of the optic disk is sharp and well made out. It becomes blurred in optic neuritis, papilledema, drusen of the optic disk.
5. Cup: The central pale area of the optic disk is called cup of the optic disk. It is obliterated in papilledema and papillitis.
6. Cup-to-disk ratio: Normal C:D ratio is about 0.2–0.4. It is increased in glaucoma and other causes of optic atrophy.
7. Neuroretinal rim: It is the part of the optic disk that is surrounding the cup. It is decreased or thin in glaucoma and in other causes of optic atrophy:
   a. Abnormalities like hemorrhages on optic disk are seen in glaucoma, papilledema, papillitis, etc.
   b. Abnormalities like neovascularization of the disk seen in diabetic retinopathy, central retinal vein occlusion (CRVO), etc.

Macula

Macula is situated about 2 disk diameters lateral to the temporal margin of the optic disk. The central part of macula is called foveola, which shows as a bright reflex called foveal reflex. Macula has to be examined for abnormalities such as macular edema, macular hole, macular hemorrhage, macular scarring and hard exudates at macula.

Vessels

Normal ratio of arteries to vein size is 2:3. Vessels of the retina have to be examined for:

1. Narrowing of arteries as in CRVO, hypertensive retinopathy.
2. Dilatation and tortuosity of veins as in CRVO, angiomatosis, papilledema.
3. Neovascularization as in diabetic retinopathy, CRVO.

Pulsations of Arteries and Veins

Arterial pulsations are always abnormal and seen in aortic regurgitation. Venous pulsations are normally seen and they are absent in papilledema.

General Background

Normally background of the retina is reddish pink in color. The background of retina has to be examined for abnormalities such as:

1. Superficial retinal hemorrhages seen in hypertensive retinopathy, diabetic retinopathy, CRVO.
2. Deep retinal hemorrhages seen in diabetic retinopathy.
3. Cotton-wool spots seen in hypertensive retinopathy, diabetic retinopathy.
4. Hard exudates seen in hypertensive retinopathy, diabetic retinopathy.

The findings of retinal examination are documented on charts meant for documenting retinal examination findings (Fig. 11.2). The chart consists of three concentric circles divided into 12 meridians and each representing 1 clock hour. The outer circle corresponds to the junction of the pars plana and pars plicata, the middle circle corresponds to ora serrata and the inner circle corresponds to equator. Macula is drawn in the center of the circle and optic disk is drawn nasal to it.

The image seen with the indirect ophthalmoscope is inverted vertically and reversed laterally. The chart is placed upside down and the findings are recorded exactly where they are seen and by this way the chart corresponds to the inverted image of the fundus.

Color codes: The color codes used in documenting the lesions are as follows:

- Retinal veins—blue
- Flat or attached retina—red

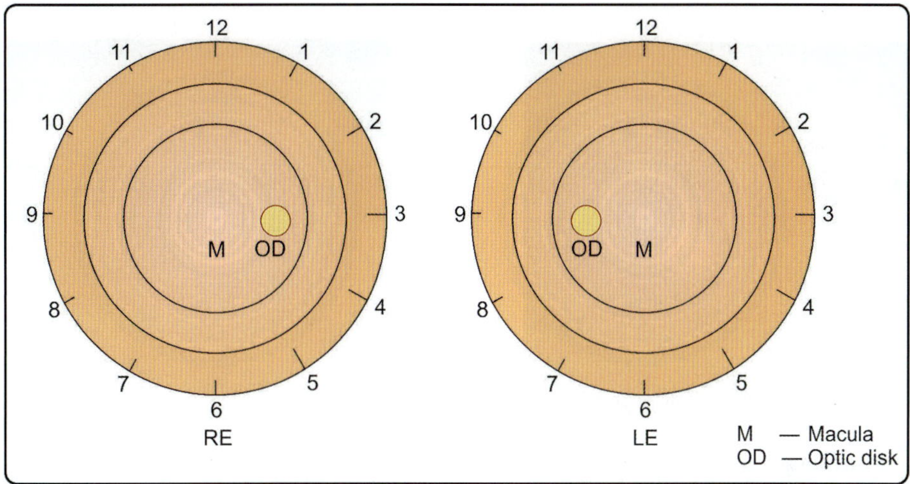

Fig. 11.2: Retinal chart (LE, left eye; M, macula; OD, optic disk; RE, right eye).

- Detached retina—blue
- Retinal break—red with blue outline
- Thin retina—red hatching with blue outline
- Vitreous opacity—green
- Retinal pigment—black
- Lattice degeneration—blue hatching with blue outline.

Fundus Examination in Common Retinal Disorders

Rhegmatogenous Retinal Detachment

Retinal detachment (RD) (Figs 11.3A to D) due to break in the sensory layer of retina allowing fluid from the vitreous cavity (synchitic or liquefied vitreous gel) to seep in between sensory retina and retinal pigment epithelium and separate them is called rhegmatogenous retinal detachment (Figs 11.4 and 11.5).

In fresh retinal detachment

- Detached retina is convex in configuration and corrugated appearance
- Detached retina undulates freely with ocular movements
- There is no shifting of fluid.

In long-standing retinal detachment

- Retinal thinning
- Secondary intraretinal cysts
- Subretinal demarcation lines
- Proliferative vitreoretinopathy.

Exudative Retinal Detachment

1. Retinal detachment caused by exudation from choriocapillaries, which seeps into the subretinal space through damaged retinal pigment epithelium thus separating it from sensory retina is called exudative retinal detachment (Fig. 11.6).
2. Retinal breaks are absent.
3. Retinal detachment configuration is convex. The detached retina is smooth, noncorrugated and bullous.
4. Shifting of fluid is the characteristic feature of exudative RD.

Tractional Retinal Detachment

1. Retinal detachment caused by tractional membranes (vitreoretinal membranes) from inflammatory or vascular causes on the surface of the retina pulling the sensory retina away from retinal pigment epithelium (RPE) is called tractional retinal detachment (Fig. 11.7).

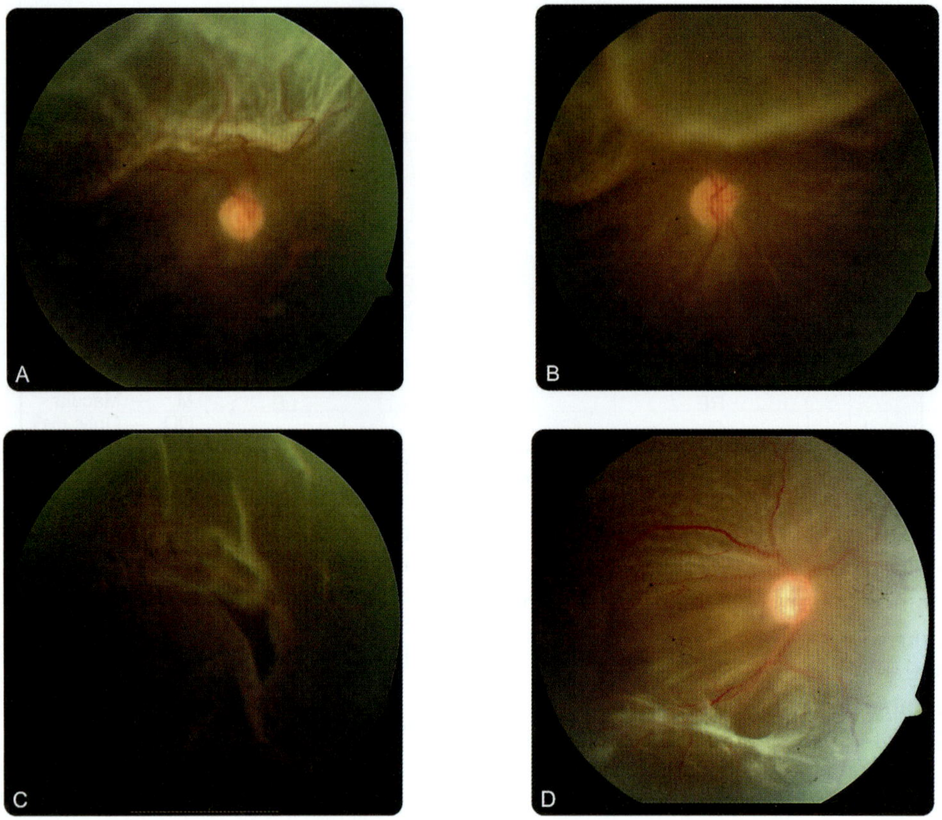

Figs 11.3A to D: Grayish, folded and raised retina seen in retinal detachment

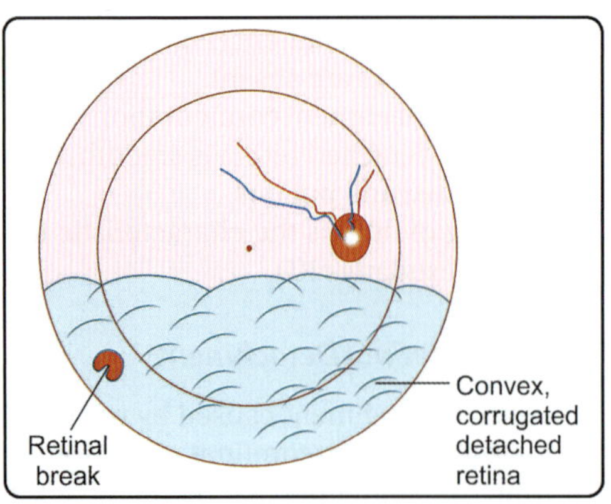

Fig. 11.4: Rhegmatogenous retinal detachment

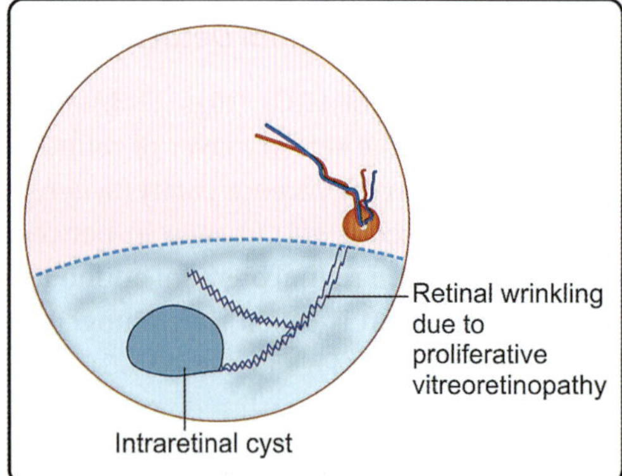

Fig. 11.5: Old rhegmatogenous detachment *(Note:* Subretinal demarcation line, intraretinal cyst, retinal wrinkling due to proliferative vitreoretinopathy).

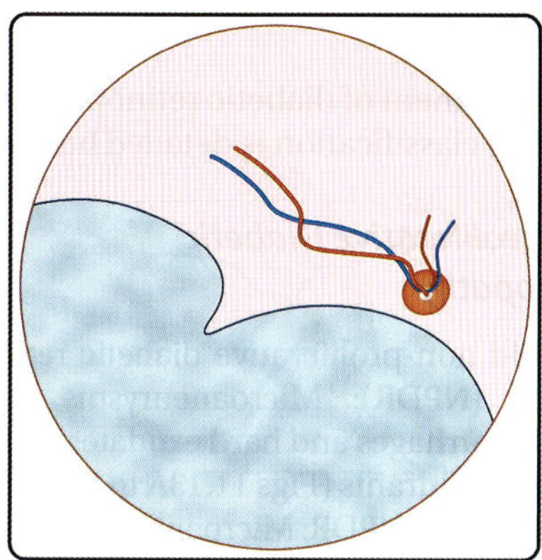

Fig. 11.6: Exudative retinal detachment *(Note:* Convex configuration of detached retina, which is noncorrugated and bullous).

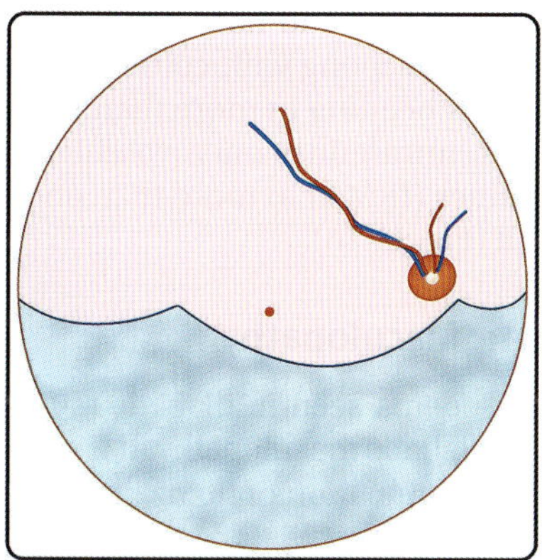

Fig. 11.7: Tractional retinal detachment *(Note:* Concave configuration of detached retina).

2. Retinal breaks are absent.
3. Retinal detachment configuration is concave.
4. Mobility of the detached retina is severely reduced.

HYPERTENSIVE RETINOPATHY

Retinopathy occurring as a result of changes in the retinal vasculature because of systemic hypertension is called hypertensive retinopathy. Arteriovenous crossing changes in a case of hypertensive retinopathy are:

1. Gunn's sign: Tapering of veins on either side of arteriovenous crossing.
2. Bonnet sign: Dilatation of the veins distal to the arteriovenous crossing.
3. Salus sign: Deflection of veins at arteriovenous crossing.

Arteriosclerotic changes seen in hypertensive retinopathy (Table 11.1) are graded as detailed below.

Table 11.1: Keith-Wagener-Barker classification

Grade	Description
I	Mild generalized arteriolar attenuation
II	Moderate to marked generalized narrowing and focal attenuation of arterioles associated with arteriovenous nipping
III	Abnormalities seen in grades I and II along with retinal hemorrhages, hard exudates and cotton-wool spots
IV	Abnormalities seen in grades I, II, III, swelling of the optic nerve head and macular star

Grade I: Increased or widening of arteriolar light reflex (Fig. 11.8).

Grade II: Copper wire appearance of the arterioles with moderate arteriovenous crossing changes (Figs 11.9, 11.10A and B).

Grade III: Silver wire appearance of the arterioles with marked arteriovenous crossing changes (Fig. 11.11).

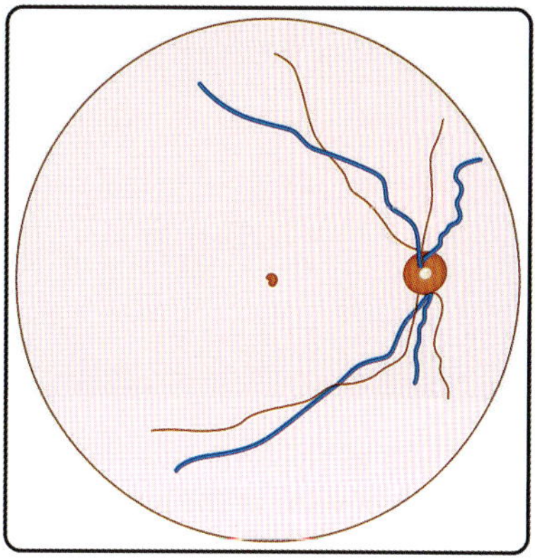

Fig. 11.8: Grade I hypertensive (HTN) retinopathy *(Note:* Narrowing of retinal arteries).

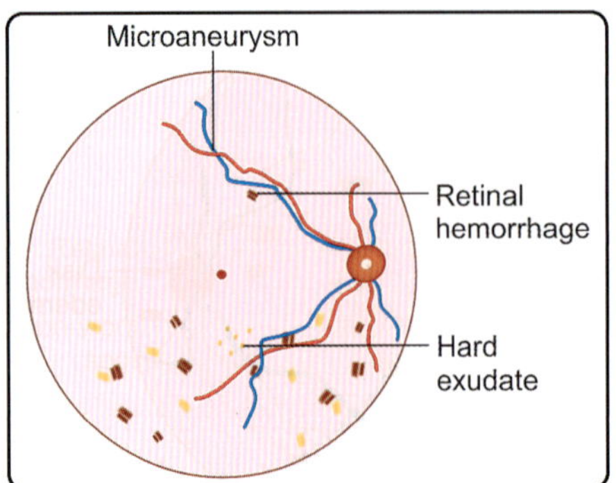

Fig. 11.14: Mild non-proliferative diabetic retinopathy *(Note:* Microaneurysms, retinal hemorrhages hard exudates in two quadrants).

plexiform and inner nuclear layers of the retina in the macula. It may be seen in NPDR or proliferative diabetic retinopathy (PDR).

Diabetic maculopathy is called clinically significant macular edema (CSME), if it has the following characteristics:

- Presence of retinal thickening within 500 μm from the center of the macula
- Presence of hard exudates within 500 μm of the center of the macula, associated with surrounding retinal thickening
- Presence of retinal thickening one disk area or larger, a part of which is within one disk diameter from the center of the macula (Figs 11.17A to C).

Proliferative Diabetic Retinopathy

The PDR is characterized by proliferation of new vessels, i.e. neovascularization at optic disk or elsewhere (Fig. 11.18).

High-risk Characteristics of Proliferative Diabetic Retinopathy

- New vessels on the optic disk (NVD) of one fourth to one third or more of the disk area
- The NVD of less than one fourth of disk area or new vessels elsewhere (NVE) with vitreous hemorrhage or preretinal hemorrhage (Fig. 11.19)
- The NVE more than half disk area with vitreous hemorrhage or preretinal hemorrhage.

CENTRAL RETINAL ARTERY OCCLUSION

Occlusion of the central retinal artery resulting in hypoxic damage of the retina is called central retinal artery occlusion (CRAO). Central retinal artery occlusion is caused by thrombosis or embolism or vasculitis of the central retinal artery. Examination of retina shows:

1. Retinal arteries are markedly narrowed with thread-like appearance with retinal veins being normal.
2. The retina appears white in color because of edema resulting in opacification.
3. Cherry-red spot at the macula.

Box carring or segmentation of blood in the retinal vessels giving raise to cattle truck appearance is seen in severe obstruction (Fig. 11.20).

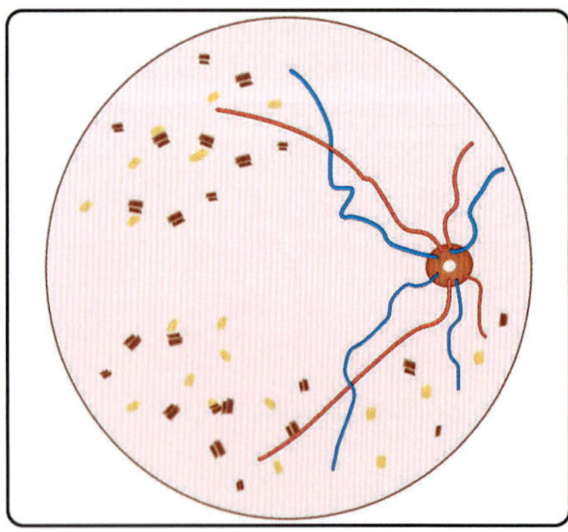

Fig. 11.15: Moderate non-proliferative diabetic retinopathy (*Note*: Microaneurysms, retinal hemorrhages, hard exudates in three quadrants).

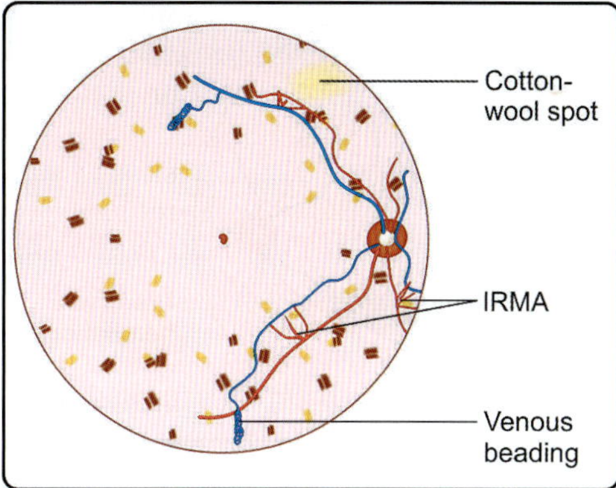

Fig. 11.16: Severe non-proliferative diabetic retinopathy *(Note:* Microaneurysms, retinal hemorrhages, hard exudates in four quadrants along with cotton-wool spots, venous beading in two quadrants and IRMA in one quadrant (4–2–1 rule).

BRANCH RETINAL VEIN OCCLUSION

Occlusion of a branch of central retinal vein resulting in involvement of the corresponding part of retina, which is supplied by that particular branch is called branch retinal vein occlusion. Superotemporal branch is commonly involved branch of the retinal vein. Rigid arteriosclerotic artery compressing on the retinal vein is the most common cause for retinal vein occlusion. Fundus picture shows:

- Dilated and tortuous vein beyond the site of occlusion
- Retinal edema and hemorrhages limited to the retina drained by affected retinal vein (Fig. 11.21).

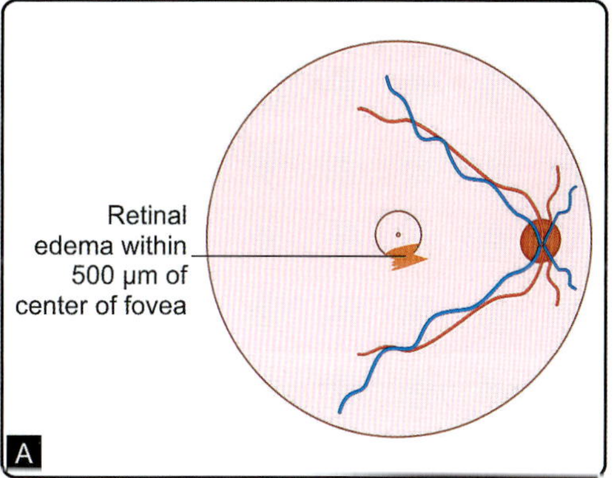

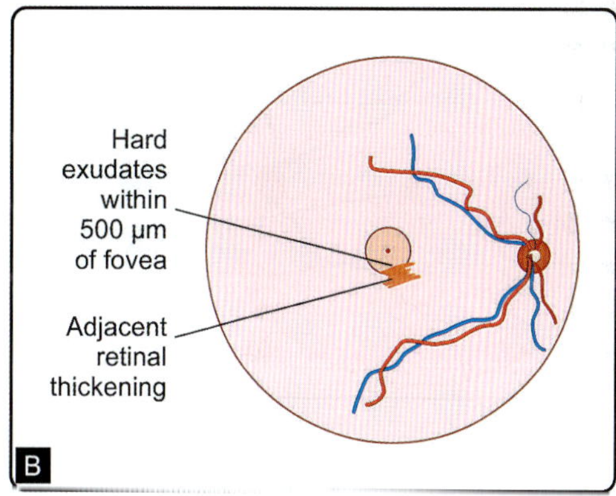

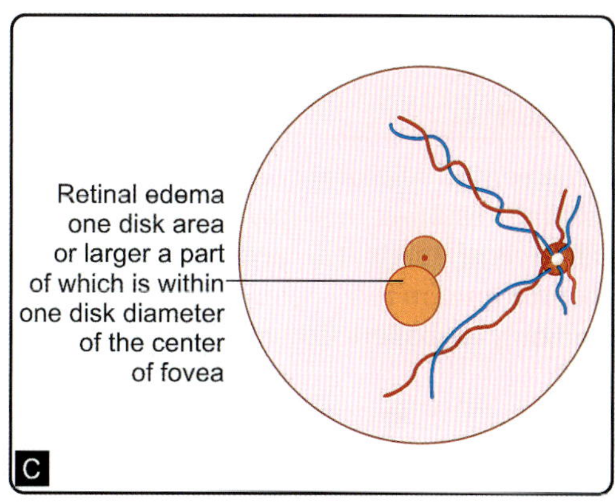

Figs 11.17A to C: Clinically significant macular edema

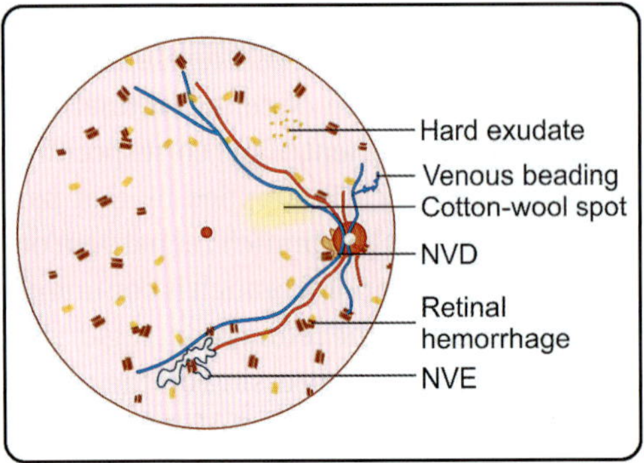

Fig. 11.18: Proliferative diabetic retinopathy (PDR) *[Note:* New vessels elsewhere (NVE) and new vessels on optic disk (NVD)].

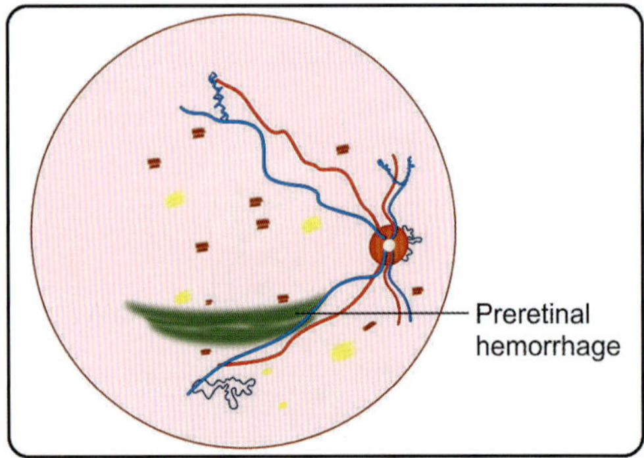

Fig. 11.19: Proliferative diabetic retinopathy (PDR) with preretinal hemorrhage

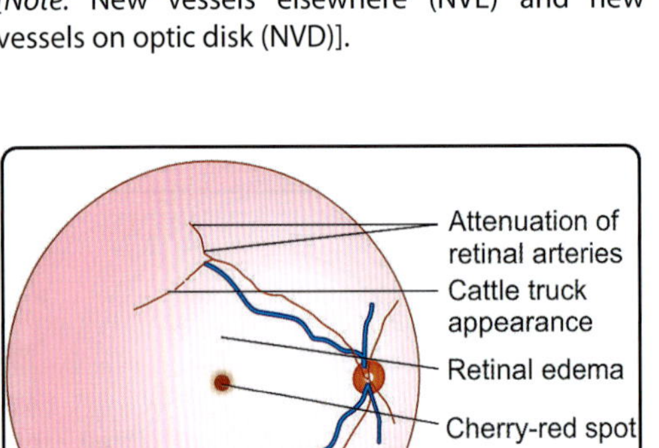

Fig. 11.20: Central retinal artery occlusion *(Note:* Attenuation of retinal arteries, cattle truck appearance, retinal edema and cherry-red spot).

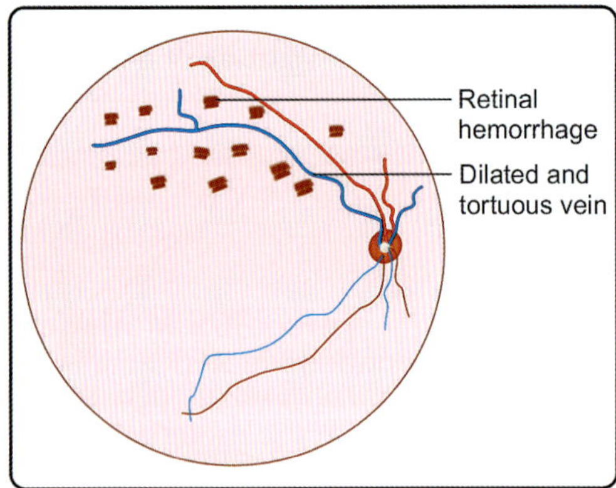

Fig. 11.21: Branch retinal vein occlusion *(Note:* Dilated and tortuous vein in the superotemporal quadrant associated with retinal hemorrhages in the affected quadrant).

CENTRAL RETINAL VEIN OCCLUSION

Occlusion/Obstruction of the central retinal vein at the lamina cribrosa and resulting in occlusion retinopathy is called central retinal vein occlusion. It is the second common retinal vascular disorder second only to diabetic retinopathy. It is of two types:

1. Non-ischemic.
2. Ischemic (Figs 11. 22A to C).

Non-ischemic Central Retinal Vein Occlusion

Non-ischemic central retinal vein (Fig. 11.23) occlusion is common of the two. It is characterized by mild to moderate decreased visual acuity. Fundus picture shows:

- Mild tortuosity of retinal veins
- Engorgement of retinal veins
- Few retinal hemorrhages.

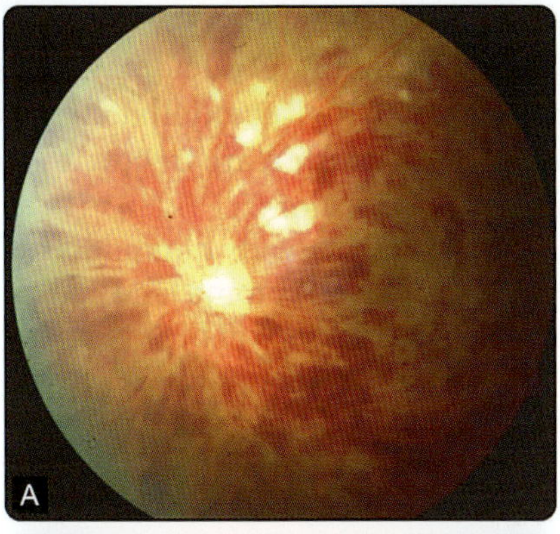

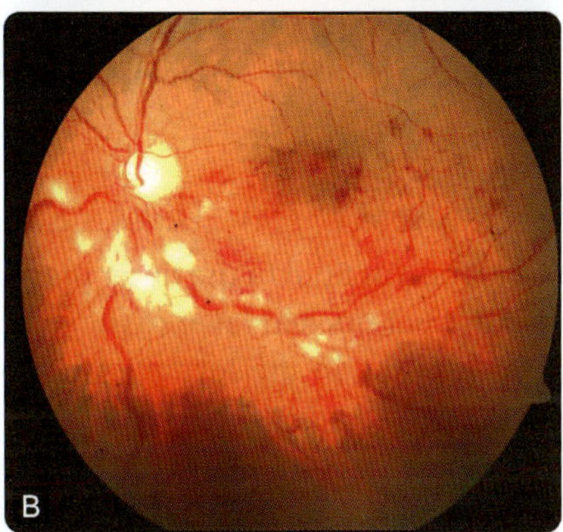

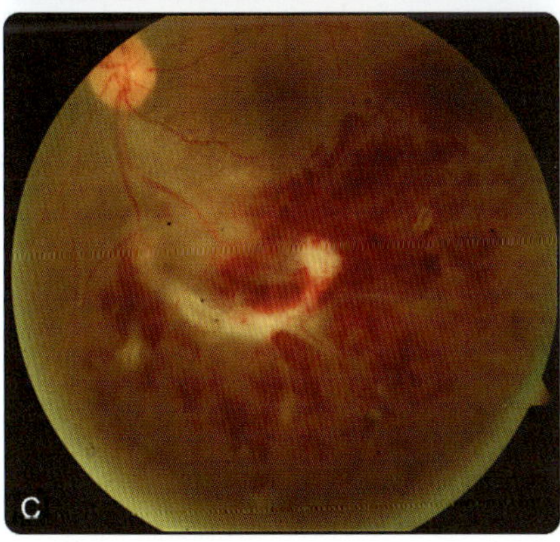

Figs 11.22A to C: A. Central retinal vein occlusion (*Note:* Tortuous retinal veins, retinal hemorrhages, cotton-wool spots in all the four quadrants and disk edema); **B.** Hemiretinal vein occlusion (*Note:* Tortuous retinal veins, retinal hemorrhages and cotton-wool spots in two inferior quadrants); **C.** Branch retinal vein occlusion [*Note:* Tortuous retinal veins, retinal hemorrhages and cotton-wool spots in one quadrant (inferotemporal)].

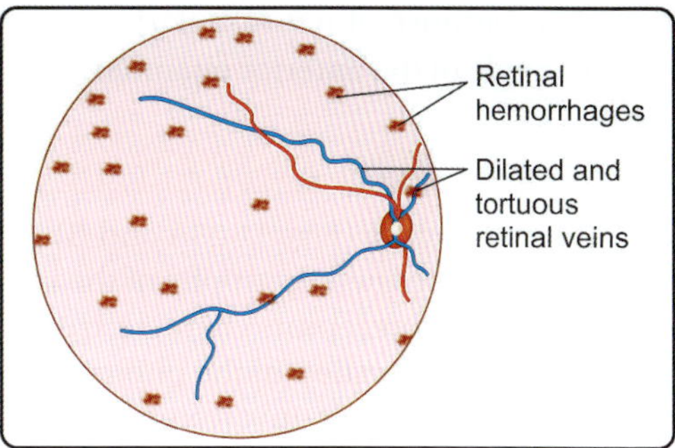

Fig. 11.23: Non-ischemic central retinal vein occlusion

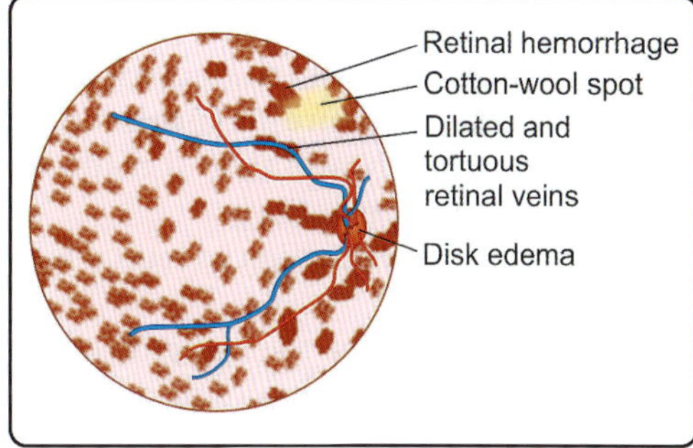

Fig. 11.24: Ischemic central retinal vein occlusion

Ischemic Central Retinal Vein Occlusion

Ischemic central retinal vein occlusion (Fig. 11.24) is characterized by marked decrease in visual acuity, relative afferent papillary defect on the affected side. Fundus picture shows:

- Retinal venous engorgement and tortuosity
- Wide spread retinal hemorrhages giving rise to tomato splashed appearance
- Cotton-wool spots
- Macular edema
- Optic disk edema.

The neovascular glaucoma also called 90 days glaucoma (as it develops within 3 months) is the most common complication occurring in ischemic central retinal vein occlusion because of neovascularization of iris and angle of the anterior chamber.

RETINITIS PIGMENTOSA

Retinitis pigmentosa (Figs 11.25A and B) is a genetically determined dystrophy of the retina affecting photoreceptors characterized by progressive degeneration of the photoreceptors with predominant involvement of the rods. Patient presents with night blindness and delayed dark adaptation. Fundus picture shows:

1. The RPE changes in the form of bony corpuscle pigmentation, characteristically perivascular in nature and beginning in the midperiphery and extend gradually anteriorly and posteriorly.
2. Narrowing or attenuation of retinal arterioles.
3. Pale waxy pallor of the optic disk with consecutive optic atrophy in advanced stages (Fig. 11.26).

CENTRAL SEROUS RETINOPATHY

Central serous retinopathy is an idiopathic disease characterized by serous detachment of the neurosensory retina in the macular region (Fig. 11.27). It is usually seen in middle-aged adults with males being more commonly affected than females. Type A personality, emotional stress and systemic hypertension are frequently associated with risk factors.

Patient presents with diminution of vision with positive scotoma and metamorphopsia. Visual acuity will be in the range of 6/9–6/12 and refraction showing hypermetropic refraction.

Fundus picture shows round or oval detachment of sensory retina at the posterior pole (Fig. 11.28). Fundus fluorescein angiography shows smokestack pattern or inkblot pattern.

CYSTOID MACULAR EDEMA

Accumulation of fluid in the outer plexiform layer and inner nuclear layer of the retina in macula resulting in the formation of cystic spaces in the macula is called cystoid macular edema. It follows a variety of diseases such as postoperative complication of cataract surgery, diabetic retinopathy, retinal vein occlusion and retinitis pigmentosa. Fundus picture shows honeycomb appearance (Fig. 11.29). Fundus fluorescein angiography shows flower petal appearance.

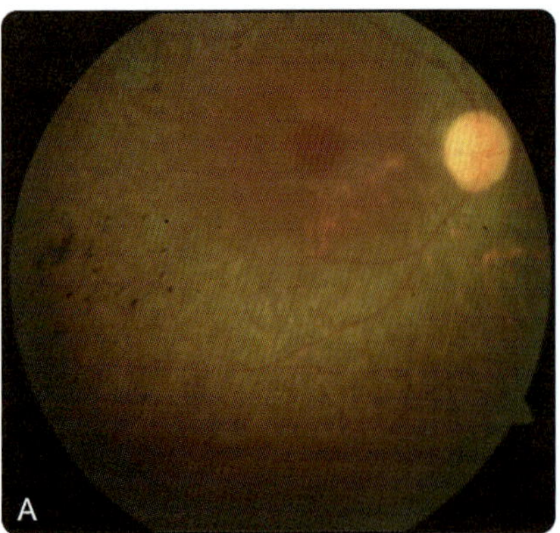

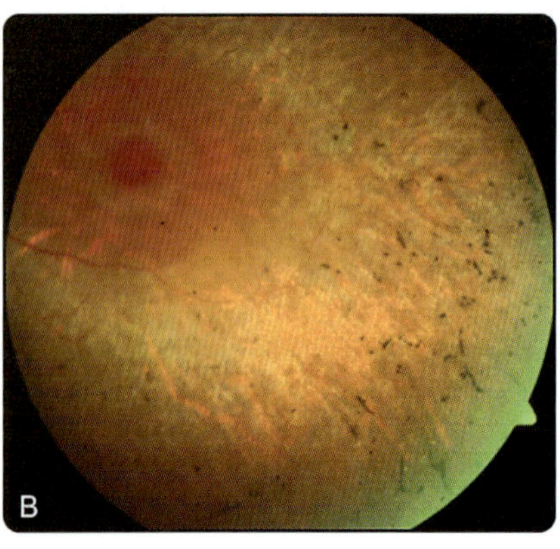

Figs 11.25A and B: Retinitis pigmentosa (*Note:* Attenuation of retinal arteries, waxy disk pallor of optic disk and bony corpuscle pigmentation).

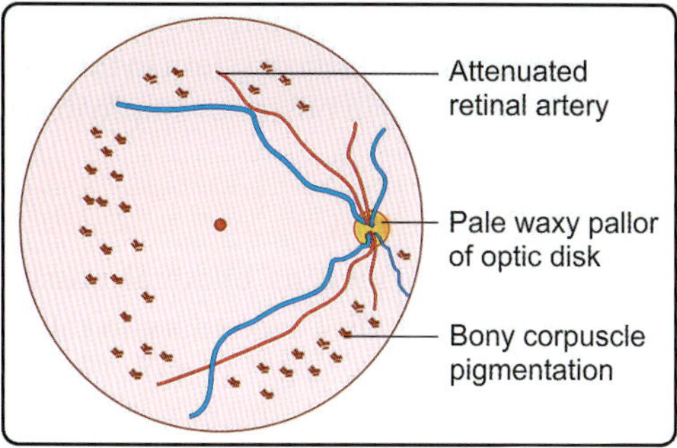

Fig. 11.26: Retinitis pigmentosa

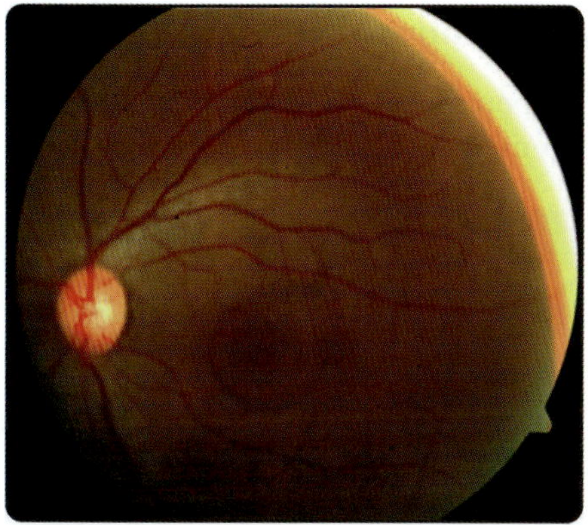

Fig. 11.27: Central serous retinopathy *(Note:* Elevation of macular area demarcated by a circular ring).

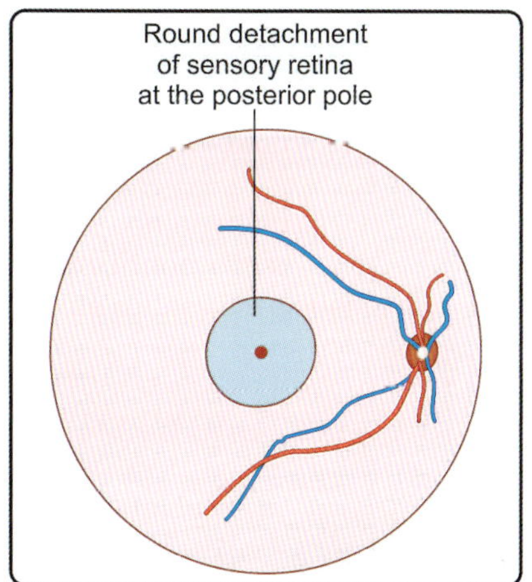

Fig. 11.28: Central serous retinopathy *(Note:* Round detachment of sensory retina at the posterior pole)

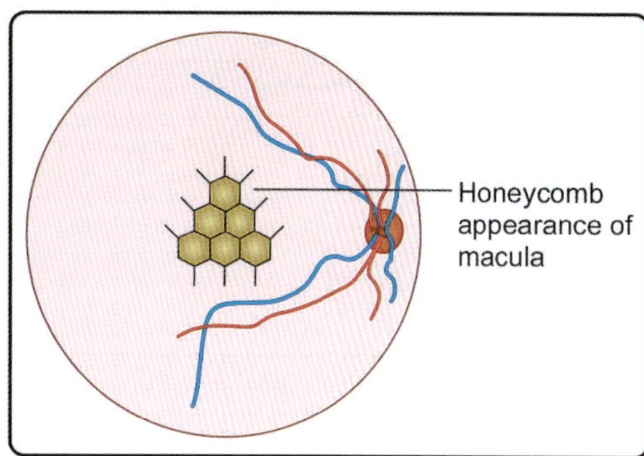

Fig. 11.29: Cystoid macular edema (*Note*: Honeycomb appearance of macula).

MYOPIA

Myopia is a clinical type of myopia characterized by degenerative changes because of rapid increase in the axial length of the eyeball. Pathological myopia is usually more than 6.0 diopters with axial length of more than 25 mm.

Fundus Changes in High Myopia

Fundus changes in high myopia include (Figs 11.30 and 11.31A to D).

Optic disk: This appears large with large physiological cup, temporal crescent or annular crescent and may show tilted appearance.

Macula: It shows foster Fuchs' spot, because of accumulation of pigment associated with subretinal neovascularization and choroidal hemorrhage. Myopic foveoschisis and macular hole are the other pathologies seen in the macula.

Background: The retina shows tessellated appearance and patches of choroidal atrophy.

Periphery of the retina: Cystoid degeneration, lattice degeneration and other retinal degenerations are seen commonly in the periphery of the retina.

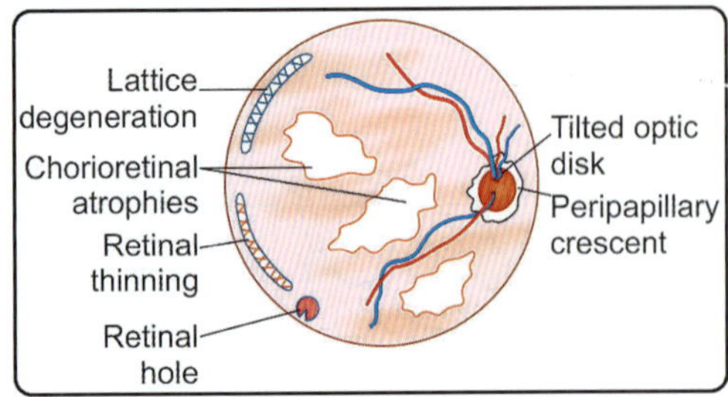

Fig. 11.30: Pathological myopia

Vitreous: It shows degenerations like vitreous liquefaction, muscae volitantes or vitreous opacities and posterior vitreous detachment.

Choroid: It shows lacquer cracks indicating breaks in the Bruch's membrane with choroidal atrophy.

Sclera: Thinning of sclera in the posterior part of the eyeball with ectasia of sclera in the posterior pole resulting in posterior staphyloma.

PAPILLEDEMA

Papilledema is defined as bilateral passive edema of the optic disk secondary to raised intracranial pressure (Fig. 11.32). Fundus picture of established papilledema is shown in Figs 11.33A and B.

Vascular Signs

- Hyperemia of optic disk
- Hemorrhages

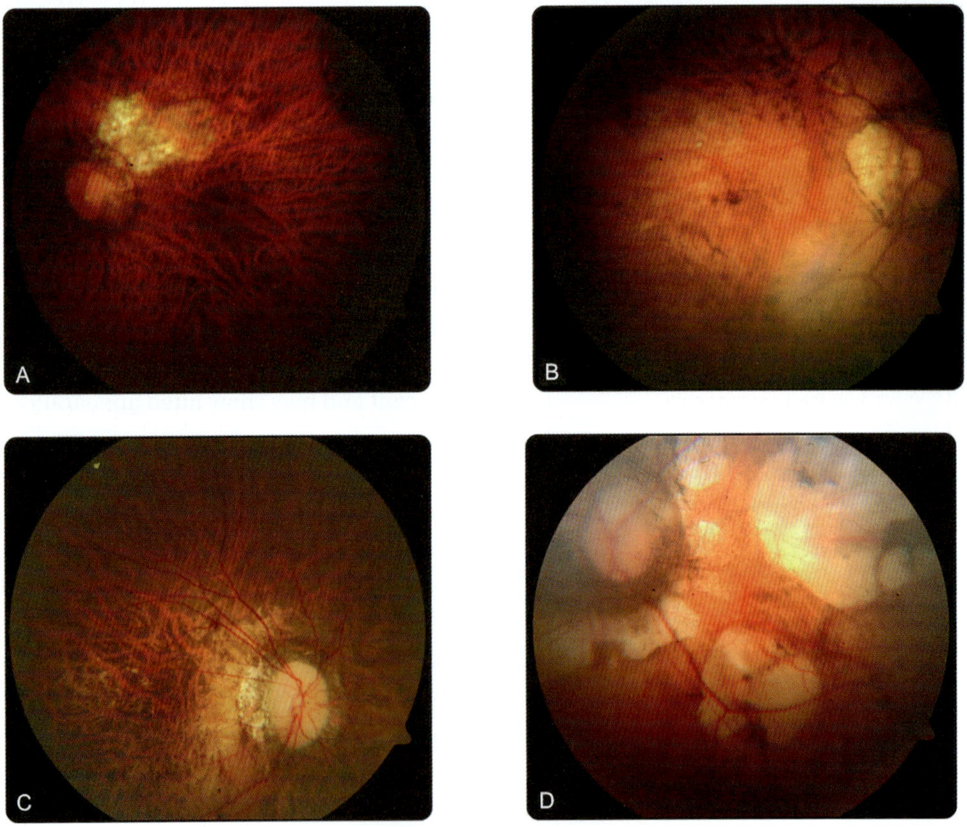

A B C D

Figs 11.31A to D: Fundus changes in pathological myopia (*Note:* Temporal crescent, tilted disk, chorioretinal atrophic patches).

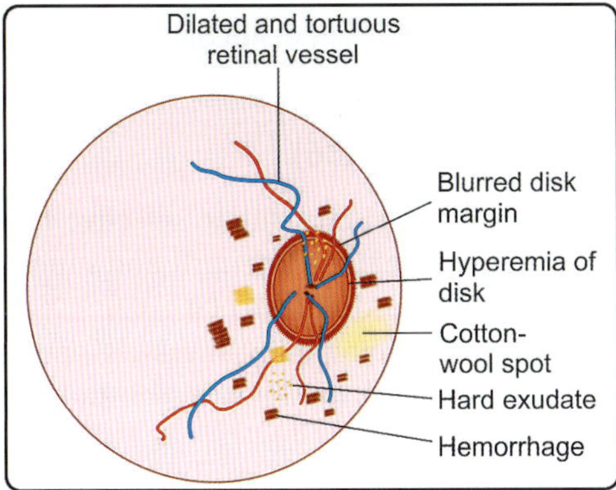

Fig. 11.32: Papilledema

- Hard exudates
- Cotton-wool spots
- Congestion of the retinal vessels.

Mechanical Signs

- Elevation of the optic disk > 3 D
- Edema of the nerve fiber layer
- Obscuration of the disk margins
- Obliteration of the physiological cup
- Folds of retina and or choroid.

OPTIC NEURITIS

Inflammation of optic nerve is called optic neuritis. Based on the ophthalmoscopic features it can be classified as:

- Papillitis
- Retrobulbar neuritis
- Neuroretinitis.

Papillitis

Papillitis shows hyperemia of optic disk, edema of optic disk < 1 mm, peripapillary hemorrhages. It has features similar to papilledema, differentiated from papilledema by marked visual loss (in papilledema vision is affected in late stage due to optic atrophy) disk edema < 1 mm or 3 D, less venous engorgement, less retinal hemorrhages, presence of posterior vitreous haze because of cells in posterior vitreous and it is usually unilateral (Fig. 11.34).

Retrobulbar Neuritis

Retrobulbar neuritis shows normal optic disk. Patient presents with marked diminution of vision, relative afferent pupillary pathway defect. It is described as a disease where neither ophthalmologist sees anything nor patient sees anything.

Neuritis

Neuroretinitis shows features of papillitis plus macular star because of hard exudates (Figs 11.35A and B).

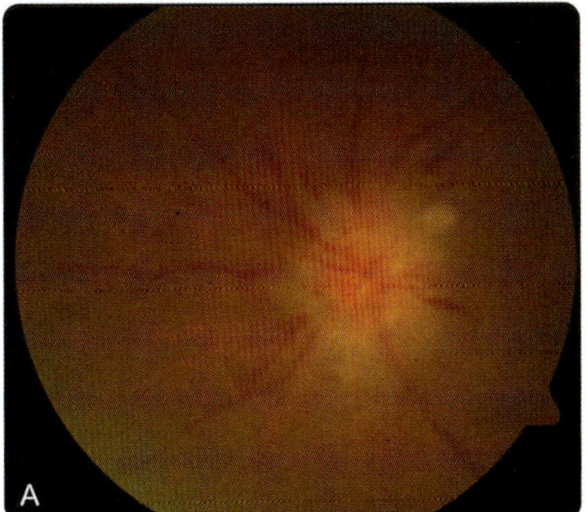

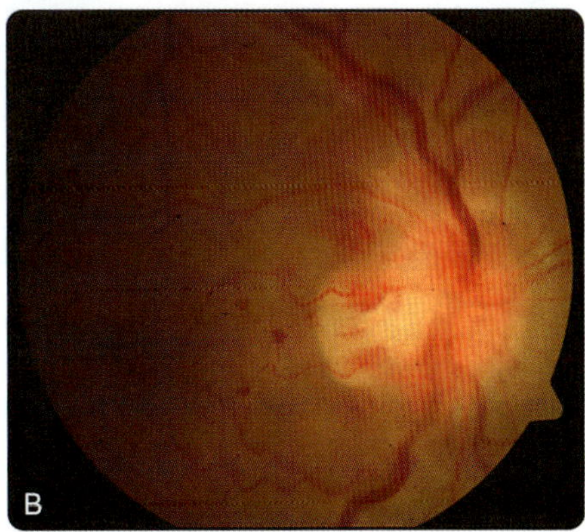

Figs 11.33A and B: Papilledema

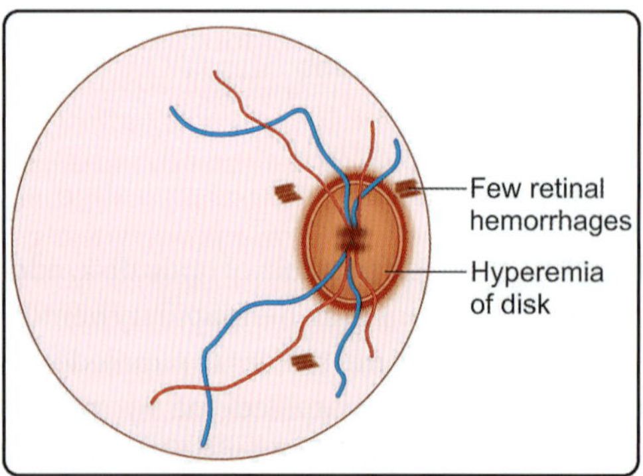

Fig. 11.34: Papillitis

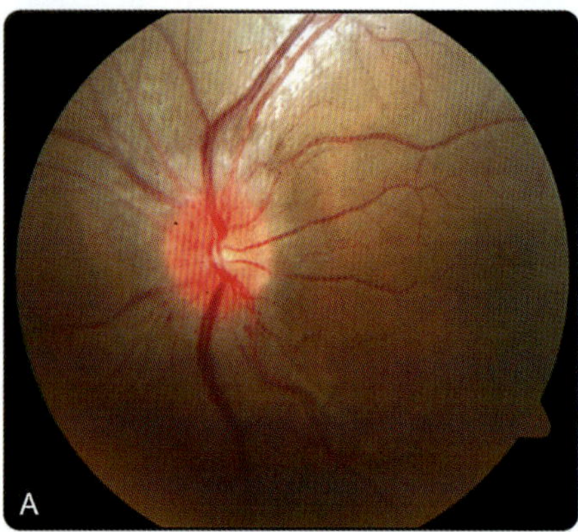

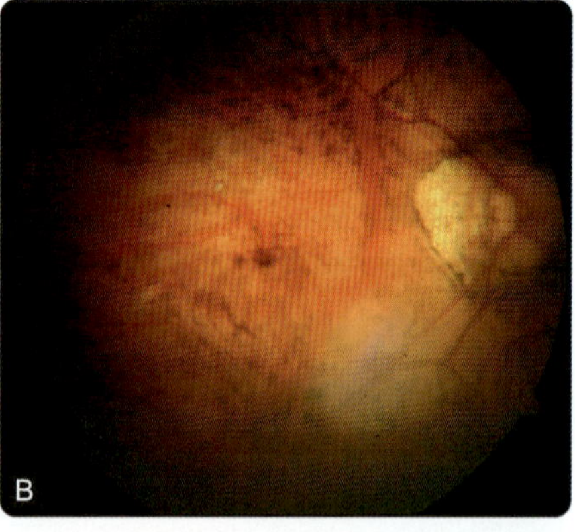

Figs 11.35A and B: Optic neuritis (papillitis) *[Note:* Optic disk shows hyperemia, edema (< 1 mm) blurring of disk margins, obliteration of physiological cup and tortuous retinal veins].

OPTIC DISK CHANGES IN GLAUCOMA

Early Glaucomatous Changes (Fig. 11.36)

1. Vertically oval cup due to selective loss of neuroretinal rim inferiorly and superiorly with cup-disk ratio of 0.4–0.6.
2. Baring of the circumlinear vessels—presence of pallor between vessel and the neuroretinal rim.
3. Asymmetry of the cup-disk ratio between the two eyes by more than 0.2.
4. Disk hemorrhages flame shaped or splinter shaped within the peripapillary retinal nerve fiber layer.
5. Peripapillary atrophy.
6. Pallor of the optic disk.

Advanced Glaucomatous Changes

1. Cup-disk ratio 0.7–0.9.
2. Thinning of neural retinal rim.
3. Nasal shifting of blood vessels.
4. Bayoneting sign: Double angulation of the retinal blood vessels giving the appearance of being broken at the disk margin is called bayoneting sign.

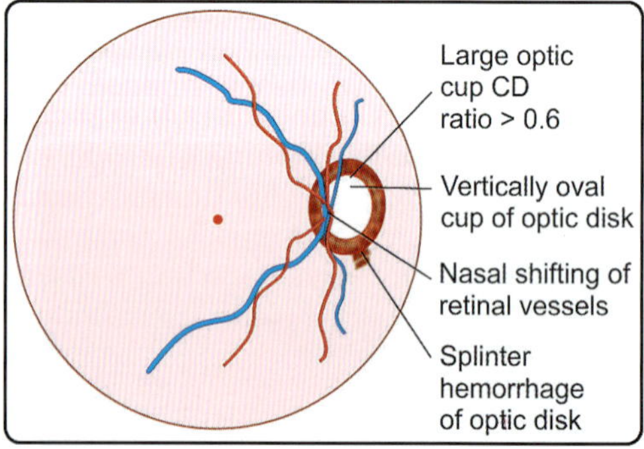

Fig. 11.36: Optic disk changes in glaucoma *(Note:* Vertically oval cup of optic disk, splinter hemorrhage of optic disk).

5. Lamellar dot sign: Visibility of the pores of the lamina cribrosa because of loss of retinal ganglion cells is called lamellar dot sign (Figs 11.37 and 11.38A and B).

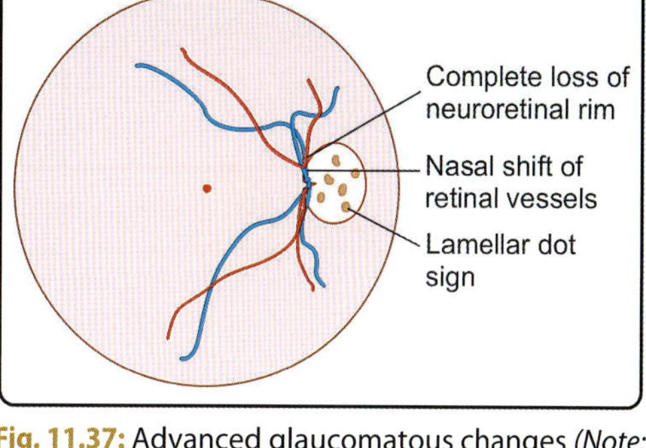

Fig. 11.37: Advanced glaucomatous changes *(Note:* Nasal shift of retinal vessels, lamellar dot sign, complete loss of neuroretinal rim).

PRIMARY OPTIC ATROPHY

Primary optic atrophy (Figs 11.39A and B) occurs without antecedent swelling of optic disk. The causes of primary optic atrophy include tumors compressing optic nerve, retrobulbar optic neuritis, hereditary optic neuropathy. Fundus picture shows:

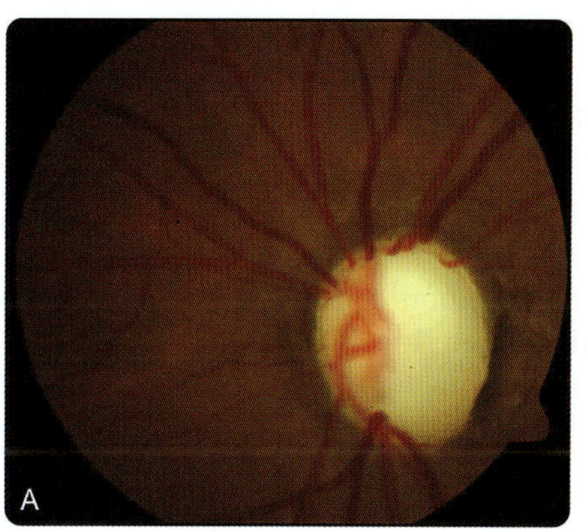

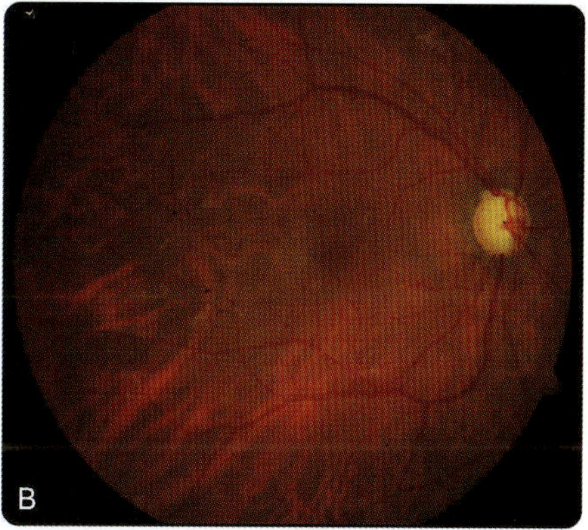

Figs 11.38A and B: Glaucomatous optic disk changes *[Note:* Marked cupping of optic disk, bayoneting sign (vessels appear of being, broken off at the margin), thinning of neuroretinal rim].

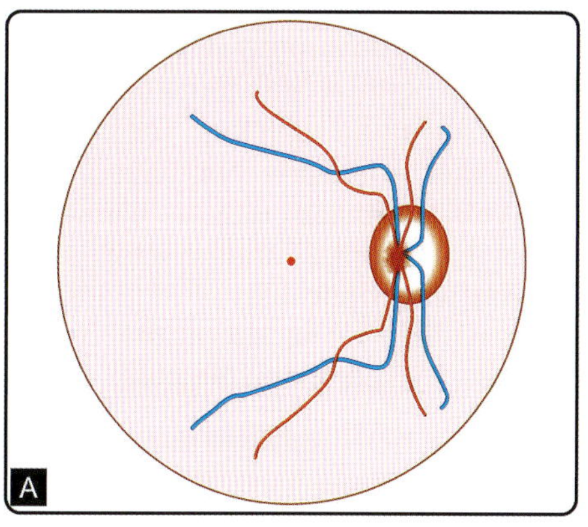

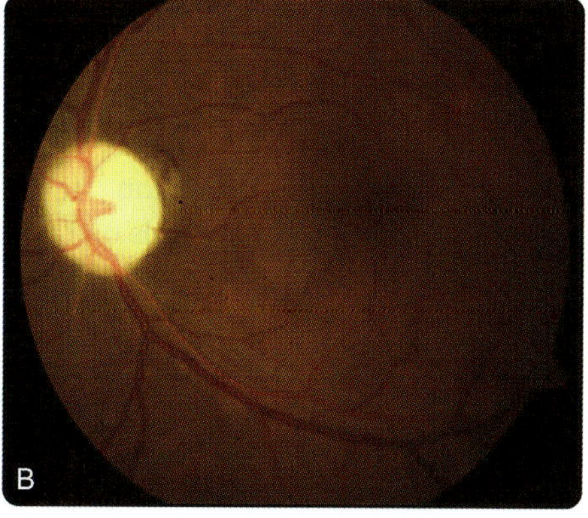

Figs 11.39A and B: Primary optic atrophy. **A.** Diagrammatic representation; **B.** Photograph *(Note:* Pale white color of the optic disk, clear margins of the optic disk and normal surrounding retina).

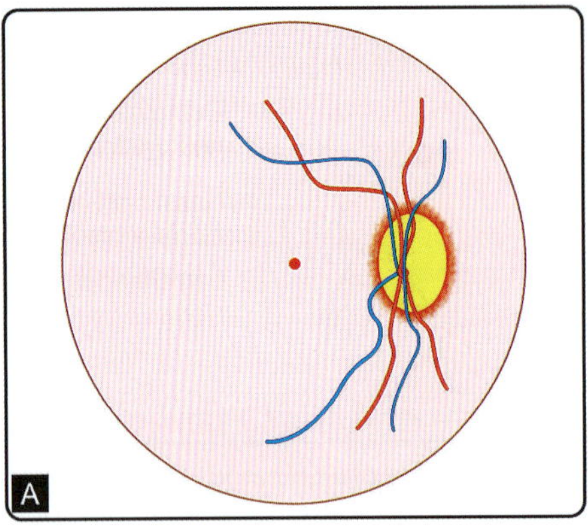

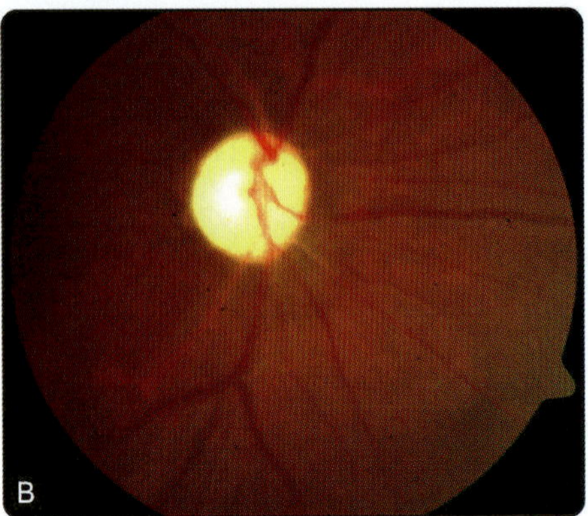

Figs 11.40A and B: Secondary optic atrophy. **A.** Diagrammatic representation; **B.** Photograph *(Note:* Dirty white color of the optic disk, blurred disk margins and perivascular sheathing of surrounding retinal vessels).

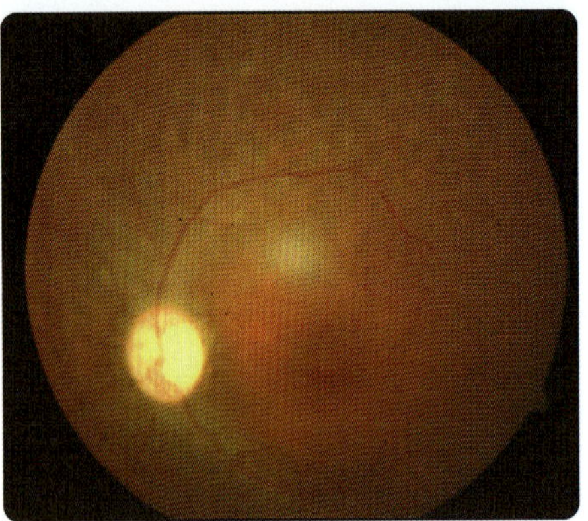

Fig. 11.41: Consecutive optic atrophy *(Note:* Yellow waxy pallor of the optic disk and attenuation of the surrounding retinal vessels).

- Pale optic disk with clear delineated disk margins
- Kestenbaum sign—reduction in the number of small blood vessels on the optic disk
- Normal retinal vessels and surrounding retina.

SECONDARY OPTIC ATROPHY

Secondary optic atrophy (Figs 11.40A and B) occurs with antecedent swelling of the optic disk.

The common causes are papilledema, papillitis, anterior ischemic optic neuropathy Fundus picture shows:

1. Dirty white optic disk with poorly delineated margins of the optic disk due to excessive gliosis.
2. Attenuation of retinal vessels and perivascular sheathing.

CONSECUTIVE OPTIC ATROPHY

Consecutive optic atrophy (Fig. 11.41) occurs due to degenerative/inflammatory/vascular lesions of surrounding retina. The causes include central retinal artery occlusion, central retinal vein occlusion, retinitis pigmentosa, pathological myopia. Fundus picture shows:

- Yellow waxy optic disk
- Surrounding retina shows the causative disease, e.g. retinitis pigmentosa.

Chapter 12

Community Ophthalmology

Chapter Outline

- Community Ophthalmology
- Blindness and Low Vision
- Blindness Statistics
- National Program for Control of Blindness (NPCB)
- Vision 2020
- District Blindness Control Society
- National Trachoma Control Program
- Xerophthalmia
- Important Dates in Ophthalmology

COMMUNITY OPHTHALMOLOGY

Community ophthalmology is the application of techniques of clinical ophthalmology in combination with the methodologies of community medicine to promote ocular health and to prevent blindness.

BLINDNESS AND LOW VISION

Blindness

Clinically, the condition in which a person is not able to perceive light is called blindness. However, the definition of blindness varies worldwide and for the purpose to ensure uniform data collection World Health Organization (WHO) has proposed a uniform definition and has defined low vision and blindness. Best corrected visual acuity in the better eye less than 3/60 (or its equivalent) or field of vision less than 10° is referred as blindness.

Low Vision

Best corrected visual acuity in the better eye in the range of 6/18–6/60 or its equivalent, or field of vision between 20° and 30° is referred as low vision grade I or mild visual impairment. Best corrected visual acuity in the better eye in the range of 6/60–3/60 or its equivalent, field of vision between 10° and 20° is referred as low vision grade II, or severe visual impairment.

Legal Blindness

Best corrected visual acuity in the better eye less than 6/60 or field of vision less than 20° is called legal blindness. It is the level of visual acuity required to become eligible for disability benefits given by government.

Economical Blindness

Economical blindness is same as legal blindness. Best corrected visual acuity in the better

Classification of Xerophthalmia

The different eye signs graded by the WHO are:

1. Night blindness (XN): It is the earliest manifestation of vitamin A deficiency. Scotopic vision, a function of rods is affected since vitamin A is an essential component of rhodopsin; pigment present in rods. Normal night vision usually returns back within 3 days of supplementing vitamin A.
2. Conjunctival xerosis (X1A) and corneal xerosis (X2): These are due to keratinization occurring in the epithelial surfaces of mucous membranes. Keratinizing metaplasia occurs in the epithelial surfaces due to deficiency of vitamin A, which is responsible for maintenance of normal epithelial architecture.
3. Bitot's spots (X1B): These are defined as collections of foamy material over an area of conjunctival xerosis consisting of desquamated-keratinized epithelial cells and saprophytic bacilli. Their presence indicates conjunctival xerosis. Bitots spots along with night blindness indicate significant vitamin A deficiency. Bitot's spots usually disappear within 2 weeks of starting treatment by vitamin A. However, in few they may persist for an indefinite time usually in the temporal quadrant of the conjunctiva because of the persisting keratinizing metaplasia caused by vitamin A deficiency.
4. Corneal ulceration/Keratomalacia involving less than one third of cornea (X3A). It is because of liquefactive necrosis of the cornea. Corneal ulcers in vitamin A deficiency show sharply demarcated punched out ulcers situated usually in the periphery of the cornea.
5. Corneal ulceration/Keratomalacia involving greater than one third of cornea (X3B).
6. Xerophthalmic fundus (XF): It is characterized by the presence of yellowish dots in the periphery of the fundus representing the loss of pigment from retinal pigment epithelium. They may cause blind spots or scotomas. It usually responds within 2 weeks of supplementing vitamin A.
7. Corneal scars secondary to xerophthalmia (XS).

Women of reproductive age with vitamin A deficiency should have a daily dose of 10,000 IU for 2 weeks. Large doses of vitamin A are contraindicated in women of reproductive age as they are contraindicated in pregnancy (Tables 12.1 and 12.2).

IMPORTANT DATES IN OPHTHALMOLOGY

World Sight Day: Second Thursday of October every year is marked as World Sight Day to draw the attention on blindness and its implications.

Table 12.1: Treatment of vitamin A deficiency

Schedule	In children, aged more than 1 year (oral vitamin A in IU)	In children less than 1 year or weight less than 8 kg (oral vitamin A in IU)	In children with severe vomiting or diarrhea
Immediately on diagnosis	200,000	100,000	Water-miscible retinyl palmitate 100,000 IU can be used instead of first dose
Next day	200,000	100,000	
2–4 week later	200,000	100,000	

Table 12.2: Supplementation of single large doses of vitamin A

Schedule	Supplementation in units
First dose at 9 month with measles vaccination	100,000 IU
Second dose at 18 month with booster dose of diphtheria, pertussis and tetanus (DPT)/ oral polio vaccine (OPV)	200,000 IU
Third dose at 24 month	200,000 IU
Fourth dose at 30 month	200,000 IU
Fifth dose at 36 month	200,000 IU

World Glaucoma Day: March 12th of every year is observed as Glaucoma Day to spread awareness regarding glaucoma, which is called silent thief of vision.

World Glaucoma Week: To maximize the awareness regarding glaucoma day is replaced by glaucoma week. It is observed between March 11th and 17th of every year.

National Eye Donation Fortnight: It is celebrated between August 25th and September 8th to encourage and to create awareness for eye donation.

National Eye Donation Day: September 8th of every year.

Bibliography

1. Agarwal, Gupta LC, Sanjeev Agarwal. Clinical Examination of Ophthalmic Cases. CBS Publishers and Distributors Pvt. Ltd.
2. Anita Panda. Clinical Examination of the Eye. CBS Publishers and Distributors Pvt. Ltd.
3. Dadapeer K. Essentials of Ophthalmology, 1st edition. New Delhi: Jaypee Brothers Medical Publishers (P) Ltd.
4. Dandona R, Dandona L. Childhood blindness in India: a population based perspective. Br J Ophthalmol. 2003;87(3):263-5.
5. Definition: visual impairment. (Expert comments: Karin van Dijk). New Vision.
6. Duke Elders. Duke-Elder's Practice of Refraction, 10th edition. Elsevier.
7. Foster A, Gilbert C, Johnson G. Changing patterns in global blindness: 1988-2008. Community Eye Health. 2008;21(67):37-9.
8. Gilbert C, Hernandez-Duran LA, Kotiankar S, et al. Prevention of childhood blindness. International Centre for Eye Health.
9. In: Dutta LC (Ed). Modern Ophthalmology, 3rd edition. New Delhi: Jaypee Brothers Medical Publishers (P) Ltd.
10. In: James F Vander, Janice A Gault (Eds). Ophthalmology Secrets in Color, 3rd edition. Elsevier.
11. In: Myron Yanoff, Jay S Duker (Eds). Ophthalmology, 2nd edition. Mosby.
12. In: Peyman, Sanders, Goldberg (Eds). Principles and Practice of Ophthalmology. vol. 3, 1st edition. New Delhi: Jaypee Brothers Medical Publishers (P) Ltd.
13. Jack J Kanski. Clinical Ophthalmology, 5th edition. Butterworth-Heinemann.
14. Jose R, Rathore AS, Rajshekar V, et al. Salient features of the National Program for Control of Blindness during the XIth five-year plan period. Indian J Ophthalmol. 2009;57(5):339-40.
15. Jose R, Rathore AS, Sachdeva S. Community ophthalmology: revisited. Indian J Community Med. 2010;35(2):356-8.
16. Jose R, Sachdeva S. Community rehabilitation of disabled with a focus on blind persons: Indian perspective. Indian J Ophthalmol. 2010;58(2):137-42.
17. Justis P Ehlers, Chirag P Shah. The Wills Eye Manual, 5th edition. Lippincott Williams & Wilkins.
18. Keerti Bhusan Pradhan. Lions Aravind Institute of Community Ophthalmology, Madurai and Partho Banerjee Community ophthalmology dimensions: Illumination. vol. 1, No. 2. Apr-Jun 2001.
19. Keith P West, Jr RD, Alfred Sommer PH. Delivery of oral doses of vitamin A deficiency and nutritional blindness. A state-of-the-art review, Nutrition policy discussion paper No. 2.
20. Khurana AK, Indu Khurana. Anatomy and Physiology of Eye, 2nd edition. CBS Publishers and Distributors Pvt. Ltd.
21. Khurana AK. Ophthalmology, 2nd edition. New Delhi: New Age International (P) Limited.
22. Khurana AK. Theory and Practice of Optics and Refraction. Elsevier.
23. Lanning B Kline, Frank J Bajandas. Neuro-Ophthalmology Review Manual, revised edition. New Delhi: Jaypee Brothers Medical Publishers (P) Ltd.
24. Mukherjee PK. Clinical Examination in Ophthalmology. Elsevier.
25. National Institute of Health and Family Welfare Documentation services National Programme for control of Blindness.

26. National Programme for Control of Blindness. Guidelines for DBCS Revised September 2005.
27. National Programme for Control of Blindness. Guidelines for State Health Society & District Health Society Revised 11th Five-Year Plan 2009.
28. Ramanjit Sihota, Radhika Tandon. Parsons' Diseases of the Eye, 20th edition. Elsevier.
29. Resnikoff S, Pascolini D, Mariotti SP, et al. Global magnitude of visual impairment caused by uncorrected refractive errors in 2004. Bull World Health Organ. 2008;86(1):63-70.
30. Samar K Basak. Essentials of Ophthalmology, 2nd edition. Current Books International.
31. Tanuj Dada, VK Dada. Secrets of ECCE and IOL. New Delhi: Jaypee Brothers Medical Publishers (P) Ltd.
32. Vision 2020: The right to sight. Global initiative for the elimination of avoidable blindness. Action plan 2006-2011.
33. World Health Organization. Global initiative for the elimination of avoidable blindness. Programme for the Prevention of Blindness and Deafness. Geneva: WHO; 1997.
34. World Health Organization. Preventing blindness in children: report of WHO/IAPB scientific meeting. Programme for the Prevention of Blindness and Deafness, and International Agency for Prevention of Blindness. Geneva: WHO; 2000.

Index

Page numbers followed by *f* refer to figure, *t* refer to table, *b* refer to box

D

E

F

G

H

I

J

K

L

M

N

O

P

R

S

T

U

V

W

X